THE LIMBIC SYSTEM

Functional Organization and Clinical Disorders

The Limbic System
Functional Organization and Clinical Disorders

Editors

Benjamin K. Doane, Ph.D., M.D.

Professor of Psychiatry
Department of Psychiatry
Dalhousie University
Victoria General Hospital
Halifax, Nova Scotia, Canada

Kenneth E. Livingston, M.D.

Professor Emeritus
Departments of Surgery
and Pharmacology
University of Toronto
The Wellesley Hospital
Toronto, Ontario, Canada

Raven Press ■ New York

Raven Press, 1140 Avenue of the Americas, New York, New York 10036

Made in the United States of America

Library of Congress Cataloging-in-Publication Data
Main entry under title:

The Limbic system.

Papers presented at the 2nd International
Neuroscience Symposium.
    Includes bibliographies and index.
    1. Epilepsy—Congresses. 2. Limbic system—
Diseases—Congresses. 3. Limbic system—Congresses.
4. Neuropsychiatry—Congresses. 5. Kindling
(Neurology)—Congresses. I. Doane, B. K. (Benjamin K.)
II. Livingston, Kenneth E. III. University of Toronto.
Continuing Medical Education. IV. International
Neuroscience Symposium (2nd : 1983 : Toronto, Ont.)
V. Title: Patterns of limbic system dysfunction.
[DNLM: 1. Epilepsy—congresses. 2. Kindling
(Neurology)—congresses. 3. Limbic System—physiology
—congresses. 4. Limbic System—physiopathology—
congresses. WL 314 L7327 1983]
RC372.L565   1985   616.8'53   85-25803
ISBN 0-88167-134-7

Preface

The concept of the limbic system introduced by James Papez in 1937 has advanced in less than 50 years from a somewhat nebulous formulation to a position of pivotal importance in our understanding of how the human brain works. In his 1937 paper, "A Proposed Mechanism of Emotion," Papez posed the question, Is emotion a magic product or is it a physiologic process? Although this question cannot yet be answered comprehensively, there is growing evidence that major substrates for the elaboration of emotion and behavior lie within the complex circuitry of the limbic system. It is now apparent that within the next few years further insight into the dynamics of the limbic system as a whole will have a further impact on medical education and health care and on many aspects of the behavioral sciences.

One of the major landmarks in the evolution of our understanding of limbic mechanisms was the experimental "discovery" and definition of the kindling phenomenon by Goddard nearly two decades ago. Since that time, clinical interest has focused particularly on the relevance of kindling to temporal lobe epilepsy (now designated as complex partial seizures). Kindling studies have contributed directly to important diagnostic and therapeutic advances in this field. However, in a larger experimental and clinical context, it seems increasingly probable that focal or generalized seizure is but one endpoint in a broad spectrum of clinical syndromes reflecting various patterns of disturbed limbic system function. A growing body of evidence, derived both from the experimental laboratory and from clinical observation, supports the view that limbic system dysfunction underlies many patterns of recurrent emotional and behavioral disturbance.

The material in this volume has been organized in four parts. Beginning with a review of the basic structural and functional organization of the limbic system, subsequent sections discuss the kindling mechanism and some of its clinical or behavioral manifestations, limbic epilepsy, and implications of our current understanding of the limbic system in psychiatry.

This volume will be of interest to those studying the basic anatomical, physiological, and biochemical aspects of the limbic system, as well as those concerned primarily with the clinical manifestations of limbic system dysfunction and their treatment.

BENJAMIN K. DOANE
KENNETH E. LIVINGSTON*

---

*Deceased.

v

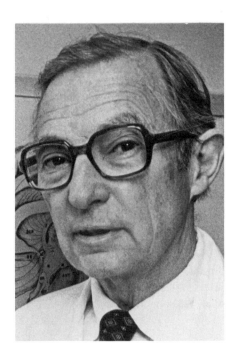

KENNETH EDWIN LIVINGSTON, M.D.
31 October 1918–21 July 1984

Note from a 1982 memorandum:

It is likely that insight into limbic mechanisms will have increasingly revolutionary effects on medical education, neurological and psychiatric health care, and on many fields of understanding in the behavioral and social sciences. More especially, insight into limbic mechanisms will influence how people empathize with one another, and introspect in relation to their own brains.

Acknowledgments

This book is a compilation of the papers presented at an international symposium that was held in Toronto under the title "Patterns of Limbic System Dysfunction: Seizures, Psychosis, and Dyscontrol." This symposium focused on the role of limbic system dysfunction in a broad spectrum of major clinical disabilities classified and treated as neurological, psychiatric, or psychological disorders.

This symposium, like the earlier one held in 1976, was largely the inspiration of Dr. Kenneth E. Livingston, whose tragic illness prevented his attendance at the 1983 symposium and subsequently led to his untimely death. In planning the 1983 meeting, it was Ken Livingston's wish to bring together individuals working in the basic and clinical sciences, not only to represent the span of interest in topics related to limbic system function and dysfunction, but to promote communication and interchange of ideas between those studying basic anatomical, physiological, and biochemical aspects of the limbic system, on the one hand, and those concerned primarily with the clinical manifestations of limbic system dysfunction and their treatment, on the other.

Those present at the symposium, whether as participants or observers, shared the opinion that the meeting largely achieved the purposes stated above. Much enthusiasm was evident throughout the meeting, although this was tempered some-what by sadness due to the real awareness of Ken Livingston's absence and ill health. It is gratifying, at least, to know that he was aware of the success of the event. Now, the publication of this book, which was also his wish, not only helps to solidify the achievements of the symposium itself but also serves as a tribute from the participants to Dr. Kenneth E. Livingston, a man whose open-minded interest and infectious enthusiasm for life and for his work will continue, through very tangible memories, to inspire those who are privileged to have known him.

The success of the symposium and the publication of its contents have been made possible only with the support of many people and organizations. I appreciate the encouragement given to me by two of those most closely associated with Ken Livingston over the years—his brother, Robert B. Livingston, and Paul MacLean. Without their help, the job of carrying through with the meeting in his absence would have been more difficult. Miss Nancy Stead, Dr. Livingston's personal secretary, worked very hard during the early stages of planning the meeting and also made very much easier my task of carrying on wihout Ken Livingston's help. Ms. Michele Lahey, Dr. Livingston's research assistant, provided invaluable as-sistance with local arrangements. Before, during, and after the symposium, Miss Doris McBride in the Department of Continuing Medical Education, the Faculty of Medicine, at the University of Toronto, worked beyond the call of duty with personal sacrifice. Within the Department of Psychiatry, Dalhousie University, thanks are due to Miss Beverly Quigley, who helped with preparations for the symposium, and to Mrs. Shelagh Parker, whose preparation of manuscripts and attention to other details, with help from Mrs. Shirley Taylor, have made this book possible.

Grateful acknowledgment is made of the financial support provided by the W. P. Scott Charitable Foundation with the personal encouragement of Mr. Michael Scott and family; Dr. Fred Lowy, Dean of Medicine at the University of Toronto; the W. Garfield Weston Foundation in Toronto; the Royal College of Physicians and Surgeons of Canada; Ciba-Geigy Pharmaceuticals; The Upjohn Company of Canada; Ayerst Research Laboratories; and Pfizer Canada Ltd.

B.K.D.

Contents

Epilogue

Contributors

R. E. Adamec
Department of Psychology
Memorial University of Newfoundland
St. John's, Newfoundland, Canada A1B 3X9

Penny S. Albright
Department of Pharmacology
University of Toronto
Toronto, Ontario, Canada M5S 1A8

David M. Bear
New England Deaconess Hospital
Boston, Massachusetts 02215

W. M. Burnham
Department of Pharmacology
University of Toronto
Toronto, Ontario, Canada M5S 1A8

W. Stephen Corrie
Departments of Neurosciences and Psychiatry
Medical College of Ohio
Toledo, Ohio 43699

Benjamin K. Doane
Department of Psychiatry
Dalhousie University
Victoria General Hospital
Halifax, Nova Scotia, B3H 2Y9 Canada

Michael Dragunow
Department of Psychology
University of Otago
Dunedin, New Zealand

Shunkichi Endo
Department of Neuropsychiatry
Nippon Medical School
Sendagi, Bunkyo-ku
Tokyo, 113 Japan

Shirley M. Ferguson
Departments of Neurosciences and Psychiatry
Medical College of Ohio
Toledo, Ohio 43699

M. Girgis
Faculty of Medicine
University of Sydney
Sydney, New South Wales, Australia 2006

P. Gloor
Montreal Neurological Institute and the Department of Neurology and Neurosurgery
McGill University
Montreal, Quebec, Canada H3A 2B4

Graham V. Goddard
Department of Psychology
University of Otago
Dunedin, New Zealand

Sadao Hirose
Department of Neuropsychiatry
Nippon Medical School
Sendagi, Bunkyo-ku
Tokyo, 113 Japan

S. J. Kish
Department of Pharmacology
University of Toronto
Toronto, Ontario, Canada M5S 1A8

K. E. Livingston*
Department of Pharmacology
University of Toronto
Toronto, Ontario, Canada M5S 1A8

Robert B. Livingston
Department of Neuroscience
University of California at San Diego
La Jolla, California 92093

*Deceased.

xiv CONTRIBUTORS

Paul D. MacLean
*Laboratory of Brain Evolution and
Behavior
National Institute of Mental Health
Bethesda, Maryland 20205*

E. Keith Macleod
*Department of Psychology
University of Otago
Dunedin, New Zealand*

Eiichi Maru
*Department of Psychology
University of Otago
Dunedin, New Zealand*

D. McIntryre
*Department of Psychology
Carleton University
Ottawa, Ontario, Canada*

Russell R. Monroe
*Department of Psychiatry
University of Maryland
Baltimore, Maryland 21201*

Haring J. W. Nauta
*Division of Neurosurgery
The University of Texas Medical Branch
Galveston, Texas 77550*

Walle J. H. Nauta
*Department of Psychology and Brain
Science
Massachusetts Institute of Technology
Cambridge, Massachusetts 02139*

H. B. Niznik
*Department of Pharmacology
University of Toronto
Toronto, Ontario, Canada M5S 1A8*

C. E. Poletti
*Massachusetts General Hospital
Harvard Medical School
Boston, Massachusetts 02114*

Robert M. Post
*Biological Psychiatry Branch
National Institute of Mental Health
Bethesda, Maryland 20205*

R. J. Racine
*Department of Psychology
McMaster University
Hamilton, Ontario, Canada L8S 4K1*

Mark Rayport
*Departments of Neurosciences and
Psychiatry
Medical College of Ohio
Toledo, Ohio 43699*

C. Stark-Adamec
*Department of Psychology
University of Regina
Regina, Sasketchewan, Canada S4S 0A2*

Michael R. Trimble
*National Hospital for Nervous Diseases
and Institute of Neurology
Queen Square
London, WC1N 3BG, United Kingdom*

Thomas W. Uhde
*Biological Psychiatry Branch
National Institute of Mental Health
Bethesda, Maryland 20205*

THE LIMBIC SYSTEM

Functional Organization and Clinical Disorders

The Limbic System: Functional Organization and
Clinical Disorders, edited by B. K. Doane and
K. E. Livingston. Raven Press, New York © 1986.

Culminating Developments in the Evolution of the Limbic System: The Thalamocingulate Division[1]

Paul D. MacLean

*Laboratory of Brain Evolution and Behavior, National Institute of Mental Health,
Bethesda, Maryland 20205*

In this chapter, I shall focus on new findings on the functions of the cingulate gyrus, which, in several respects, represents the culminating development of the limbic system, or, as one might say, the highest level of the Papez circuit (65). Cingulate, meaning girdle, applies to the part of the limbic lobe engirdling the corpus callosum. Figure 1 shows how Campbell (10) depicted the distribution of the cingulate cortex in his classical study of 1905.

As is well known, the cingulate gyrus has long been a major interest of Ken Livingston. Before returning to contemporary history, it is necessary to delve into

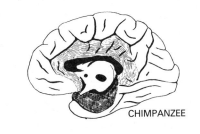

CHIMPANZEE

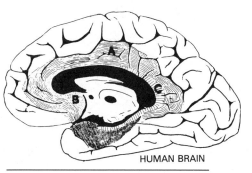

HUMAN BRAIN

FIG. 1. Medial surface of chimpanzee and human brain. This redrawn figure from Campbell's (10) classical study of 1905 shows only the shading he used for the great limbic lobe of Broca. Shading with concentric lines **(A)** identifies most of the exposed cingulate cortex; stipple **(B)** and radiate shading **(C)**, respectively, overlies paragenual and retrosplenial cingulate cortex. (From MacLean, refs. 49, 52; redrawn from Campbell, ref. 10.)

[1]This chapter is dedicated to the memory of Kenneth E. Livingston.

1

ancient history and review how three forms of behavior that most clearly mark the evolutionary dividing line between reptiles and mammals found representation in the cingulate gyrus. These three forms of behavior are (a) nursing, in conjunction with maternal care; (b) audiovocal communication for maintaining maternal–offspring contact; and (c) play. This behavioral triad is basic to the family way of life of mammals. Significantly, the cingulate gyrus and its subcortical connections appear to have no recognizable counterpart in the reptilian brain (11). Based on this comparative anatomical observation, Clark and Meyer speculated that the functions subserved by the cingulate circuit "must have a relation to forms of cerebral activity which are not to be found in any vertebrates other than mammals" (11, p. 342). Apropos of the topic of this volume, the findings to be discussed are relevant not only to a prospectus of future research on the limbic system (51), but also to certain psychological disorders referred to in the subtitle of the volume.

EVOLUTIONARY CONSIDERATIONS

Comparative neuroanatomical findings, together with studies of ontogeny, phylogeny, and paleontology, provide evidence that the human forebrain has evolved and expanded to its great size while retaining commonalities of three neural assemblies that reflect an ancestral relationship to reptiles, early mammals, and late mammals (44). Greatly different in chemistry and structure and, in an evolutionary sense, eons apart, these three major formations of the forebrain constitute an amalgamation of three brains in one—a triune brain (Fig. 2) (41,42). In reptiles, birds, and mammals, the use of histochemical methods for identifying acetylcholinesterase and dopamine has been particularly valuable for identifying corresponding structures of the protoreptilian forebrain. Commonly known as basal ganglia, these structures include the olfactostriatum (olfactory tubercle and nucleus accumbens), together with the corpus striatum (caudate and putamen; see ref. 13, p.

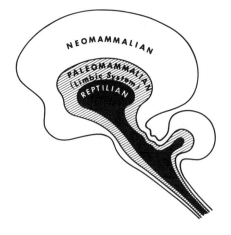

FIG. 2. Evolutionary triune development of the primate brain. Three neural assemblies of the forebrain (labeled) reflect, both neuroanatomically and chemically, an ancestral relationship to reptiles, early mammals, and late mammals. The limbic system would be a synonymous term for the "paleomammalian" brain. (From MacLean, ref. 40.)

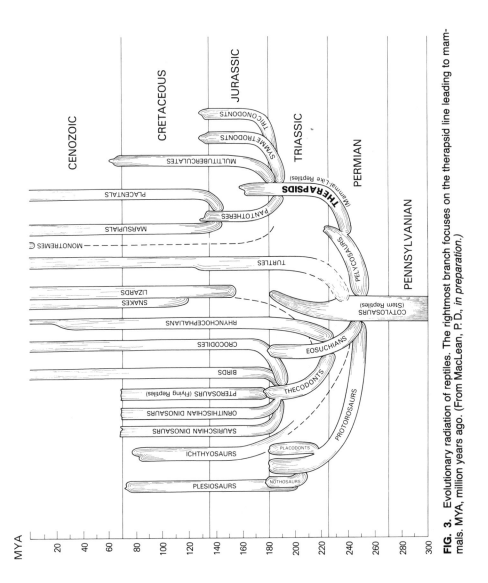

FIG. 3. Evolutionary radiation of reptiles. The rightmost branch focuses on the therapsid line leading to mammals. MYA, million years ago. (From MacLean, P. D., *in preparation.*)

360), globus pallidus, and satellite collections of gray matter. The entire mass may be referred to as the striatal complex or, in comparative terms, the reptilian complex (R-complex) (44). All except parts of the pallidum belong to the telencephalon. The forebrain assembly identified with early mammals corresponds to the so-called limbic system, which comprises the great limbic lobe of Broca and structures of the brainstem with which it has primary connections (37). In reptiles and birds the pallial areas with similarities to limbic cortex are rudimentary and only partially represented. The "neomammalian brain" may be defined as the neocortex and structures of the brainstem with which it is primarily connected. (Some anatomists regard the subcortical ganglionic structures in the dorsal ventricular ridge of reptiles and birds as "neocortex.")

The lineage of mammals can be traced back 250 million years ago to the mammal-like reptiles or so-called therapsids (Fig. 3). Long before the dinosaurs, the therapsids populated Pangaea (92) (Fig. 4: 1) in great numbers. Their remains have been found in every continent, including Antarctica, which broke off from the great southern continent called Gondwanaland (81) (Fig. 4: 2). Some of the therapsids, known as cynodonts and believed to be the antecedents of mammals, resembled dogs and wolves (Fig. 4: 3). It should be emphasized that, in addition to this general appearance, the jaws and teeth and other cranial features were approaching the mammalian condition.

COMPARATIVE ASPECTS OF REPTILIAN BEHAVIOR

What can be inferred about the behavior of the therapsids? This question was addressed in a recent conference on the mammal-like reptiles (74). There is no evidence yet whether or not the therapsids were egg laying, and, relevant to the question of whether or not they exhibited parental behavior, there is only one finding suggesting such a possibility.

Late in triassic times the therapsids became extinct. If a cooling trend or alternating wet and arid conditions existed, it is possible that some forms transitional with mammals retained their eggs and developed placenta-like membranes. Somewhere along the line, scales became replaced by hairs and associated sweat glands. Milk glands are believed to have developed from sweat or sebaceous glands. The advanced therapsids were hard of hearing. Two small bones in the jaw joint (Fig. 4: 4) had not yet migrated into the middle ear to become the malleus and incus that afforded more acute hearing in mammals. The therapsids may have been mute like most of today's lizards and also cannibalistic. If they were mute, this may have had survival value for the young because if the latter had called attention to themselves by vocalization, their parents might have searched them out and eaten

---

FIG. 4. Illustrations relevent to the ecology and biology of the mammal-like reptiles. **1**: Pangaea. **2**: Gondwanaland. **3**: Two representative carnivorous therapsids (**A**, *Lycaenops*; **B**, *Thrinaxodon*) illustrating their mammal-like features. **4**: **A** and **A′**, diagram emphasizing two bones of the therapsid jaw joint (the quadrate above and articular below) that become, respectively, the incus and malleus of the mammalian ear (**B**). (Drawings based on various sources; from MacLean, P. D., *in preparation*.)

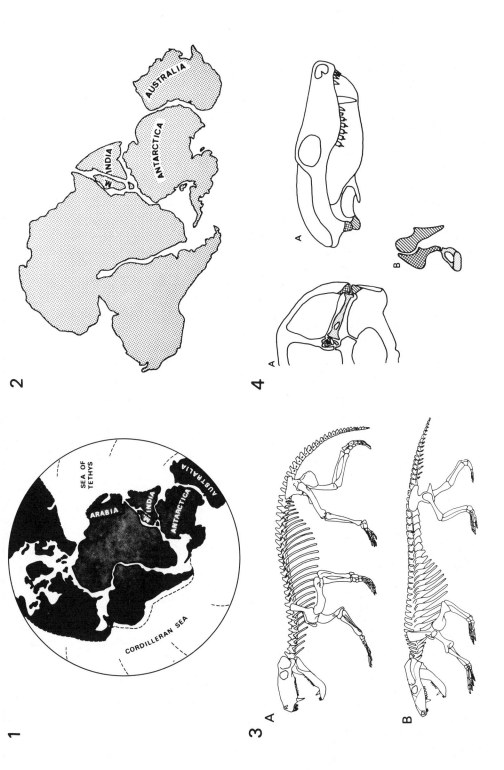

1

2

3 A

B

4

them. It is believed that the tiny *transitional* mammals lived on the dark floor of the forest and may have been nocturnal. Under such conditions, it is evident how the development of audiovocal communication would have greatly helped to maintain maternal–offspring contact. The separation call (alias, isolation call) characteristic of mammals possibly represents the most primitive and basic mammalian vocalization.

Neurobehavioral Work on Lizards

There are no existing reptiles that are phylogenetically in line with the therapsids. The primitive therapsids were so lizard-like in structure that the paleontological name for one of them is *Varanosaurus*, after the monitor lizard, of which the Komodo dragon is an outstanding example. Consequently, for this and other reasons, in our comparative neurobehavioral studies involving reptiles we have focused on lizards.

For neurobehavioral work it is essential to be as knowledgeable as possible about the behavioral profile (ethogram) of the species under study. If different aspects of the behavioral profile were likened to a mountain range seen from a distance, then the behavioral profile of reptiles, birds, and mammals would appear as two main ranges (50). In one range are peaks and subpeaks identified with the chain of activities in an animal's daily *master routine* and *subroutines*. In the other range are four main patterns of behavior used by all land vertebrates in prosematic (nonverbal) communication (44). Known alternatively as displays, the four main forms in lizards are referred to as signature, territorial, courtship, and submissive displays.

In analyzing the behavior of lizards, one can identify more than 25 forms of behavior that are also typical of mammals (44,45). Most notably lacking is the family-related, behavioral triad consisting of (a) nursing, in conjunction with maternal care, (b) audiovocal communication for maintaining maternal–offspring contact, and (c) play (46,49,50,52). As a further preface to the work on the thalamocingulate division of the limbic system, emphasis should be given to a striking behavioral contrast between lizards and mammals. Most lizards lay their eggs and then go away and leave them to hatch on their own. The hatchlings come into the world prepared to do everything that they have to do except to procreate (6). Infant mammals, on the contrary, are totally dependent on nursing and maternal attention. Any prolonged separation from the mother is calamitous, a situation that again calls attention to the importance of the separation call for maintaining maternal–offspring contact.

The Striatal Complex

A major purpose of our comparative neurobehavioral studies has been a clarification of the functions of the striatal complex. The traditional neurological view holds that the striatal complex is primarily part of the motor systems under the control of the motor cortex. This view has prevailed despite the knowledge (based on both clinical findings and animal experiments) that large dissolutions of parts of the striatal complex may be present without apparent loss of motor function (44,47). It has been our purpose to learn whether or not experiments on animals engaged in measurable forms of species-typical behavior might reveal functions of the striatal complex that would not otherwise be apparent.

Without going into detail, I will simply note here that our comparative studies have demonstrated that in animals as diverse as lizards (22) and monkeys (43,47,48), the striatal complex plays an essential role in the evocation and performance of displays.

Other evidence is developing that the striatal complex is basically implicated in linking together an animal's daily master routine and subroutines.

EVOLUTION AND DIFFERENTIATION OF CINGULATE CORTEX

Before delving into the part played by the thalamocingulate division in the behavioral triad under consideration, it is relevant to both ongoing and future research to consider questions pertaining to the evolution and differentiation of the cingulate cortex.

In mammals with well-formed gyri, it may be said as a generalization that the features of the cingulate cortex are found within the limiting borders of the cingulate sulci. As Kappers et al. (3, p.1592) have commented, "It is remarkable that the sagittal fissures, which bound this region dorsally, remain constant to a considerable extent throughout the mammalian series, not only morphologically but also in their relation to the underlying cytoarchitectonic fields." Specifically, with regard to the Nissl and myelin picture, Campbell (10, p. 282) observed that all "the facts" indicate that like the hippocampal gyrus, the cingulate gyrus is "invested by cortex of great phylogenic age." These convolutions (Fig. 1) form a massive part of the great limbic lobe of Broca (7). It was Broca's special contribution to demonstrate that the limbic lobe is found as a common denominator in the brains of all mammals (7) (see Fig. 5).

According to Smith (78), Reichert in 1859 introduced the word "pallium" for the purpose of distinguishing the covering of the cerebral hemispheres from underlying structures of the brainstem. The term pallium, rather than cortex, is usually applied to the outer cerebral gray matter in reptiles and birds in which the layering of neural elements is either lacking or rudimentary. Figure 6 shows the traditional parcellation of three main pallial areas in the reptilian brain. Due to an influential paper by Smith (78) in 1901, there has been the tendency to regard the general pallium as the anlage of the neocortex. Smith referred to the "pyriform" (original spelling) and hippocampal areas as the "old pallium," whereas he introduced the name "neopallium" as a term for the rest of the mantle. Here we find a precedent for including more of the cerebral mantle, including the cingulate cortex, under the designation neocortex than is justified (see below). Raymond Dart (14), a former student of Smith, proposed a dual origin of the neopallium: Using the reptilian brain as a prototype, he argued that general pallium represented an

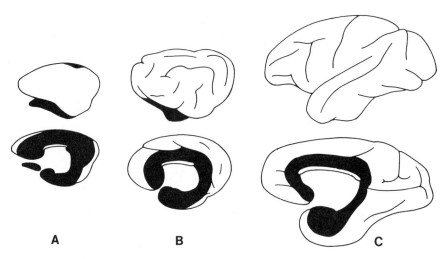

FIG. 5. Limbic lobe *(shaded)* in three familiar animals. The drawings are illustrative of Broca's observation that the limbic lobe surrounding the brainstem is a common denominator of the brains of all mammals. (From MacLean, ref. 38.)

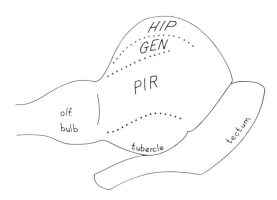

FIG. 6. Three main pallial areas of the reptilian brain. The piriform (PIR) and hippocampal (HIP) areas are regarded as rudimentary forms of the like-named areas in mammals. The general (GEN) pallium has commonly been regarded as the anlage of the neocortex. See text for a different interpretation. Other labels: olf. bulb, olfactory bulb; tectum refers to optic tectum. (From MacLean, *forthcoming book.*)

outgrowth, respectively, from the "pyriform" and hippocampal areas. Here was the germ of the concept of "successive waves of circumferential differentiation" as developed by Abbie (2, pp. 532–533) and later elaborated upon by Sanides (75) in terms of a concentric growth ring hypothesis.

Transitional Nature of Cingulate Cortex

Although recognizing the transitional nature of the parahippocampal cingulate cortex, Abbie (1,2), like Smith and Dart, referred to it as neopallium. Sanides

(75), however, in giving emphasis to its transitional features, characterized it by the Vogts' term *proisocortex* (91a).

The classification of cortex according to Maximilian Rose, of the Vogt School, would be compatible with the growth ring hypothesis. Based on his embryological studies, Rose (72, p. 67) concluded that most of the cerebral cortex can be subdivided into three principal types consisting of two, five, or seven layers, which he referred to as "bi-, quinque-, und, septemstratificatus." The two-layered cortex included the so-called archicortex. Rose characterized most cingulate and adjacent areas as "quinquestratificatus." Since he considered such cortex to be transitional between the first and third types, he had referred to it in earlier studies as *meso-cortex* (72), a terminology that Yakovlev (96, p. 331) and collaborators (97, p. 629) subsequently applied to transitional cingulate cortex. Among the distinguishing features of mesocortex (proisocortex) is a deeply staining layer II containing a distinctive type of tufted cell with dendrites spreading into layer I, but having only "weak" basal dendrites (75), or, according to Vogt and Peters (87, p. 623), "only one basally projecting dendrite." Sanides (75) also gives special emphasis to the "bandlike layer V" of the anterior cingulate cortex.

Since most of the cingulate cortex represents a mesocortical outgrowth from the hippocampus, it is of interest to consider what might have been the cerebral changes in the transition from mammal-like reptiles to mammals. Unfortunately, there are currently available only a few cranial endocasts of therapsids (53,74). The casts indicate that the cerebral hemispheres of intermediate therapsids were relatively long and narrow, as is typical of extant reptiles. The endocasts of transitional mammals reveal a widening of the hemispheres. The conformation is suggestive of rodent brains in which an alkylating agent has been used to prevent the greater part of the neocortex and cingulate cortex from developing during gestation (53). In such brains the greatly reduced cingulate cortex occupies a position that would correspond to the parahippocampal part of the "general pallial" area in Fig. 6.

Four Main Cingulate Areas

The brain of the domestic rabbit *(Oryctolagus cuniculus)*, belonging to the order Lagomorpha, serves to illustrate features of four main areas of cingulate cortex. For this purpose, I use the description by Rose and Woosley (71), including, however, their infralimbic area along with their so-called anterior limbic, cingular, and retrosplenial areas (Fig. 7A).

Infralimbic Area

The infralimbic area corresponds approximately to Brodmann's (8) area 25 and to Rose's (73) *Regio infradiata* (aα) (Fig. 7A–C). Lying rostrodorsal to the *taenia tecta*, it extends from the level of the knee of the corpus callosum to almost the frontal pole, forming a strip that lies medial to the rostral extension of the lateral ventricle. Although the molecular layer (layer I) is as wide or wider than that of other cingulate areas, the cortical layers are thin and do not show a definite layering.

The outer margin of layer II is uneven, and, as is characteristic of cingulate cortex, the cells stain more deeply than those of the underlying layers.

It should be emphasized that this cortex is of special interest because of its close relationship to the olfactory apparatus and possible functional involvement in nursing and the separation call. Recently, reciprocal connections have been found between nerve cells in this area and the vagal solitary nucleus (28,84). The same reciprocal relationship applies to the anterior limbic area next to be described.

Anterior Limbic Area

The anterior limbic area corresponds to areas 32 and 24 of Brodmann and the dorsal part of the infraradiate region (bα + cα) of Rose (73) (cf. Fig. 7). The prelimbic area of the Krettek and Price (29) map for the rat is coextensive with area 32. The superficial elements of layer II are dark staining. There is no distinct border between the cells of layers II and III until the precentral agranular neocortex is approached. The typically small cells of these layers are distinctly larger than the so-called granular cells of the cingular area. There is no discernible granular layer IV. Layer V is about the thickness of layers II and III combined and contains larger cells that are distinctly pyramidal in shape. Layer VI is characterized by deeply staining fusiform cells. At the junction with the neocortex, the cells of this layer appear to pile up into multiple concentric rows.

The Cingular Area

Proceeding in a caudal direction, one finds that the cingulate cortex changes rather abruptly in character at about the level of the anterior thalamic nuclei. The superficial layers appear more prominent because the elements are more deeply stained, and the cortex also assumes a dysgranular appearance because of an incipient intermingling of granule-like cells with the cells of layer III. Rose and Woolsey's cingular area occupies a considerable extent of the posterior limbic cortex, corresponding approximately to Brodmann's area 23, together with his areas 29d and 29c (Fig. 7A,B). The cortex of this region is distinguished by the presence of a thin granular layer IV separating the supragranular layers II and III from the infragranular layers V and VI.

Retrosplenial Area

The parasplenial and retrosplenial regions comprise the retrosplenial area of Rose and Woolsey (71), corresponding to Brodmann's areas 29a and 29b (Fig. 7B).

--➤

FIG. 7. Parcelation, according to different authors, of cytoarchitectural areas of the cingulate cortex in the brain of a lagomorph and a rodent. **A, B, C** represent, respectively, partially redrawn figures of rabbit brain from J. Rose and Woolsey (71), Brodmann (8), and M. Rose (73). **D** shows one scheme for the rat (87). See text for other details. Abbreviations: Cg, cingular area; CC, (r)ostral and (s)plenial corpus callosum; H, hippocampus; IL, infralimbic area; IR, IR, regio infra radiata; La, anterior limbic region; Of, orbitofrontal area; P or Ps, postsubicular area; Prag, precentral agranular area; Rs, retrosplenial area; tt, taenia tecta; RSg, granular retrosplenial area.

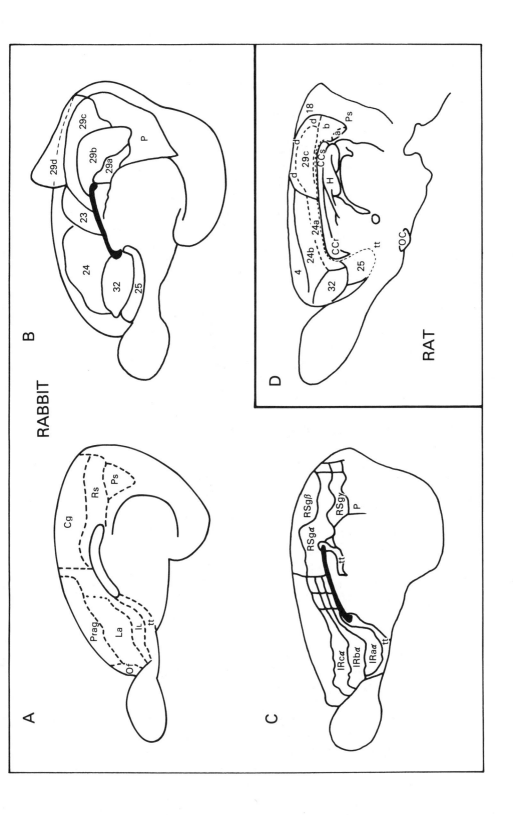

RABBIT

A

Cg
Rs
Ps
Prag
La
IL
tt
Of

B

29d
29c
29b
29a
23
24
32
25
P

C

RSgα
RSgβ
RSgγ
P
tt
IRcα
IRbα
IRaα
tt

D

18
d
d
d
b
a
29c
CCs
Ps
H
24a
24b
CCr
4
tt
32
25
OC
O

RAT

Examination in a rostrocaudal direction of supracallosal, parasplenial cortex reveals a thinning of the second layer and a progressive piling up of granular cells in layer III. This is area 29b. Behind the level of the splenium, such cells almost totally occupy the width of cortex usually identified as layers II and III. Immediately below this wide granular layer are layers V and VI. This area corresponds to Brodmann's 29a. Inferiorly, and toward the presubiculum, superficial dark-staining cells practically disappear, and this part of the retrosplenial cortex acquires a distinctive appearance because of the lining up in horizontal rows of small irregular cells that give the appearance of the warp and weave of a silken garment. According to Rose and Woolsey (71), this distinctive area would correspond to Brodmann's area 29e, 27b, and 48 that he referred to as *area retrosubicularis* (area 48) in other mammals.

Cingulate Cortex of Rodents

In view of the neurobehavioral work on rodents to be described, it may prove relevant to future research to be cognizant of how the cytoarchitectural picture in this order of mammals may differ significantly in one respect from the description given above. As was noted, the cingular area (area 23) in the rabbit is characterized by a thin granular layer IV below layers II and III. On the contrary, as Vogt and Peters (87) have pointed out, area 23 in the rat is "actually a transitional region between areas 24 and 29, where the granularity is forming in layers II-III, and not in layer IV." Moreover, area 29d included in Rose and Woolsey's cingular area is dysgranular. Accordingly, Vogt and Peters (87) contend that area 23 does not exist in the rat.

Cingulate Cortex in Primates

The question has also been raised as to whether or not the cingular area (area 23) exists in primates. In his areal scheme for subdividing the cingulate cortex, M. Rose (72) does not include the posterior cingulate cortex in primates as a meso-cortical area. Rather, he regarded this cortex as fully developed cortex with the basic seven layers (septemstratificatus). Other authors, however, both on the basis of cytoarchitecture and thalamic connections, are inclined to regard the posterior cingulate cortex as transitional in character.

Human Cingulate

Figure 1 shows Campbell's (10) depiction of the different cytoarchitectural areas that he delineated in the limbic lobe of the human brain. The concentric shading overlies most of the cingulate gyrus, which spans the corpus callosum like a great arc. He noted first of all that on the basis of fiber-stained material, "it will be granted immediately that the [cingulate cortex] is deserving of separate represen-tation on a cerebral map" (p. 184). Specifically, he explains, "Perhaps the chief distinguishing feature of this type of cortex is that it contains absolutely no large

evenly-medullated [sic] fibres like those seen in the central convolutions and calcarine region, and indeed practically none of medium calibre; they are all fine and
wavy, and in most cases varicose, hence the pallor of the cortex when compared
with that of *adjoining fields*" (p. 184) (italics added).

In his book on the connections of the primate brain, Krieg (30, p. 219) states,
"The cortex of the cingulate gyrus is regarded by all close students of cortical
architectonics as a distinct type, set off from all other cortex . . ." At the same time
he points out that posterior cingulate cortex "so nearly resembles parietal cortex
that M. Rose has excluded it from the cingulate type." Nevertheless, Krieg insists,
it retains "the cingular stamp." Presumably he had reference to the same kind of
observation made by Campbell on the basis of fiber-stained sections—namely, that
not only the anterior, but also the posterior cingulate gyrus appears pale when
compared with the supracingulate cortex. This situation seems to apply generally
to the primate brain, as one can satisfy oneself by examining the brains of such
animals as the pygmy marmoset, squirrel monkey, and on upward.

As evident in Fig. 1, Campbell (10) recognized only three areal divisions of the
cingulate gyrus. The letters B and C label two subareas that stand out prominently
in the human brain. He defined the area marked B as a 5- to 10-mm strip in the
paragenual region that *extends inferiorly as far as the medial root of the olfactory
nerve.* He described this area as being characterized by deeply staining elongated
pyramidal cells in the deep layers. He delineated the parasplenial region labeled C
as a 5- to 10-mm strip of cortex covered over, in part, by a band of myelinated
fibers that represent the continuation of the *lamina medullaris superficialis* overlying the subicular cortex of the temporal region. The so-called *induseum griseum*
extending the length of the corpus callosum represents a rudimentary continuation
of the hippocampus. It is covered by the thin part of the *lamina medullaris*, whereas
the narrow strip of gray matter lateral to it and overlain by the thick part of the
band corresponds to the subiculum and its perforating fibers. The classically recognized retrosplenial cortex lies adjacent to the subicular cortex in the supracallosal
and parasplenial areas within the region labeled C. According to Flechsig (18), the
entire region is one of the first cortical areas to become myelinated.

As evident by the region labeled A, Campbell did not draw a distinction between
the anterior and posterior cingulate areas, which were subsequently identified by
Brodmann as areas 24 and 23. These two areas are clearly distinguished by the
presence in the latter of a distinct granular layer IV, and the border between them
is marked roughly by a line extending from the central sulcus to the corpus
callosum. Brodmann's areas 24 and 23 correspond approximately to the regions
labeled LA and LC by von Economo and Koskinas (17). These last authors also
recognized a retrosplenial area, corresponding to Brodmann's area 29, which they
labeled LD.

Based on their studies of both cytoarchitecture and thalamic connections in the
rabbit and cat, Rose and Woolsey (71, p. 33) went so far as to state: "There is no
reason to assume that the retrosplenial and cingular fields should be separate

regions, as is widely accepted. They are certainly related and it seems reasonable to combine them both in one posterior limbic region."

Nonhuman Primates

In cytoarchitectonic studies, Lorente de Nó (35) emphasized that reliance on the Nissl and myelin picture may lead to faulty conclusions and that Golgi-stained material for identifying plexi, types of cells, and cellular connections is also necessary. Brent Vogt (86) recently noted that except for Cajal's (68) studies on the interhemispheric cortex of the rodent, there exist no extensive Golgi studies on the cingulate cortex of other species. Vogt (86) himself has provided a description of the Golgi picture of the retrosplenial cortex in the macaque.

In infrahuman primates generally, the four main areas of the cingulate gyrus can be differentiated on the basis of the criteria that have been discussed. The posterior cingulate cortex with a resemblance to the medial parietal neocortex shows a significant difference insofar as it is distinctly paler because of the lesser myelination of the radiate fibers. Moreover, the granular layer is thinner and lies nearer to the surface, signifying also that the supragranular layers are more poorly developed than in the supracingulate cortex.

Finally, recent findings with improved neuroanatomical techniques lend further assurance to original findings that the posterior cingulate and retrosplenial areas in primates, are, as in the case of nonprimate mammals, innervated by the anterior thalamic nuclei (see below).

Other Comparative Aspects

It is also relevant to future research that there is both anatomical (12,22a,54,70) and electrophysiological (56,64,84a) evidence of visual inputs to the retrosplenial area. Some of the original cytoarchitectural observations of Campbell (10) are of interest in the light of such findings. He noted that the retrosplenial area is unusually extensive in pig and that in the depth of the stem of the parasplenial sulcus (corresponding to the rostral stem of the calcarine in primates), the retrosplenial cortex can be easily confused with the primary visual cortex. In his words, "[C]are must be exercised not to confound it with the visual, for in sections stained for nerve fibres, a linear arrangement occurs, which a superficial observer might mistake for a line of Gennari" (p. 275). Cajal (68) himself, in his earlier observations, mistook the retrosplenial cortex in rodents for the visual cortex. Regarding the question of some kind of visual function, it is pertinent to mention that in such visually deficient animals as the ground shrew and the bat, the retrosplenial area is poorly developed (72).

Whales (Cetacea)

Apropos of the subsequent focus on the role of the cingulate gyrus in maternal behavior, vocalization, and play, it is of interest to comment on the development and structure of this convolution in whales. The behavioral triad in question is remarkably expressed in this order of mammals. The cingulate part of the limbic lobe is well developed. The Nissl picture of the cingulate cortex has recently been described and illustrated by Morgane et al. (58). Given a familiarity with the rodent brain, it is surprising to find that in these animals that separated from the land mammals some 60 or more million years ago (21,26), one can detect in the main cingulate areas many of the same diagnostic features. In Golgi studies, Morgane et al. (57) observed that cells of layer II generally are characterized by the presence of "extraverted neurons" resembling the primitive type in the hedgehog by having four or more dendritic processes extending into the molecular layer and possessing no basilar dendrites.

CONNECTIONS AND FUNCTIONS OF THALAMOCINGULATE DIVISION

Based both on connectional and functional neuroanatomical considerations, the limbic system can be parceled into three main corticosubcortical subdivisions. As indicated in Fig. 8, two telencephalic nuclear groups located in the amygdala and

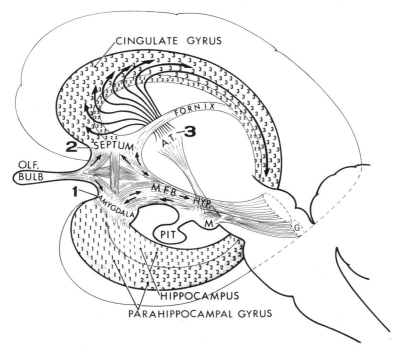

FIG. 8. Three major subdivisions of the limbic system. The small numerals 1, 2, and 3 overlie, respectively, the amygdaloid, septal, and thalamocingulate divisions. The corresponding large numerals identify connecting nuclei in the amygdala, septum, and anterior thalamus. Abbreviations: AT, anterior thalamic nuclei; G, tegmental nuclei of Gudden; HYP, hypothalamus; M, mammillary bodies; MFB, medial forebrain bundle; PIT, pituitary; OLF, olfactory. (From MacLean, ref. 42.)

the septum are centers for two of these subdivisions. The amygdala division has been shown to be involved in feeling and expressive states essential for self-preservation (namely, the search for food, feeding, fighting, and self-protection), whereas the septal division has been found to be implicated in feeling and expressive states conducive to procreation (42,44).

Thalamic Connections

The thalamocingulate division is so referred to because the afferent supply to the mesocortical areas derives from the thalamus. Since the focus of this chapter is on the functions of this subdivision, reference should be made to a clarification of thalamocingulate afferents provided by recent neuroanatomical studies. A major new finding pertains to the anterior limbic area that was formerly believed to be innervated primarily by the anterior medial and anterior ventral nuclei. Leonard's (32) finding that the medial frontal cortex in the rat, including the anterior limbic cortex, is innervated by the medial dorsal (MD) nucleus and probably also by the anterior medial (AM) nucleus has now been confirmed by others (29,89). In the monkey it also appears that the anterior cingulate cortex is co-innervated by MD (4,88) and (AM) (4) and that, in addition, it receives afferents from a number of the intralaminar nuclei (4,88). In both primate and nonprimate animals, the bulk of the projections of the anterior thalamic nuclei appears to co-innervate the posterior cingulate cortex, including the retrosplenial area. The most detailed information derives from horseradish peroxidase and autoradiographic studies on the cat (69). In summarizing these connections, it should be pointed out that the posterior part of Rose and Woolsey's retrosplenial area in the cat and other carnivores includes Brodmann's area 30. This dorsal "dysgranular" area forms a quarter-moon-shaped border around the ventral retrosplenial granular (area 29). The anterior dorsal nucleus projects almost entirely to the ventral granular area, i.e., area 29. The anterior medial nucleus has heavier projections to this area than to the anterior limbic area, whereas the anterior ventral nucleus has a greater projection to the dorsal "dysgranular" area (area 30) than to the cingular area (area 23). The lateral dorsal nucleus lying just caudolateral to the anterior group and peripheral to the internal medullary lamina is a neothalamic nucleus and projects more extensively to the posterior cingulate than to the anterior cingulate cortex (69). The limbic cortex of the so-called infralimbic area appears to receive fibers from nucleus reuniens (71).

Regarding olfactory connections with the limbic cortex, it appears to be the rule that secondary olfactory projections end in the outer half of layer I, whereas tertiary afferents terminate in the lower half of layer I. A parallel situation would seem to apply to the cingulate mesocortex. According to Oscar Vogt's (90) scheme of 1910, the molecular layer may be subdivided into layers 1a, b, and c. According to the comment by B. Vogt et al. (89), Ia is the primary site of termination of fibers from the anterior thalamus. In the anterior limbic area (areas 32 and 24) the authors found that lesions of the medial dorsal nucleus (complicated by damage also to the anterior medial nucleus) terminated in layers Ia and Ib, whereas callosal fibers were distributed to layers Ib and Ic. In the cat Robertson and Kaitz (69) observed that the projections from the anterior thalamic group terminate in the outer half of layer I and in the superficial layers (layers II and III). The lateral dorsal nucleus, in keeping with its neothalmic origins, projects to granular layer IV; terminal labeling also appears in layer I and part of layer III contiguous with layer IV (69).

Based largely on Cajal's findings with the Golgi method (68), it was generally believed until recently that the cingulum constituted primarily a pathway of projection from the cingulate cortex. In studies involving nerve degeneration, Domesick (15) found, in agreement with Krieg's (30) earlier findings in the rat that the cingulum is largely composed of thalamocingulate fibers. The fibers of projection, on the contrary, penetrate the corpus callosum and proceed lateralwards around the stria terminalis to enter the lateral thalamic peduncle of the thalamus. In the cat, Kaitz and Robertson (25) found that in most instances cingulate cortical areas project back to the same thalamic nuclei from which they receive connections. The notable exception was that the dorsal dysgranular retrosplenial cortex is the only cingulate area that projects to the anterior dorsal nucleus (25). As was mentioned, this nucleus innervates mainly the ventral granular retrosplenial area.

Cingulate Role in Maternal Behavior and Play

On the basis of acute experiments performed on anesthetized animals, evidence had accumulated between 1936 and 1950 that stimulation of the anterior cingulate gyrus elicited autonomic-related responses, including pupillary, cardiovascular, respiratory, gastrointestinal, and urinary changes (see refs. 24, 67 for review). No integrated forms of behavior, however, had been identified with the cingulate convolution until John Stamm's studies on the rat, which were reported in 1955 (80). Most notably, he found that ablation of the supracallosal cingulate cortex resulted in such severe deficits in maternal behavior that only 12% of the pups survived (80). Scoring of maternal behavior in the rat includes observations on nest building, nursing, and retrieval of the young. Later, Slotnick (76) confirmed and extended Stamm's findings, demonstrating *inter alia* that cingulate ablations also interfered with parental behavior of male rats.

We ourselves observed deficits in maternal behavior in a different kind of an experiment designed to assess the performance of species-typical behavior of hamsters reared from birth without the neocortex (46,59). Operations were performed on hamster pups 1 to 2 days of age under cryoanesthesia. The neocortex was eliminated either by heat applied to the skull or by aspiration. Littermates used for controls were treated in exactly the same manner except there was no destruction of brain tissue. A checklist based on an extensive ethogram was used to record the day-to-day behavior development of both the experimental animals and their littermates used as controls. Special tests were used for obtaining measurements of such species-typical behavior as mating, species-preference behavior, territorial defense, scent marking, and the like (59).

The maturation of the hamsters without neocortex resembled that of their litter-mates with respect to weight gain, physical development, and the time of appearance of hamster-typical behavior (Figs. 9A,B). For example, they appeared normal with respect to thermotaxis, nest building, digging, seed cracking, food pouching, hoarding, tunnel blocking, scent marking, showing species preference, territorial defense, and circadian rhythm (59). They developed play fighting at the expected time. The males showed some alteration in copulatory ability, but successfully impregnated females. The females devoid of neocortex had a regular estrus cycle, were normally receptive to males, conceived, gave birth to young, and successfully

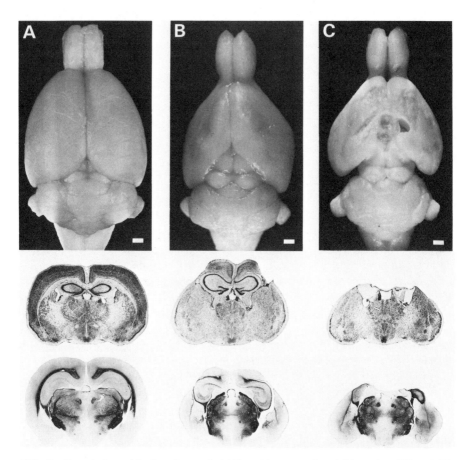

FIG. 9. Dorsal view of brains of a control **(A)** and two experimental hamsters **(B)** and **(C)**. Representative sections through diencephalon at rostral (cell stain) and caudal levels (fiber stain) are shown underneath. **B:** Brain of female deprived postnatally of all the neocortex except a remnant at frontal pole. The preserved cingulate cortex is seen above the hippocampus. The fibrous zonal layer (not visible at this magnification) helps to identify the lateral border of the cingulate cortex. **C:** Brain of another female with additional loss of cingulate cortex and part of the underlying hippocampus. *White bars* correspond to 1 mm. (From Murphy et al., ref. 59.)

reared them. If, however, in addition to the neocortex, the cingulate limbic cortex was aspirated (Fig. 9C), the pups did not engage in playful behavior at the expected or later time, and females as adults showed marked deficits in maternal behavior. The latter findings were to be expected because of the prior-described experiments on rats. In our study I was particularly struck by the absence of play, because in observations on lizards I had never detected anything resembling playful behavior. Regarding the maternal and play deficits, it was as though the animals with the additional loss of cingulate cortex had regressed in the direction of reptiles.

Findings with Respect to the Separation Call

As was noted, audiovocal communication for maintaining maternal–offspring contact represents the third constituent of the behavioral triad. All mammals that have been examined thus far have been found to produce separation calls. Possibly serving as a protection against predators such as owls, the separation calls of several small rodents are in the ultrasonic range. As illustrated by the spectrograms of a squirrel monkey, macaque, and human infant shown in Fig. 10, the separation calls of primates are characterized by a slowly changing tone. This commonality, Newman (60) points out, "suggests that the mechanisms controlling infant cry patterns have had a conservative evolutionary history."

For investigating the cerebral representation of the separation call, Newman and MacLean (61) have used squirrel monkeys. By 1 year of age the separation call of these New World monkeys is almost as stable as a fingerprint (83) and can be regularly elicited under laboratory conditions. Moreover, the call can be reliably differentiated from the more than 30 other vocalizations identified with these monkeys (94). In our work we used two types of squirrel monkeys, which are informally referred to as gothic and roman because of the peaked and rounded shape of the circumocular patch above the eye (Fig. 11). The chromosomes of these two varieties of squirrel monkey show certain karyotypic differences. The gothic and roman types can be just as readily distinguished by their separation calls, which, respectively, have a downward and upward deflection at the termination of the call (93) (Fig. 12).

Methods

Our studies on cerebral localization have involved testing the effects of subcortical and cortical lesions on the structure and production of the isolation call. Preoperative criterion performance requires that a monkey produce 20 spontaneous isolation calls within a period of 15 minutes while caged within a sound-reducing chamber. Animals that fail postoperatively to achieve criterion are tested for an additional 15 minutes so as to disclose whether or not they are capable of producing isolation calls, as is normally expected, in response to conspecific calls. At other times and under different conditions the monkeys are tested for their ability to produce the other main types of squirrel monkey vocalizations. Standard equipment is used for recording and performing the spectrographic analysis of the calls.

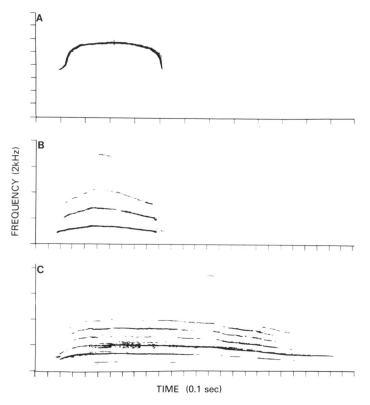

FIG. 10. Spectrograms of separation (isolation) calls of squirrel monkey, macaque, and human infant. In primates such calls have the basic pattern of a slowly changing tone. (After Newman, ref. 60.)

Effects of Brainstem Lesions

In the first series of experiments we identified a region at the junction of the thalamic and midbrain tegmentum, destruction of which either eliminates or alters the normal structure of the call (61). Bilateral lesions of the central tegmental tract or of the ventral periaqueductal gray in the midbrain interfered with the production of the call (61).

Results of Cortical Abaltion

Given these findings, what structures in the telencephalon might be involved in the regulation of the isolation call? In an attempt to answer this question, our first experiments focused on the medial frontal region. In 1945 Wilbur Smith (79) reported for the first time that stimulation of the anterior cingulate gyrus in anesthetized rhesus monkeys resulted in vocalization. Kaada (24) confirmed and extended these findings, commenting that the vocalizations "resembled those which a monkey daily emits in its cage, varying from low cooing sounds to high pitched

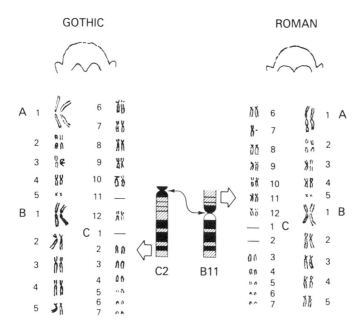

FIG. 11. Contrasting ocular patches of so-called gothic- and roman-type monkeys (shown diagrammatically in left and right upper parts of figure). The two types of monkeys show consistent behavioral differences in their displays (39) and separation calls (see Fig. 12). In addition to these behavioral differences, the two types of squirrel monkeys have karyotypic differences. Their 44 chromosomes are divided into groups A, B, and C on the basis of the length and position of the centromeres. As illustrated by the enlargement at center of Figure, Ma et al. (36) postulate that the difference between the two types of monkeys is due to a pericentric inversion of the B11-C2 chromosomes.

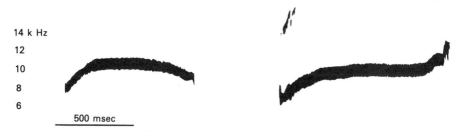

FIG. 12. Distinctive spectrograms of gothic- and roman-type monkeys. Horizontal time line corresponds to 500 msec. (From MacLean, ref. 52.)

sounds and cries." The effects could be obtained only by stimulation of a restricted area of the anterior cingulate cortex in lightly anesthetized monkeys. Ward's (91) negative results were probably due to deeper anesthesia. Dua and MacLean (16) elicited vocalization by stimulating of a corresponding area in awake sitting squirrel monkeys. In this same species Jürgens and Ploog (23) elicited "chirping calls" (a group of calls containing the "isolation peep") by stimulating of the subcallosal cingulate gyrus. In awake, sitting macaques, Robinson (70a) elicited "kōō" calls (which he compared to the separation call) by stimulation of the anterior cingulate gyrus.

In the light of such findings we have examined the effects of extensive and limited ablation of the frontal limbic and neocortex on the isolation call (52,55). Bifrontal lobectomy *rostral* to the cingulate sulcus has no effect on the call. Bilateral elmination of the frontal lobes rostral to the knee of the corpus callosum and the lateral ventricles, on the contrary, results in an enduring elimination of the call.

Bilateral aspiration of the anterior supplementary area (face area) results only in a transitory elimination of the isolation call, with full recovery occurring within 9 weeks. Recovery has also occurred following bilateral aspiration of the anterior cingulate, pregenual cingulate, and subcallosal cingulate cortex together with the adjacent medial frontal cortex. If, however, the ablation also includes the posterior part of the gyrus rectus, there is an enduring elimination of spontaneous isolation calls (52,61a).

Comment

Kirzinger and Jürgens (27) recently reported a study in which they investigated the effects of various frontal ablations on the spontaneous vocal repertoire of squirrel monkeys. They found that ablations of the anterior cingulate cortex, the neocortical face area, and the posterior supplementary area had no effect on the production or structure of vocalizations. They reported, however, that ablations of the "anterior supplementary" area resulted in reduced vocalization that was primarily attributable to a "drastic reduction of the isolation peep." It is our understanding that their postoperative observations did not extend beyond 4 weeks. As was mentioned, following aspiration of the corresponding area we observed full recovery of the call within 9 weeks.

In experiments on macaques, Sutton et al. (82) found that ablation of various neocortical areas had no effect on conditioned koo calls, but that following bilateral ablations involving the anterior cingulate and subcallosal cingulate cortex, postoperative calls were weak and infrequent in the test situation.

We are unaware of cases in the great apes or in humans in which there has been operative or naturally occurring destruction confined to the rostral limbic and adjacent medial frontal cortex. In humans a few cases have been described in which occlusion of the anterior cerebral artery resulted in akinetic mutism and in which the infarction was said to be largely confined to the cingulate gyrus (5,9,63). Alterations of speech have not been reported in cases in which cingulate lesions were produced for the purpose of alleviating psychiatric illness; it would appear that in most cases such lesions have been largely in the anterior supracallosal cingulate region. Penfield and Jasper (66) observed that stimulation of the anterior cingulate cortex both interrupts speech and prevents the initiation of speech.

CONCLUDING COMMENTS

It is beginning to appear on the basis of comparative neurobehavioral studies that the cingulate subdivision of the limbic system is implicated in three forms of behavior that characterize the evolutionary transition from reptiles to mammals— namely, (a) nursing, in conjunction with maternal care; (b) audiovocal communication for maintaining maternal–offspring contact; and (c) playful behavior. Significantly, there is no evident counterpart of this subdivision in the reptilian brain.

In discussing a few implications of these findings, I will only touch on the first two aspects of the family-related behavioral triad. It would be impossible in a limited space to deal in addition with the unique role of play in the evolution of mammals, particularly as it has contributed to human acculturation not only with respect to games and sports, but also in regard to creative associations inspired by wit and humor in the various arts and sciences.

As was noted, the reptilian hatchling and new born mammal are poles apart with respect to parental dependence. For mammals the separation of the sucklings from the mother is calamitous. Because of the fatal consequences of separation, nature appears to have assured that maternal–offspring separation in mammals induces severe distress comparable to pain. It is evident that the distress of separation continues later in life to affect affiliated individuals, as illustrated by the production of separation calls by adult members of a group. Apropos the pain of separation and the distressful nature of the isolation call, it is of timely interest that opiate receptors are found in high concentration in the primate cingulate cortex (95). In agreement with what other workers have observed in nonprimate mammals, Newman et al. (62), in our laboratory, found that small doses of morphine sulfate eliminate the isolation call of squirrel monkeys, whereas the antagonist naloxone reinstates the calls. Years ago Foltz and White (19) reported that anterior cingulate lesions alleviated withdrawal symptoms in addicted subjects. Such considerations suggest that the thalamocingulate division may be implicated in the generation of "separation feelings," which are conducive to drug addiction. The possibility exists that, more than the fleeting effects of euphoria, those suffering from opiate addiction seek release from an ineffable feeling of isolation and alienation.

Although parental behavior has been shown to occur in rodents deprived of their endocrine glands (77), the neuroendocrine system plays a fundamental role in nursing and rearing the young. Woods et al. (95a) provided evidence in the rabbit that a locus near the junction of the anterior limbic cortex and septum projects to the paraventricular nucleus, which controls the release of oxytocin, which in turn induces contractions of the myoepithelial cells of the mammary glands. How, one might ask, does feedback from these contractions influence the mood and calling of a mother separated from its young? In this context, one is reminded of the restlessness and the day-long calling of a mare for its foal or a ewe for its lamb. In the light of such neuroendocrine mechanisms, what is the possibility that some forms of depression seen clinically in women may represent separation reactions *in vacuo*?

Prior to the present day armamentarium of psychotherapeutic agents, Ken Livingston (33,34), who early in life had been influenced by his father's interest in pain mechanisms and the alleviation of pain, was among those (e.g., refs. 31 and 85) who sought to learn whether or not small lesions of the anterior cingulate gyrus might alleviate the mental suffering of psychotic or otherwise hopelessly distressed patients. In recent years he became interested in the phenomenon of limbic kindling as a possible pathophysiological mechanism underlying persisting psychological disturbances that might be amenable to pharmacological treatment.

As noted earlier, the anterior medial nucleus and the medial dorsal nucleus have overlapping projections to the rostral cingulate limbic and medial frontal neocortex. Significantly, such connections indicate how the most recently prefrontal cortex is linked to the cingulate convolution inferred to be involved in parental care, the isolation call, and play. Years ago, Franzen and Meyers (20) reported some heuristic observations, indicating that ablation of the prefrontal cortex in monkeys had a deleterious effect on maternal behavior and also reduced play.

It may be imagined that originally a parental concern for the young amounted to a sense of responsibility. Through the higher reaches of the brain, represented by the prefrontal cortex and its union with the thalamocingulate division, we might imagine that a parental concern for the young eventually generalizes to other members of the species, a psychological development that amounts to an evolution from a sense of responsibility to what we call conscience. Thanks to these same reaches of the brain, we may rise out of our feeling of isolation from Ken Livingston because of his illness, and rejoice, instead, in the joy and exhuberance with which he strived to make this a happier world in which to play out our hopes for future generations.

ACKNOWLEDGMENTS

I am most grateful to Mrs. Katherine V. Compton and Mr. Robert E. Gelhard for technical help in preparing this manuscript. I thank Dr. John D. Newman for providing me the spectrograms for Fig. 12.

REFERENCES

1. Abbie, A. A. (1940): Cortical lamination in the Monotremata. *J. Comp. Neurol.*, 72:428–467.
2. Abbie, A. A. (1942): Cortical lamination in a polyprotodont marsupial, Parameles nasuta. *J. Comp. Neurol.*, 76:509–536.
3. Ariëns Kappers, C. U., Huber, G. C., and Crosby, E. C. (1936): *The Comparative Anatomy of the Nervous System of Vertebrates, Including Man*, 2 Vols. Macmillan Co., New York.
4. Baleydier, C., and Mauguiere, F. (1980): The duality of the cingulate gyrus in monkey. Neuroanatomical study and functional hypothesis. *Brain*, 103:525–554.
5. Barris, R. W., and Schuman, H. R. (1953): Bilateral anterior cingulate gyrus lesions. *Neurology (Minneap.)*, 3:44–52.
6. Bellairs, A. (1970): *The Life of Reptiles*, 2 Vols. Universe Books, New York.
7. Broca, P. (1878): Anatomie comparée des circonvolutions cérébrales. Le grand lobe limbique et la scissure limbique dans la série des mammifères. *Rev. Anthrop.*, 1:385–498.
8. Brodmann, K. (1909): *Vergleichende Lokalisationslehre der Grosshirnrinde in ihren Prinzipien dargestellt auf Grund des Zellenbaues*. Barth, Leipzig.

9. Buge, A., Escourolle, R., Rancurel, G., and Poisson, M. (1975): Mutisme akinetique et ramollissement bicingulaire. 3 observations anatomo-cliniques. *Rev. Neurol.*, 131:121–137.
10. Campbell, A. W. (1905): *Histological Studies on the Localization of Cerebral Functions.* University Press, Cambridge.
11. Clark, W. E. LeG., and Meyer, M. (1950): Anatomical relationships between the cerebral cortex and the hypothalamus. *Br. Med. Bull.*, 6:341–345.
12. Conrad, C. D., and Stumpf, W. E. (1975): Direct visual input to the limbic system: Crossed retinal projections to the nucleus anterodorsalis thalami in the tree shrew. *Exp. Brain Res.*, 23:141–149.
13. Crosby, E. C., Humphrey, T., and Lauer, E. W. (1962): *Correlative Anatomy of the Nervous System.* Macmillan Co., New York.
14. Dart, R. A. (1935): The dual structure of the neopallium: its history and significance. *J. Anal. (British)*, 69:3–19.
15. Domesick, V. B. (1970): The fasciculus cinguli in the rat. *Brain Res.*, 20:19–32.
16. Dua, S., and MacLean, P. D. (1964): Localization for penile erection in medial frontal lobe. *Am. J. Physiol.*, 207:1425–1434.
17. Economo, C. von, and Koskinas, G. N. (1925): *Die Cytoarchitektonik der Hirnrinde des erwachsenen Menschen.* J. Springer, Berlin.
18. Flechsig, P. (1921): Die myelogenetische Gliederung der Leitungsbahnen des Linsenkernes beim Menschen. Ber Verh. sachs. Akad. Wiss. Leipzig. *Methem.-phys. Klasse*, 73:295–302.
19. Foltz, E. L., and White, L. E. (1957): Experimental cingulumotomy and modification of morphine withdrawal. *J. Neurosurg.*, 14:655–673.
20. Franzen, E. A., and Myers, R. E. (1973): Neural control of social behavior: Prefrontal and anterior temporal cortex. *Neuropsychologia*, 11:141–157.
21. Gingerich, P. D., Wells, N. A., Russell, D. E., and Shah, S. M. (1983): Origin of whales in epicontinental remnant seas: New evidence from the early Eocene of Pakistan. *Science*, 220:403–406.
22. Greenberg, N. B., MacLean, P. D., and Ferguson, J. L. (1979): Role of the paleostriatum in species-typical display behavior of the lizard *(Anolis carolinensis). Brain Res.*, 172:229–241.
22a. Itaya, S. K., Hoesen, G. W. van, and Jenq, C. B. (1981): Direct retinal input to the limbic system of the rat. *Brain Res.*, 226:33–42.
23. Jürgens, U., and Ploog, D. (1970): Cerebral representation of vocalization in the squirrel monkey. *Exp. Brain Res.*, 10:532–554.
24. Kaada, B. R. (1951): Somato-motor, autonomic and electrocorticographic responses to electrical stimulation of 'rhinencephalic' and other structures in primates, cat and dog. A study of responses from the limbic, subcallosal, orbito-insular, piriform and temporal cortex hippocampus-fornix and amygdala. *Acta Physiol. Scand.*, 24:1–285.
25. Kaitz, S. S., and Robertson, R. T. (1981): Thalamic connections with limbic cortex. II. Corticothalamic projections. *J. Comp. Neurol.*, 195:527–545.
26. Kesarev. V. S., Malofeyeva, L. I., and Trykova, O. V. (1977): Ecological specificity of cetacean neocortex. *J. Hirnforsch.*, 18:447–460.
27. Kirzinger, A., and Jurgens, U. (1982): Cortical lesion effects and vocalization in the squirrel monkey. *Brain Res.*, 233:299–315.
28. Kooy, D. van der, McGinty, J. F., Koda, L. Y., Gerfren, C. R., and Bloom, F. E. (1982): Visceral cortex: A direct connection from prefrontal cortex to the solitary nucleus in rat. *Neurosci. Lett.*, 33:123–127.
29. Krettek, J. E., and Price, J. L. (1977): The cortical projections of the medial dorsal nucleus and adjacent thalamic nuclei in the rat. *J. Comp. Neurol.*, 171:157–192.
30. Krieg, W. J. S. (1947): *Connections of the cerebral cortex.* I. The albino rat. C. Extrinsic connections. *J. Comp. Neurol.*, 86:267–394.
31. Le Beau, J. (1952): The cingular and precingular areas in psychosurgery (agitated behaviour, obsessive compulsive states, epilepsy). *Acta Psychiatr. Neurol. Scand.*, 27:305–316.
32. Leonard, C. M. (1969): The prefrontal cortex of the rat. I. Cortical projection of the mediodorsal nucleus. II. Efferent connections. *Brain Res.*, 12:321–343.
33. Livingston, K. E. (1953): Cingulate cortex isolation for the treatment of psychoses and psychoneuroses. *Proc. Assoc. Res. Nerv. Ment. Dis.*, 21:374–378.
34. Livingston, K. E. (1975): Surgical contributions to psychiatric treatment. In: *American Handbook of Psychiatry, Treatment*, edited by D. X. Freedman and J. E. Dyrud, pp. 548–563. Basic Books, Inc., New York.

35. Lorente de Nó, R. (1934): Studies on the structure of the cerebral cortex: I. The area entorhinalis. *J. Psychol. Neurol.*, 45:381–438.

36. Ma, N. S. F., Jones, T. C., Thorington, R. W., and Cooper, R. W. (1974): Chromosome banding patterns in squirrel monkeys *(Saimiri sciureus). J. Med. Primatol.*, 3:120–137.

37. MacLean, P. D. (1952): Some psychiatric implications of physiological studies on frontotemporal portion of limbic system (visceral brain). *Electroencephalogr. Clin. Neurophysiol.*, 4:407–418.

38. MacLean, P. D. (1954): Studies on limbic system ("visceral brain") and their bearing on psychosomatic problems. In: *Recent Developments in Psychosomatic Medicine*, edited by R. Cleghorn and E. Wittkower, 495 pp. Sir Isaac Pitman & Sons, Ltd., London.

39. MacLean, P. D. (1964): Mirror display in the squirrel monkey, *Saimiri sciureus. Science*, 146:950–952.

40. MacLean, P. D. (1967): The brain in relation to empathy and medical education. *J. Nerv. Ment. Dis.*, 144:374–382.

41. MacLean, P. D. (1970): The triune brain, emotion, and scientific bias. In: *The Neurosciences Second Study Program*, edited by F. O. Schmitt, pp. 336–349. Rockefeller University Press, New York.

42. MacLean, P. D. (1973): A triune concept of the brain and behavior. In: *The Hincks Memorial Lectures*, edited by T. Boag and D. Campbell, pp. 6–66. University of Toronto Press, Toronto.

43. MacLean, P. D. (1975): Role of pallidal projections in species-typical display behavior of squirrel monkey. *Trans. Am. Neurol. Assoc.*, 100:29–32.

44. MacLean, P. D. (1975): On the evolution of three mentalities. *Man-Environment Systems*, 5:213–224. Reprinted in : *New Dimensions in Psychiatry; A World View*, Vol. 2, edited by S. Arieti and G. Chrzanowski, 1977, pp. 305–328. John Wiley & Sons, New York.

45. MacLean, P. D. (1978): Why brain research on lizards? In : *The Behavior and Neurology of Lizards*, edited by N. Greenberg and P. D. MacLean, pp. 1–10. U.S. Government Printing Office, Washington, D.C., DHEW Publication, No. (ADM) 77–491.

46. MacLean, P. D. (1978): *A Mind of Three Minds: Educating the Triune Brain*. Seventy-seventh Yearbook of the National Society for the Study of Education, pp. 308–342. University of Chicago Press, Chicago.

47. MacLean, P. D. (1978): Effects of lesions of globus pallidus on species-typical display behavior of squirrel monkeys. *Brain Res.*, 149:175–196.

48. MacLean, P. D. (1981): Role of transhypothalamic pathways in social communication. In: *Handbook of the Hypothalamus*, Vol. 3, edited by P. Morgane and J. Panksepp, pp. 259–287. Marcel Dekker, Inc., New York.

49. MacLean, P. D. (1982): The co-evolution of the brain and family. In: *Anthroquest*, The L. S. B. Leakey Foundation News, No. 24, Winter/1982, pp. 1 and 14–15 (The L. S. B. Leakey Foundation, Pasadena, CA).

50. MacLean, P. D. (1982): On the origin and progressive evolution of the triune brain. In: *Primate Brain Evolution: Methods and Concepts*, edited by E. Armstrong and D. Falk, pp. 291–316. Plenum Press, New York.

51. MacLean, P. D. (1985): Editorial: Evolutionary psychiatry and the triune brain. *Psychol. Med.*, 15:219–221.

52. MacLean, P. D. (1985): Brain evolution relating to family, play, and the separation call. *Arch. Gen. Psychiatry*, 42:405–417.

53. MacLean, P. D. (1986): Neurobehavioral significance of the mammal-like reptiles (therapsids). In: *The Ecology and Biology of Mammal-like Reptiles*. Smithsonian Institution Press, Washington, DC. (in *press*).

54. MacLean, P. D., and Creswell, G. (1970): Anatomical connections of visual system with limbic cortex of monkey. *J. Comp. Neurol.*, 138:265–278.

55. MacLean, P. D., and Newman, J. D. *(in preparation)*.

56. MacLean, P. D., Yokota, T., and Kinnard, M. D. (1968): Photically sustained on-responses of units in posterior hippocampal gyrus of awake monkey. *J. Neurophysiol.*, 31:870–883.

57. Morgane, P. J., Jacobs, M. S., and Galaburda A. (1985): Evolutionary morphology of the dolphin brain. In: *Dolphin Behavior and Cognition: Comparative and Ecological Aspects*, edited by R. Buhr, R. Schusterman, J. Thomas, and F. Wood. L. Oxford Univ. Press, New York.

58. Morgane, P. J., McFarland, W. L., and Jacobs, M. S. (1982): The limbic lobe of the dolphin brain: A quantitative cytoarchitectonic study. *J. Hirnforschung*, 23:465–552.

59. Murphy, M. R., MacLean, P. D., Hamilton, S. C. (1981): Species-typical behavior of hamsters deprived from birth of the neocortex. *Science*, 213:459–461.
60. Newman, J. D. (1985): The infant cry of primates: An evolutionary perspective. In: *Infant Crying: Theoretical and Research Perspectives*, edited by B. M. Lester and C. F. Z. Boukydis, pp. 307–323. Plenum Press, New York.
61. Newman, J. D., and MacLean, P. D. (1982): Effects of tegmental lesions on the isolation call of squirrel monkeys. *Brain Res.*, 232:317–339.
61a. Newman, J. D., and MacLean, P. D. (1985): Importance of medial frontolimbic cortex in the production of the isolation call of squirrel monkeys. *Neurosci. Abstr.* 11(Pt. 1):495.
62. Newman, J. D., Murphy, M. R., and Harbaugh, C. R. (1982): Naloxone-reversible suppression of isolation call production after morphine injections in squirrel monkeys. *Soc. Neurosci. Abstr.*, 8:940.
63. Nielsen, J. M., and Jacobs, L. L. (1951): Bilateral lesions of the anterior cingulate gyri. *Bull. Los Angeles Neurol. Soc.*, 16:231–234.
64. O'Leary, J. L., and Bishop, G. H. (1938): Margins of the optically excitable cortex in the rabbit. *Arch. Neurol. Psychiatry (Chicago)*, 40:482–499.
65. Papez, J. W. (1937): A proposed mechanism of emotion. *Arch. Neurol. Psychiatry (Chicago)*, 38:725–743.
66. Penfield, W., and Jasper, H. H. (1954): *Epilepsy and the Functional Anatomy of the Human Brain*. Little, Brown & Co., Boston.
67. Pool, J. L. (1954): The visceral brain of man. *J. Neurosurg.*, 11:45–63.
68. Ramon ý Cajal, S. (1955): *Studies on the Cerebral Cortex (Limbic Structures)*. Translated from the Spanish by L. M. Kraft. Lloyd-Luke Ltd., London, and Year Book Publishers, Chicago.
69. Robertson, R. T., and Kaitz, S. S. (1981): Thalamic connections with limbic cortex. I. Thalamocortical projections. *J. Comp. Neurol.*, 195:501–525.
70. Robertson, R. T., Kaitz, S. S., and Robards, M. J. (1980): A subcortical pathway links sensory and limbic systems of the forebrain. *Neurosci. Lett.*, 17:161–165.
70a. Robinson, B. W. (1967): Vocalization evoked from forebrain in *Macaca mulatta*. *Physiol. Behav.*, 2:345–354.
71. Rose, J. E., and Woolsey, C. N. (1948): Structure and relations of limbic cortex and anterior thalamic nuclei in rabbit and cat. *J. Comp. Neurol.*, 89:279–348.
72. Rose, M. (1927): Gyrus limbicus anterior and Regio retrosplenialis. (Cortex holoprotoptychos quinquestratificatus). Vergleichende Architektonik bei Tier und Mensch. *J. Psychol. Neurol.*, 35:65–173.
73. Rose, M. (1931): Cytoarchitektonischer Atlas der Grosshirnrinde des Kaninchens. *J. Psychol. Neurol. (Leipzig)*, 43:353–440.
74. Hotton III, N., MacLean, P. D., Roth J. J., and Roth, E. C. *The Ecology and Biology of Mammal-like Reptiles*. Smithsonian Institution Press, Washington, DC. *(in press)*.
75. Sanides, F. (1969): Comparative architectonics of the neocortex of mammals and their evolutionary interpretation. *Ann. NY Acad. Sci.*, 16:404–423.
76. Slotnick, B. M. (1967): Disturbances of maternal behavior in the rat following lesions of the cingulate cortex. *Behaviour*, 24:204–236.
77. Slotnick, B. M. (1975): Neural and hormonal basis of maternal behavior in the rat. In: *Hormonal Correlates of Behavior*, Vol. 2, edited by B. Eleftheriou and R. Sprott, pp. 585–656. Plenum Press, New York.
78. Smith, G. E. (1901): Notes upon the natural subdivision of the cerebral hemisphere. *J. Anat. Physiol.*, 35:431–454.
79. Smith, W. K. (1945): The functional significance of the rostral cingular cortex as revealed by its responses to electrical excitation. *J. Neurophysiol.*, 8:241–255.
80. Stamm, J. S. (1955): The function of the median cerebral cortex in maternal behavior of rats. *J. Comp. Physiol. Psychol.*, 48:347–356.
81. Suess, E. (1904): The face of the earth (Das antlitz der erde). Translated by H. B. C. Sollas, pp. 417–420. Clarendon Press, Oxford.
82. Sutton, D., Larson, C., and Lindeman, R. C. (1974): Neocortical and limbic lesion effects on primate phonation. *Brain Res.*, 71:61–75.
83. Symmes, D., Newman, J. D., Talmage-Riggs, G., and Lieblich, A. K. (1979): Individuality and stability of isolation peeps in squirrel monkeys. *Anim. Behav.*, 27:1142–1152.

84. Terreberry, R. R., and Neafsey, E. J. (1983): Rat medial frontal cortex: A visceral motor region with a direct projection to the solitary nucleus. *Brain Res.*, 278:245–249.
84a. Thompson, J. M., Woolsey, C. N., and Talbot, S. A. (1950): Visual areas I and II of cerebral cortex of rabbit. *J. Neurophysiol.*, 13:277–288.
85. Tow, M. P., and Whitty, C. W. M. (1953): Personality changes after operations on the cingulate gyrus in man. *J. Neurol. Neurosurg. Psychiatry*, 16:186–193.
86. Vogt, B. A. (1976): Retrospenial cortex in the rhesus monkey: A cytoarchitectonic and Golgi study. *J. Comp. Neurol.*, 169:63–98.
87. Vogt, B. A., and Peters, A. (1981): Form and distribution of neurons in rat cingulate cortex: areas 32, 24, and 29. *J. Comp. Neurol.*, 195:603–625.
88. Vogt, B. A., Rosene, D. L., and Pandya, D. N. (1979): Thalamic and cortical afferents differentiate anterior from posterior cingulate cortex in the monkey. *Science*, 204:205–207.
89. Vogt, B. A., Rosene, D. L., and Peters, A. (1981): Synaptic termination of thalamic and callosal afferents in cingulate cortex of the rat. *J. Comp. Neurol.*, 201:265–284.
90. Vogt, O. von (1910): Die myeloarchitektonische Felderung des menschlichen Stirnhirns. *J. Psychol. Neurol.*, 15:221–232.
91. Ward, A. A. (1948): The cingulate gyrus: Area 24. *J. Neurophysiol.*, 11:13–23.
91a. Vogt, C., and Vogt, O. (1919): Allgemeine Ergebnisse unserer Hiruforschung. *J. Psychol. Neurol. (Lpz.)*, 25:279.
92. Wegener, A. L. (1915): *Die Entstehung der Kontinente und Ozeane.* F. Vieweg, Braunschweig.
93. Winter, P. (1969): Dialects in squirrel monkeys: Vocalization of the roman arch type. *Folia primatol.*, 10:216–229.
94. Winter, P., Ploog, D., and Latta, J. (1966): Vocal repertoire of the squirrel monkey *(Saimiri sciureus)* its analysis and significance. *Exp. Brain Res.*, 1:359–384.
95. Wise, S. P., and Herkenham, M. (1982): Opiate receptor distribution in the cerebral cortex of the rhesus monkey. *Science*, 218:387–389.
95a. Woods, W. H., Holland, R. C., and Powell, E. W. (1969): Connections of cerebral structures functioning in neurohypophysial hormone release. *Brain Res.*, 12:26–46.
96. Yakovlev, P. I. (1948): Motility behavior and the brain. Stereodynamic organization and neural coordinates of behavior. *J. Nerv. Ment. Dis.*, 107:313–335.
97. Yakovlev, P. I., Locke, S., Koskoff, D. Y., and Patton, R. A. (1960): Limbic nuclei of thalamus and connections of limbic cortex. *Arch. Neurol.*, 3:620–641.

The Limbic System: Functional Organization and
Clinical Disorders, edited by B. K. Doane and
K. E. Livingston. Raven Press, New York © 1986.

Hemispheric Asymmetries in Emotional Function: A Reflection of Lateral Specialization in Cortical-Limbic Connections

David M. Bear

New England Deaconess Hospital, Boston, Massachusetts 02215

Structures traditionally assigned to the limbic lobe—the amygdala, hippocampus, and cingulate—are presumed to be bilaterally symmetrical. Since asymmetry appears to be a common feature of many neuroanatomical structures below the cortical level—e.g., the thalamus—it may well be the case that subtle lateralizing features will eventually be uncovered in these limbic structures.

However, in this chapter I would like to explore another possibility: that hemispheric specialization in the human brain has led to important asymmetries in cortical connections to these limbic structures. Evidence for this possibility may be drawn from clinical, anatomical, and physiological studies in the higher primates and man.

Following a brief review of findings that argue for lateralization in human emotional functions, I shall summarize another group of converging investigations that points to the existence of alternative, complementary pathways into limbic structures from the primate's most important neocortical sensory analyzer, the visual system. Finally, I shall propose reasons for believing that these parallel "dorsal" and "ventral" sensory-limbic pathways have been extensively altered by lateral cortical asymmetries.

LATERALIZATION OF EMOTIONAL FUNCTION IN MAN

The appearance of deficits after lateralized lesions—e.g., aphasia following left hemisphere infarction—provides strong evidence for asymmetry in function. The first described and perhaps still the most striking alteration in "emotional functioning" is the phenomenon of anosognosia, or denial of illness, produced by lesions in the right hemisphere (1). At first, the affected patient may not acknowledge the existence of gross impairments such as paralysis on the left side of his body. Subsequently, he may come to acknowledge the deficit but minimize the severity or importance of the defects.

29

This emotional indifference cannot be attributed to simple sensory unawareness by the left hemisphere, which may visualize the affected limbs and is repeatedly reminded verbally of the deficits. Instead, damage to particular structures in the right hemisphere appears to prevent appropriate emotional orientation, and without this orientation there is both sensory inattention and emotional unconcern. Many patients at one stage of the illness do verbally acknowledge their deficits, but they may treat them facetiously or derisively (2). Patients with right hemisphere lesions also selectively fail to appreciate, or they may distort, accounts of illness in others (3).

This lack of concern has been related to an absence of significant depression, noted clinically or psychometrically, among patients suffering right hemisphere lesions (4). A neuroendocrine marker of depression, the incomplete suppression of plasma cortisol by oral dexamethasone, may also fail to develop in patients with neglect (5).

The lack of appropriate concern in patients with right hemisphere lesions often extends beyond the illness to include financial difficulties, interpersonal conflicts, and other physical injuries. I would like to suggest that the fundamental deficit, of which denying the illness may only be a special case, is a failure in emotional surveillance. The patient is not detecting the most important threat to the self, and therefore he does not sustain attention, mount emotional concern, or initiate appropriate strategies for elimination of this problem (6).

Other studies are consistent with a dominant role of the right hemisphere in emotional surveillance and especially in the search for threatening situations. Films of surgical dissections were judged more horrible (7) and led to greater changes in heart rate (8) when projected to the right hemisphere of normal subjects. The galvanic skin response to ipsilateral electric shock was diminished or abolished by right hemisphere but not left hemisphere lesions (9). Selective anesthetization of the right hemisphere by intracarotid sodium amytal led to euphoric unconcern, whereas inactivation of the left hemisphere, leaving the intact right hemisphere to appreciate deficits in language and motor function, produced tears and sadness (10,11). Although there are fewer direct observations implicating the right hemisphere in scanning for positive emotional stimuli, the right hemisphere patient is typically indifferent rather than overzealous or even appropriately motivated to pursue positive emotional goals.

We now turn to a different class of emotional functions involved in the social communication of affects. Tachistoscopic observations in normal subjects consistently show the right hemisphere superior in detection of facial emotion (12,13). Dichotic listening studies in normal subjects (14), and discrimination testing following lateralized lesions (15), document greater sensitivity of the right hemisphere to nonverbal auditory cues of emotion. In the expression of emotion, dominance of the right hemisphere is suggested by the greater emotional expressivity of the left lower face (16,17) and the loss of emotional prosody (18,19) after right-sided lesions.

In the past, different aspects of emotional communication have been investigated in separate patients employing different methodologies. To clarify the neurological mechanisms and their possible localizations, Benowitz et al. (20) employed a quantitative, standardized test of the nonverbal perception of emotions (Profiles of Nonverbal Sensitivity). This instrument assesses multiple modalities of affect recognition in the same subject by requiring discrimination of brief emotional vignettes presented through face, body, or nonverbal vocal "channels" (21).

As illustrated in Fig. 1, patients with radiologically verified right hemisphere lesions were severely impaired in emotional discrimination over all channels, whereas the left hemisphere subjects did not differ significantly from the well-standardized control mean (20). Discrimination of facial emotion was most sensitive to a right hemisphere lesion. Testing of the isolated hemispheres in split-brain subjects yielded consistent lateralization of these functions. Furthermore, preliminary analysis of these data, in agreement with a study employing localized electrocortical stimulation (22), specifically implicates the right temporal lobe in reading facial emotion.

These observations thus provide additional evidence of lateralization and right hemisphere predominance for multiple emotional functions. However, to elucidate the underlying mechanisms that may account for lateralization as well as intrahemispheric localization, I suspect that we must keep in mind the diversity of these functions, as reflected, for example, in the distinction between emotional surveillance and affect communication. Despite the heterogeneity of function, unitary formulations of a fundamental processing difference between right and left hemispheres have been suggested. Some of the proposed dichotomies are summarized in Table 1.

These characterizations are impressionistically consistent with observation. However, in addition to confounding a diversity of emotional functions, they do not

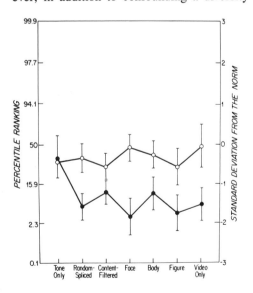

FIG. 1. Nonverbal sensitivity following lateralized cerebral injury. *Tone only:* all auditory channels. *Video only:* all visual channels. *Random spliced:* scrambled speech segments. *Content filtered:* distorted speech passage. *Figure:* face and body shown. Brackets represent standard error of the mean; (●) right hemisphere damage ($n = 7$); (○) left hemisphere damage ($n = 4$).

TABLE 1. *Characterizations of functional asymmetry*

Dimension	Right hemisphere	Left hemisphere
Emotionality	Affective, emotional	Cognitive, neutral
Emotional/attentional bias	Concerned, vigilant	Unconcerned, inattentive
Cognitive preference	Spatial, simultaneous, holistic	Temporal, sequential, analytic
Focus	Peripheral, incidental	Central, intentional
Response style	Impulsive	Reflective

lead directly to mechanistic, anatomical, or evolutionary explanations of asymmetries. It is at this point that I should like to consider the possible underlying role of cortical connections to limbic structures in the two hemispheres.

CORTICAL-LIMBIC CONNECTIONS

The importance of cortical connections to and from the limbic system, and possible hemispheric asymmetries in these connections, was suggested to me by interictal emotional changes frequently encountered in patients with temporal lobe epilepsy (23,24). These observations led to the present hypotheses, and I hope that they may serve a similar heuristic function for the reader. However, the anatomical suggestions below are not logically dependent on these data.

Three studies involving different methodologies found distinctions in interictal behavior produced by right versus left temporal lobe epileptic foci. Flor-Henry (25), reviewing assigned psychiatric diagnoses in psychotic temporal lobe epileptics, reported a preponderance of mood and affective disorders with right-sided foci; thought disorder ("schizophreniform psychosis") was statistically more frequent with foci in the left temporal lobe. In the investigation by McIntyre et al. (26), utilizing developmental tests of conceptual style derived from studies of adolescent aggresivity, right temporal lobe epileptics produced an "impulsive" aggressive pattern compared with the controlled "reflective" profile of the left temporal lobe epileptics.

Bear and Fedio (24) constructed questionnaires sampling specific behaviors previously reported in temporal lobe epilepsy. Patients with either right or left unilateral foci, based on self-ratings or on the evaluation of observers, demonstrated the distinctive behaviors to a quantitatively equivalent extent (Fig. 2, vertical axis). However, principal components analysis revealed a qualitative dichotomy within the set of 18 traits. An emotive cluster involved overt display of mood or affect, such as euphoria, sadness, aggressivity, and altered sexual behavior; "ideative" traits included religiosity, philosophical interest, sense of personal destiny, paranoid concerns, and hypergraphia.

As illustrated by their position on the horizontal axis of Fig. 2, right temporal epileptics demonstrated more emotive characteristics, whereas those with left temporal lobe foci showed ideative traits. The emotive-ideative dimension separated the groups without overlap (24).

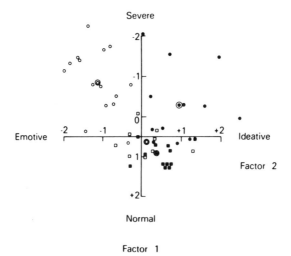

Factor 1

FIG. 2. Behavior in lateralized temporal lobe epilepsy. *Factor 1*: intensity of behavioral changes. *Factor 2*: quality of behavioral changes. (○), Right temporal lobe epileptics; (●) left temporal lobe epileptics; (□) neurological contrast group; (■) control group; circled values represent group means.

Based on contrasting features of the Klüver-Bucy syndrome and behavior changes in temporal lobe epilepsy, I have suggested that the interictal behavior syndrome reflects enhanced affective associations resulting from increased functional connectivity between sensory association cortices and limbic structures, such as the amygdala, within the temporal lobe. For example, the kindling effect of a discharging epileptic focus may bring about fortuitous sensory-limbic connections that are the converse of sensory-limbic disconnections effected by temporal lobectomy or amygdalectomy (24). Recent demonstration of enhanced autonomic responses to visual stimuli in temporal lobe epileptics is consistent with this mechanism (27).

With regard to laterality, we may then ask whether the differences between right and left temporal lobe epileptics reflect disparate patterns of enhanced connections to limbic structures within the two hemispheres. For example, the ideative traits associated with a left hemisphere focus may represent deepened emotionality reflected in abstract thought or writing, whereas the emotive-impulse profile of the right temporal lobe epileptic suggests a more immediate affective investment of ongoing sensory events leading to rapid alteration in mood or drive discharge.

Let us, then, consider the pattern of cortical sensory connections to the limbic system, which may be influenced by hemispheric asymmetries. Vision is the most extensively represented sensory system in the primate cortex, and the anatomy and physiology of visual-limbic connections are the best understood. For our purpose, I should like to stress the evidence for two separate, complementary cortical-visual systems with independent limbic connections; these may be designated ventral or temporal-frontal as opposed to dorsal or parietal-frontal. Figure 3 is a highly

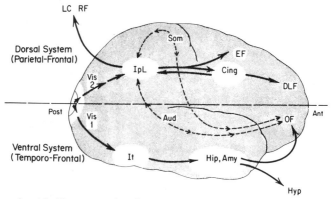

FIG. 3. Two visual limbic systems in primate brain and human right hemisphere: (LC) locus coeruleus; (RF) reticular formation; (Vis) visual; (Ipl) inferior parietal lobule; (It) inferotemporal visual cortex; (Som) somesthetic; (Aud) auditory; (Cing) cingulate; (EF) frontal eye fields; (DLF) dorsolateral frontal cortex; (OF) orbital frontal cortex; (Hip) Hippocampus; (Amy) amygdala; (Hyp) hypothalamus; (Ant) anterior; (Post) posterior. (Analogous pathways for somesthetic and auditory limbic processing are suggested.)

TABLE 2. *Cortical visual–limbic systems*

	Ventral (temporofrontal) system	Dorsal (parietofrontal) system
Pathway	Area 17 → 18, 19 → inferotemporal → visual cortex → amygdala, hippocampus → orbital frontal cortex	Area 17 → 18, 19 → ? → inferior parietal lobule → cingulate → dorsolateral frontal cortex
Visual functions	Central object vision; "stimulus equivalence"; object recognition independent of spatial placement in visual field	Spatial vision, especially peripheral; "foveal sparing"; recognition and spatial placement of relevant stimuli; initiation of saccadic eye movement
Limbic functions	Drive-relevant responses in foveal vision; acquisition and storage of visual–emotional associations	Surveillance of environmental for drive-relevant stimuli; arousal, attention, and spatial orientation (attention or command functions)
Processing characteristics	Sequential temporal relations, critical for establishing sensory-reinforcement linkages; effector circuits for weighing alternative drive responses in light of SR memory and constructing appropriate strategies	Simultaneous, spatial surveillance with precise positional encoding required for orientation; effector circuits for rapid arousal, saccadic eye and body movements, emotional activation

schematic diagram of the pathways and Table 2 summarizes characteristics of the two systems.

Converging evidence suggests that the ventral or temporal visual-limbic route is a foveal system for recognition of objects by multiple attributes independent of their exact position within the visual field (28). The powerful projections between inferotemporal visual cortex and temporal-limbic structures are crucial for both appropriate drive responding and new stimulus-response learning (28,29). In addition to the extensive hypothalamic projections from amygdala and hippocampus, it would appear that a major limbic-motor association field for the ventral system is the orbital frontal cortex, which is strongly connected to the rostral temporal lobe by the uncinate fasciculus; lesions of the orbital-frontal lobe produce learning deficits similar to those resulting from temporal-limbic lesions (29).

By contrast, the dorsal or parietal visual-limbic route involves polysynaptic projections from the circumstriate belt to the inferior parietal lobule, within which (areas PG and PF) approximately one-third of cells are light-sensitive (30). The majority of these have peripheral receptive fields that spare the fovea (31,32). There is a unique limbic input from the cingulate gyrus (33,34) and reciprocal connections from inferior parietal lobule to cingulate. Somesthetic-kinesthetic input reaches the inferior parietal lobule from the superior parietal lobule (32,34).

Many observations implicate the inferior parietal lobule in detection and spatial localization of drive-relevant stimuli (30,32). In addition to efferents from inferior parietal lobule to reticular activating nuclei, locus ceruleus, and frontal eye fields, the dorsal-limbic structures may preferentially project to dorsolateral prefrontal cortex (30,32,34). This system appears to mediate, whether through attention or command, emotional arousal and rapid selective orientation to stimuli that are drive pertinent (30,32).

Before considering the implications of these contrasting systems for hemispheric specialization, let me suggest an intrahemispheric structure-function correlation. Lesions of the dorsal system involving inferior parietal lobule, cingulate, and specifically the dorsal prefrontal cortex, might be expected to interfere with spatial surveillance, orientation, and emotional arousal resulting in spatial learning deficits, neglect, apathy, or abulia. By contrast, ventral lesions, whether involving the temporal lobe (Klüver-Bucy syndrome) or—particularly—orbital prefrontal cortex, would selectively prevent access to previously learned emotional associations, including acquired socialized responses. In the presence of unopposed dorsal structures, the ventral lesion could produce a transient, reflexive release of, for example, sexual or aggressive responses to environmental stimuli, without consideration of learned (delayed) consequences. These predictions nicely fit the striking dichotomy between dorso-lateral and orbital-frontal personality changes described in man (35).

Some additional processing characteristics of the two systems are presented in Table 2. It would appear that in the monkey brain, these systems exist in parallel in each hemisphere, the parietal "surveillance" system detecting relevant stimuli which are subsequently foveated and brought into the temporal "learning and emotional responding system." I would now like to propose that the development and progression of specific hemispheric asymmetries in man may be related to lateralized specializations of these systems.

HEMISPHERIC ASYMMETRY IN CORTICAL-LIMBIC CONNECTIONS

A greater posterior extent of the planum temporale in the left hemisphere was the first proven hemispheric asymmetry (36). More recently, Galaburda et al.

(37,38) have related this finding to volumetric increase in a specific cytoarchitectonic area (Tpt) at the left parietotemporal junction.

The representation of this left hemispheric specialization in Fig. 4 suggests a possible functional significance. Geschwind (39) identified a unique requirement of human language, probably unmet by the lower primate brain, for learning and storage of extensive nonlimbic sensory-sensory (i.e., visual-auditory) associations. These are essential, for example, to see an object and retrieve its name or to learn a phonetic alphabet. Anatomically, the volume of cortex including Wernicke's area and extending into the parietal lobe (angular gyrus) would be ideally situated to mediate such intersensory associations. Electrophysiologic recordings from Tpt in monkeys include units responding to multiple sensory modalities (40).

One may speculate about the evolutionary steps that led to the development and progression of this asymmetric sensory-sensory association system. Of course, the development of communication beyond emotional signaling will eventually have powerful survival advantages for a socialized species. However, the original evolutionary "experiment" in the left hemisphere may not have involved communication, but the cross-modal or modality-independent representation of stimuli, which allows for identification and generalization of learning beyond a single modality. Thus, all the "facts" about snakes can be stored and retrieved whether one sees, hears, or touches one.

We may compare this "new" cross-modal learning system to the older, polymodal system which, I suspect, characterizes the parietotemporal cortex of the lower primate brain and the human right hemisphere: A topographic representation of the world in which visual, somesthetic, or auditory stimuli are arrayed in spatial register for the purpose of rapid attention and orientation through any sensory channel. For all the advantages of cross-modal learning and language that the left parietotemporal system may bring, just this spatial representation and surveillance

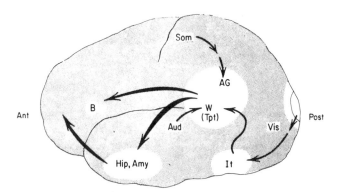

FIG. 4. Sensory limbic connections in human left hemisphere: (W) Wernicke's area; (Tpt) temporoparietotemporal architechtonic area; (AG) angular gyrus; (B) Broca's area. (Other abbreviations as in Fig. 3.)

function would be sacrificed. As a result of the polysynaptic intermodal associations developed in the left parietotemporal system, one might also predict a loss of emotional immediacy and decrements in encoding and retrieving complex stimuli within a single modality (Table 3).

Table 3 is an attempt to relate some of the well-established superiorities of the left hemisphere to its distinctive sensory-limbic connection system. In brief, my suggestion is that the dorsal limbic surveillance system (Fig. 3, Table 2) has been replaced by an intermodal ventral learning system (Table 3). The importance of the angular gyrus in retrieving an auditory representation of a visual stimulus, i.e., in confrontation naming, is clear (39). Furthermore, the unique result of destruction of the left angular gyrus, Gerstmann's syndrome, may be interpreted as disruption of somesthetic associations with learned intermodal conceptual schema, e.g., writing or finger naming. The role of Wernicke's area in auditory-visual association is supported by the development of alexia in Wernicke's aphasia. Furthermore, a recent study suggests a special role of the auditory system in the formation of many cross-modal linkages, since congenitally deaf individuals are deficient in forming visual-somesthetic associations (41). I suspect this is why the congenitally deaf are rarely effective readers.

Mathematical and linguistic operations involve centrally perceived (foveated) stimuli that are sequentially processed and learned; these characteristics are the hallmarks of the ventral-limbic system (Table 2), and left temporal lobe lesions disrupt these functions (42).

The abilities above are traditionally labeled cognitive. However, it could be predicted that the left ventral limbic system would also mediate affective investment or "cathexis" of linguistic concepts, cross-modal abstractions, and intellectual reflection (24) (Table 3).

One might consider some of the superiorities of the right hemisphere as resulting from functions compromised by left hemisphere specialization. I would suggest

TABLE 3. *Limbic connections within left hemisphere*

Pathway	Convergence of visual, auditory, and somesthetic associations at parietotemporal junction, a cross-modal integrating system that includes Wernicke's area and the angular gyrus; projection to temporal limbic structures such as the hippocampus; direct projections to ventral premotor cortex (i.e., Broca's area) via arcuate fasciculus
Cognitive functions	Formation and retrieval of nonspatial intermodal associations; importance of angular gyrus in naming; Gerstmann's syndrome as somesthetic-kinesthetic feedback related to learned cross-modal schemata; Wernicke's area and alexia
Limbic functions	
Mnemonic	Learning based on temporal (sequential) rather than topographic associations of stimuli in separate modalities (i.e., auditory, visual); language
Emotional	Affective investment of intermodal abstractions—words, verbal concepts; love of intellectual reflection

that the preservation of two structural features could account for a "secondary dominance" of the right hemisphere in several emotional and cognitive functions (Table 4).

Independent dorsal (parietofrontal) limbic connections in the right hemisphere would allow for superior emotional surveillance, through scanning of external and internal milieus in multiple modalities for drive-relevant stimuli. An analogous, though more complex, specialized function is scanning the stored environment, i.e., memory, for the most drive-salient situations. In cognitive terms, the spatial superiority of the right hemisphere may result from the hard-wired, topographic interleafing of sensory modalities, especially visual and somesthetic, necessary for rapid orientation. The importance of extrafoveal, peripheral scanning, and simultaneous processing of many sectors of space may have led to a related superiority of the right frontal lobe in "incidental" learning (43).

A specialized feature of the right ventral (temporofrontal) system may be the retention of independent connections between each cortical sensory system and the limbic system (39) (Fig. 3, Tables 2,4). In terms of emotional function, these intramodal sensory-limbic links may allow for a more immediate or powerful affective reaction to stimuli (44) characterized, for example, by larger autonomic responses (8). The decoding of emotional signals within a single sensory modality, i.e., vocal intonation or facial expression, might best be accomplished by the direct sensory limbic connections of this system.

Ventral limbic structures such as the hippocampus and the amygdala are crucial for memory as well as affective responses. Some memory tasks are best performed by intramodal encoding of a complex stimulus: i.e., retaining the visual location of a randomly located dot, or the haptic representation of an abstract shape, or an auditory record of a novel melody. In these situations, the right hemisphere has superiority (42). Of course, stimuli that may be encoded linguistically, i.e., employing intermodal associations—should be better stored by the left hemisphere. However, the same melodic sequence that must be retained by the naive listener as

TABLE 4. *Secondary dominant functions of the right hemisphere resulting from retained limbic connections*

Retained structure	Emotional functions	Cognitive functions
Dorsal: parietofrontal system	Drive surveillance—internal and external milieu: emotionally appropriate arousal—recognition of threats, pursuit of drive goals	Spatial (topographic) representation; attention peripheral surveillance; "incidental" learning
Ventral: temporofrontal system with independent sensory limbic connections	Primary affective and autonomic response within each sensory modality; decoding and transmission of unimodal affective signals	Memory for complex unimodal stimuli

an intramodel, auditory memory trace could be recoded by the musician in abstract, i.e., musical notation. The proposed asymmetry in ventral sensory-limbic connections does, then, predict a right to left hemisphere shift in functional superiority, depending on the strategy of memorization, which has been observed (45).

Let me briefly suggest some further testable implications of the structure-function correlations proposed in Table 4. Within the right hemisphere, an anterior to posterior distribution of expressive to receptive functions in emotional communication has been proposed (18). Table 4 suggests an additional dorsal to ventral specialization. It would be consistent with this parcellation of functions that neglect, unconcern, and denial of illness—failures of emotional surveillance—be associated with right parietal and perhaps dorsal-frontal lesions, whereas the reading of facial emotions—a task involving foveal visual-limbic associations—be associated with the right temporal lobe. There is evidence for these selective localizations (20,22).

Another potential implication concerns developmental deficits in emotional functions. We know that acquired lesions of the right hemisphere may impair emotional processing. In all probability, congenital abnormalities, including inherited dystrophies of the right hemisphere, might be expected to produce abnormality of emotional functions analogous to dyslexia, which has been associated with malformation of language association cortex in the left hemisphere (46). Recently, my colleagues, Drs. Mesulam and Weintraub, examined several socially awkward children with adequate verbal functions but spatial and constructional deficits implicating the right hemisphere; in some cases a similar pattern was found in a parent. Of particular interest was the failure of the "emotional dyslexic" to maintain eye-contact, i.e., to foveate the social partner. If the distinction between peripheral and central emotional-visual systems were valid, this finding would lead to further mechanistic and anatomical implications.

Most psychiatrists consider dreaming an emotional function. Within a dream, one may experience visual scenes portraying emotionally charged conflicts, either flight from danger or pursuit of a sought-after drive object. There are rapid conjugate movements of the eyes and autonomic responses. Whereas the role of brainstem structures in coordinating these events in dreaming has been extensively studied (47), little attention has been directed to cortical involvement. Furthermore, a convincing biological rationale for rapid eye movement (REM) sleep or dreaming has not been proposed.

Drawing on the analyses above, I would suggest that dreaming may be a nocturnal activation—perhaps a critically important priming—of the dorsal emotional surveillance circuits now specialized in the right hemisphere. This system may not have to deal with catastrophic emotional problems during a typical waking day, but under the cover of powerful inhibition on spinal motoneurons, the right parietal scanning circuits could play out a form of emotional war game at night. If this activation of the surveillance circuits were prevented, a falloff in attention and emotional control—the most consistent consequences of REM deprivation—might be expected.

Damage to the right parietal lobe would be expected to reduce or alter dreaming; and this has been reported (48). On the other hand, cessation of dreaming is not a consequence of temporal lobectomy. The preservation of dream reports in split-brain patients (49) does not exclude specialized involvement of the right parietal lobe since the isolated left hemisphere would learn of both eye movements and emotional activation from the brainstem.

I should like to conclude with some potential therapeutic implications of these ideas. It is important to stress how impaired the patient with right hemisphere damage may be by unconcern, unrealistic assessment of emotional priorities, and failures in emotional communication. In rehabilitation of aphasic patients with left hemisphere injuries, the use of melodic intonation (50) or visual-gestural association (51) may successfully enlist abilities of the right hemisphere. Following right hemisphere injury, I suspect we must repeatedly tell the verbal hemisphere about the tendency to neglect, minimize, and socially misperceive, and present verbal "sequential" strategies, which the patient may apply for correction. Steps in emotional perception and communication may have to be explicitly rehearsed. Because visual scanning is so often defective, optical devices to bring the left world into the right visual field might be helpful. Techniques to maximize alertness and attention, i.e., warning lights or buzzers, might optimize therapy.

Pharmacological methods of increasing activation might also be considered. Although the right hemisphere stroke patient may not appear depressed, many alerting and arousal systems utilize biogenic amines as neurotransmitters. One should not assume that tricyclic antidepressants would have the same effects as catechol- or indole-amine agonists, since their chronic effects may include a reduction of transmission in aminergic systems (52). The dosage and timing of psychotropic agents may prove critical, since alterations in receptors such as denervation supersensitivity, or acquired subsensitivity can be expected (53). In the future, one might consider therapeutic implications of both neurochemical asymmetries (54) and distinctions between transmitters utilized by the dorsal- versus the ventral-limbic systems. For example, biogenic amines are clearly involved in emotional arousal, presumably mediated by the dorsal system, whereas acetylcholine may be specially relevant to the ventral learning structures (i.e., hippocampus) (55).

REFERENCES

1. Babinski, J. (1914): Contribution a l'etude des troubles mentaux dans l'hemipledie cerebrale (anosagnosia). *Rev. Neurol.*, 27:845.
2. Gainotti, G. (1972): Emotional behavior and hemispheric side of the lesion. *Cortex*, 8:41.
3. Wechsler, A. F. (1973): The effect of organic brain disease on recall of emotionally charged versus neutral narrative texts. *Neurology*, 23:130.
4. Gasparrini, W. G., Satz, P., Heilman, K., and Coolidge, F. L. (1978): Hemispheric asymmetries of affective processing as determined by the Minnesota Multiphasic Personality Inventory. *J. Neurol. Neurosurg. Psychiat.*, 41:470.
5. Finkelstein, S., Baldessarini, R., Arana, G., Benowitz, L., Levine, D., Bear, D., Sweet, E., and Buonanno, F. (1982): Dexamethasone suppression test in stroke. *Ann. Neurol.*, *(in press)*.
6. Bear, D. M. (1979): Personality changes associated with neurologic lesions. In: *Textbook of Outpatient Psychiatry*. Edited by A. Lazare. Williams and Wilkins Co., Baltimore, MD.

7. Dimond, S. J., Farrington, L., and Johnson, P. (1976): Differing emotional responses from right and left hemispheres. *Nature*, 261:690.
8. Dimond, S. J., and Farrington, L. (1977): Emotional response to films shown to the right and left hemisphere of the brain measured by heart rate. *Acta Psychol.*, 241:255.
9. Heilman, K. M., Schwartz, H. D., and Watson, R. T. (1978): Hypoarousal in patients with the neglect syndrome and emotional indifference. *Neurology*, 28:229.
10. Terzian, H. (1964): Behavioral and EEG effects of intracarotid sodium amytol injections. *Acta neurochir.*, 12:230.
11. Rossi, G. F., and Rosadini, G. (1967): Experimental analysis of cerebral dominance in man. In: *Brain Mechanisms Underlying Speech and Language*, p. 167. Edited by C. H. Milikin and F. L. Darley. Grune and Stratton, Inc., New York-London.
12. Rizzolatti, G., Umlita, C., and Berlucchi, G. (1971): Opposite superiorities of the right and left cerebral hemispheres in discriminative reaction time to physiognomical and alphabetical material. *Brain*, 94:431.
13. Ley, R. G., and Bryden, M. P. (1979): Hemispheric differences in processing emotions and faces. *Brain Lang.*, 7:127.
14. Carmon, A., and Nachson, I. (1973): Ear asymmetry in perception of emotional and nonverbal stimuli. *Acta Psychol.*, 37:351.
15. Heilman, K. M., Scholes, R., and Watson, R. T. (1974): Auditory affective agnosia. *J. Neurol. Neurosurg. Psychiatry*, 38:69.
16. Sackeim, H. A., Gur, R. C., and Savoy, M. C. (1978): Emotions are expressed more intensely on the left side of the face. *Science*, 202:424.
17. Borod, J., and Caron, H. (1980): Facedness and emotion related to lateral dominance, sex, and expression type. *Neuropsychologia*, 18:237.
18. Ross, E. D., and Mesulam, M. M. (1979): Dominant language functions of the right hemisphere? *Arch. Neurol.*, 36:144.
19. Tucker, D. M., Watson, R. T., and Heilman, K. M. (1977): Discrimination and evocation of affectively intoned speech in patients with right parietal disease. *Neurology*, 27:947.
20. Benowitz, L. I., Bear, D. M., Mesulam, M. M., Rosenthal, R., Zaidel, E., and Sperry, R. W. (1980): Nonverbal sensitivity following lateralized cerebral injury. *J. McLean Hosp.*, 384:146.
21. Rosenthal, R., Hall, J. A., DiMatteo, M. R., Rogers, P. L., and Archer, D. (1979): *Sensitivity to Nonverbal Communication: The PONS Test*. Johns Hopkins Press, Baltimore, MD.
22. Ojemann, G., Fried, I., Mateer, C., Wohns, R., and Fedio, P. (1980): Organization of visual function in human nondominant cortex: Evidence from electrical stimulation. *Neurosci. Abstr.*, 6:418.
23. Waxman, S. G., and Geschwind, N. (1975): The interictal behavior syndrome of temporal lobe epilepsy. *Arch. Gen. Psychiat.*, 32:1580.
24. Bear, D. M., and Fedio, P. (1977): Quantitative analysis of interictal behavior in temporal lobe epilepsy. *Arch. Neurol.*, 34:454.
25. Flor-Henry, P. (1969): Schizophrenic-like reactions and affective psychoses associated with temporal lobe epilepsy. *Am. J. Psychiat.*, 126:400.
26. McIntyre, M., Pritchard, P. B., and Lombroso, C. T. (1976): Left and right temporal lobe epileptics: A controlled investigation of some psychological differences. *Epilepsia*, 17:377.
27. Bear, D. M., and Schenk, L. (1981): Increased autonomic responses to neutral and emotional stimuli in patients with temporal lobe epilepsy. *Am. J. Psychiat.*, 138:843.
28. Gross, C. G., Bender, D. B., and Gerstein, G. L. (1979): Activity of inferior temporal neurons in behaving monkeys. *Neuropsychologia*, 17:215.
29. Mishkin, M. (1972): Cortical visual areas and their interaction. In: *The Brain and Human Behavior*, Edited by A. G. Karczman and J. C. Eccles. Springer-Verlag, New York.
30. Mountcastle, V. B., Lynch, J. C., Georgopoulosa, A., Sakata, H., and Acuna, C. (1975): Posterior parietal association cortex of the monkey: Command functions for operations within extrapersonal space. *J. Neurophysiol.*, 38:871.
31. Mountcastle, V. B., Motter, B. C., and Anderson, R. A. (1980): Some further observations of the functional properties of neurons in parietal lobe of the waking monkey. *Behav. Brain Sci.*, 3:520.
32. Lynch, J. C. (1980): The fuctional organization of posterior parietal association cortex. *Behav. Brain Sci.*, 3:485.
33. Mesulam, M. M. (1980): An anatomical basis for the functional specialization of the parietal lobe in directed attention. *Behav. Brain Sci.*, 3:510.

34. Mesulam, M. M., Van Hoesen, G., Pandya, D., and Geschwind, N. (1977): Limbic and sensory connections of the inferior parietal lobule (Area PG) in the rhesus monkey. *Brain Res.*, 136:393.
35. Blumer, D., and Benson, D. F. (1975): Personality changes with frontal and temporal lobe lesions. In: *Psychiatric Aspects of Neurologic Disease*, p. 151. Edited by D. F. Benson and D. Blumer. Grune and Stratton, Inc., New York.
36. Geschwind, N., and Levitsky, W. (1968): Human brain: Left-right asymmetries in temporal speech area. *Science*, 161:186.
37. Galaburda, A. M., Sanides, F., and Geschwind, N. (1978): Human brain: Cytoarchitectonic left-right asymmetries in the temporal speech region. *Arch. Neurol.*, 35:812.
38. Galaburda, A. M., LeMay, M., Kemper, T. L., and Geschwind, N. (1978): Right-left asymmetries in the brain. *Science*, 199:852.
39. Geschwind, N. (1965): Disconnexion syndromes in animals and man. *Brain*, 88:237.
40. Leinonen, L., Hyvarinen, J., and Sovijarai, A. R. (1980): Functional properties of neurons in the temporo-parietal association cortex of awake monkey. *Exp. Brain Res.*, 39:203.
41. Buffery, A. W. H., and Locke, M. (1981): Cerebral hemispheric asymmetry for cross-modal verbal skill in deaf and hearing children: *Abstracts, Fourth International Neuropsychology European Conference, INS Bulletin, June, 1981.*
42. Milner, B. (1971): Interhemispheric differences in the localization of psychological processes in man. *Br. Med. Bull.*, 27:272.
43. Luria, A. R., and Simernitskaya, E. G. (1977): Interhemispheric relations and the functions of the minor hemisphere. *Neuropsychologia*, 15:175.
44. Hecaen, H., and Angelergues, R. (1963): *La Cecite Psychique*, Masson et Cie, Paris.
45. Bever, T. G. and Chiarello, R. J. (1974): Cerebral dominance in musicians and nonmusicians. *Science*, 185:357.
46. Galaburda, A. M., and Kemper, T. L. (1979): Cytoarchitectonic abnormalities in developmental dyslexia: A case study. *Ann. Neurol.*, 6:94.
47. Hobson, J. A., and McCarley, R. W. (1977): The brain as a dream state generator: An activation-synthesis hypothesis of the dream process. *Am. J. Psychiat.*, 134:1335.
48. Humphrey, M. E., and Zangwill, O. L. (1951): Cessation of dreaming after brain injury. *J. Neurol. Neurosurg. Psychiatry*, 14:322.
49. Hoppe, K. D. (1977): Split brains in psychoanalysis. *Psychoanal. Q.*, 46:220.
50. Sparks, R., Helms, N., and Albert, M. (1974): Aphasia rehabilitation resulting from melodic intonation therapy. *Cortex*, 10:303.
51. Gardner, H., Zurif, E., Barry, L., and Baker, E. (1976): Visual communication in aphasia. *Neuropsychologia*, 14:275.
52. Maas, J. W. (1979): Neurotransmitters in depression: Too much, too little or too unstable. *Trends Neurosci.*, 2:306.
53. Crews, F. T., and Smith, C. B. (1978): Presynaptic alpha-receptor subsensitivity after long-term antidepressant treatment. *Science*, 202:322.
54. Oke, A., Keller, R., Mefford, I., and Adams, R. N. (1978): Lateralization of norepinephrine in human thalamus. *Science*, 200:1411.
55. Drachman, D. (1977): Memory and cognitive function in man: Does the cholinergic system have a specific role? *Neurology*, 27:783.

The Limbic System: Functional Organization and
Clinical Disorders, edited by B.K. Doane and
K.E. Livingston. Raven Press, New York © 1986.

Circuitous Connections Linking Cerebral Cortex, Limbic System, and Corpus Striatum

Walle J. H. Nauta

*Department of Psychology and Brain Science, Massachusetts Institute of Technology,
Cambridge, Massachusetts 02139, and Mailman Research Center, McLean Hospital,
Belmont, Massachusetts 02178*

Concepts evolved over the past four or five decades tend to subdivide the cerebral hemisphere of mammals into three great domains. The outermost and largest of these is formed by the neocortex (or isocortex in O. Vogt's terminology), a fairly uniformly six-layered cortex whose extensive subcortical connections, distributed throughout the length of the brainstem and spinal cord, are established almost exclusively by the internal capsule–cerebral peduncle. A second conceptual realm of the forebrain is constituted by the limbic system, a collective and functionally neutral term denoting an heterogeneous group of neural structures arranged along the medial edge of the cerebral hemisphere (*limbus* is Latin for margin) and having at its core the allocortical hippocampus and the largely subcortical amygdala. Together these form the principal telencephalic origin of the medial forebrain bundle and, thus, the hemisphere's main link with a continuum of interconnected subcortical structures that begins in the septum and extends caudalward from there through the hypothalamus and midbrain to upper levels of the rhombencephalon (see ref. 22 for a survey of subcortical limbic circuitry). A third major subdivision of the cerebral hemisphere is represented by the corpus striatum, the massive core of the hemisphere composed of the striatum (caudate nucleus and putamen) and the globus pallidus, each reciprocally associated with a smaller satellite structure (respectively, the substantia nigra and the subthalamic nucleus). Remarkably, the efferent pathways originating from the corpus striatum for the most part remain enclosed within the forebrain, but some descending lines extend into the midbrain, in particular to the superior colliculus and to tegmental regions, including the pedunculopontine nucleus (for a review of these connections see ref. 23).

Traditionally, and not without good clinical, physiological, and anatomical reason, the neocortex is considered to embody the highest levels of sensory analysis and integration, as well as certain of the more differentiated components of motor function. Last, but not least, it is regarded as the principal substrate of thought processes. The limbic system, by contrast, is viewed as the main cerebral representative of the internal milieu, expressing its functions in the form of states of affect and motivation. And finally, the corpus striatum is generally considered a somatic motor mechanism.

Useful as the notion of a tripartite composition has been—and still is—as a first approach to the functional organization of the cerebral hemisphere, it cannot entirely satisfy the mind. At the current stage of knowledge it is no longer easily conceivable that great categories of brain function can be localized so exclusively to one or the other subdivision of the brain. Among the prime reasons to suspect a need for some qualification of the tripartition concept is an anatomical one: In recent decades the three cerebral subdivisions have become more vaguely rather than more sharply delineated from each other, and, furthermore, an increasing number of cross-connections between them have been and are being reported. Moreover, their respective efferent circuitries, until quite recently thought to be almost entirely separate of each other, are now known to intersect, converge, or blend in a variety of loci. For example, only little more than 20 years ago both limbic system and corpus striatum were believed to be largely or even entirely unconnected with the cortex. Anatomical studies done since that time, however, have revealed that all or nearly all of the neocortex is connected with both mechanisms, either, as in the case of the corpus striatum, by corticofugal fibers originating throughout the expanse of the neocortex (1,18,35,36) and distributed directly to both caudate nucleus and putamen or, as in the case of the limbic system, by way of variously complex sequences of cortico-cortical connections, which ultimately converge on ventral and medial regions of the temporal cortex (16,26), which in turn project to the amygdala as well as to the entorhinal area, the major cortical source of afferents to the hippocampus (33,34).

The cortical conduction line to the amygdala is reciprocated, in part at least, by direct amygdalofugal projections to the inferior temporal (19,21) and prefrontal cortex (15,19,25; see also Nauta and Domesick, ref. 22). No similarly direct reciprocity has been discovered in the cortico-striate connection, but it nonetheless has long seemed certain that the striatum can affect the functions of the motor cortex at least, by way of its exit route leading sequentially over the pallidum and anterior parts of the ventral thalamic nucleus. More recently, however, evidence has appeared of a second and parallel conduction line, likewise leading over the pallidum and thalamus, by which the striatum could be thought to expand its influence beyond the motoric to other functional realms of the neocortex, as well as to the limbic system. The evidence at issue suggests an instance of serial linkage of all three of the main subdivisions of the cerebral hemisphere: limbic system to corpus striatum to neocortex. Since a documented description of the relevant experimental findings has been published elsewhere (9), the following account, for the most part, will be presented in the form of a summarizing survey.

LIMBIC INNERVATION OF THE STRIATUM

Recent studies in the rat with the aid of the autoradiographic fiber-tracing method (17) have led to the conclusion that the anterior striatal half (the large part rostral to the level at which the anterior commissure crosses the midplane) can be subdivided into (a) a larger ventral and medial region including, but far exceeding, the nucleus accumbens and olfactory tubercle, and (b) a somewhat smaller dorsolateral region. The reason for the distinction is that the former, ventromedial striatal subdivision is characterized by being densely innervated by several substantial and partially overlapping afferent fiber systems, each originating either from a limbic structure such as the hippocampus, amygdala, or cingulate cortex, or from a structure implicated in the circuitry of the limbic system: the ventral tegmental area or the prefrontal cortex. The remaining, anterodorsolateral striatal sector, by contrast, receives only sparse inputs of limbic origin and is, instead, heavily projected upon by the sensorimotor cortex. The contrast between these two subdivisions of the anterior striatum is epitomized by Fig. 1 in which the limbic-afferented striatal region (for the sake of convenience to be called "limbic striatum") is indicated by a variety of line and stipple patterns. Three systems of limbic afferents are each distributed throughout the extent of the region, namely: the projections from, respectively, the amygdala, the prefrontal cortex, and the ventral tegmental area, the last-mentioned one representing the region's dopaminergic innervation. The dorsolateral striatal region largely avoided by limbico-striatal inputs but densely innervated by the sensorimotor cortex ("nonlimbic striatum") has been left open.

The evidence that the striatum—or at least its rostral half—is composed of a limbic-innervated and a "nonlimbic" district naturally raised the question whether

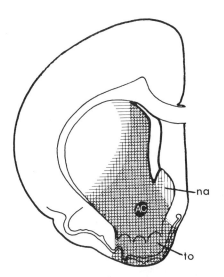

FIG. 1. Frontal section through the anterior half of the striatum of the rat. The region shaded by various line-and-stipple patterns is the ventromedial, limbic system-innervated striatal sector; note that it includes the nucleus accumbens (na) and olfactory tubercle (to). Separately indicated are the projections from the ventral tegmental area *(vertical lines)*, prefrontal cortex *(horizontal lines)*, and amygdala *(stipple).* Omitted from the figure are the additional projections to this striatal sector from the hippocampus (limited to the nucleus-accumbens region medial to the anterior commissure) and cingulate cortex (confined to a narrow vertical column along the lateral ventricle). Abbreviations used in this and all following figures: abl, basolateral amygdaloid nucleus; AC, anterior commissure; bns, bed nucleus of stria terminalis; CC, crus cerebri; cgs, central grey substance; CI, capsula interna; CP, caudatoputamen; dp, dorsal pallidum; ep, entopeduncular nucleus (internal pallidal segment); F, fornix; FCC, frontocingulate cortex; H, hippocampus; hl, lateral habenular nucleus; ht, hypothalamus; md, mediodorsal thalamic nucleus; na, nucleus accumbens; rt, nucleus reticularis thalami; SM, stria medullaris; SMC, sensorimotor cortex; sn, substantia nigra; st, subthalamic nucleus; to, olfactory tubercle; va, nucleus ventralis anterior thalami; vp, ventral pallidum; vta, ventral tegmental area.

this dualism might not be reflected somehow in the distribution of the massive striatofugal projection to the globus pallidus. Phrased in more general terms, the question would ask: Could the two striatal districts be the respective origins of two separate and distinct striatal exit lines?

Further study yielded an affirmative answer to this question. Comparison of a large number of cases (in each of which a small injection of tritiated leucine had been placed in one or the other striatal locus and the resulting radioactive fiber labeling had been registered autoradiographically) clearly showed that the limbic-afferented striatal region projects exclusively to an only recently identified ventral component of the globus pallidus,[1] the so-called *ventral pallidum*. The "nonlimbic" striatal sector projects to a larger pallidal division, here to be called *dorsal pallidum*, that occupies most of the globus pallidus as conventionally outlined in histological sections of the rat brain. For the purpose of the present account, this subdivision of the globus pallidus into two distinct parts needs some further comment.

THE VENTRAL PALLIDUM

The ventral pallidum was first described by Heimer and Wilson (13) in the rat as an extension of the globus pallidus, stretching ventrally and rostrally beneath the anterior commissure. Its identification as a pallidal subdivision of the infracommissural forebrain region was originally based on cytological characteristics, as well as on the finding that it receives a massive striatal projection originating in particular from the nucleus accumbens (24,37,38). Its pallidal nature was further documented by evidence that it also shares with the main mass of the globus pallidus a substantial projection from the subthalamic nucleus (28) as well as the histochemical characteristics of a high iron content (14,31) and a strong enkephalin-like (10,11,32) and glutamic acid decarboxylase-like immunoreactivity (2).

Despite these similarities, the ventral pallidum must be viewed as distinct from the main, conventionally recognized, retro- and supracommissural mass of the globus pallidus. A principal reason for this distinction is histochemical: Whereas both the ventral pallidum and the main mass of the globus pallidus are infiltrated by a dense plexus of enkephalin-positive fibers, the ventral pallidum contains an additional and almost equally dense plexus of substance P-positive fibers that extends over only a short distance into the main pallidal mass. For a proper understanding of the criteria followed in defining the ventral pallidum for the purposes of the present account, a brief elaboration of this last point is necessary.

It is important to note that intrapallidal enkephalin and substance P are not intrinsic to the globus pallidus proper, but are associated with the striatopallidal projection. As first observed by Fox et al. (3) in Golgi material, striatopallidal fibers enmesh the dendrites of pallidal neurons individually in sleeve-like plexuses. The characteristic histological picture reflecting this junctional arrangement in

---

[1]In the brains of rodents and carnivores the term *globus pallidus* refers exclusively to the external or lateral pallidal segment, the internal or medial pallidal segment being represented in such forms by the entopeduncular nucleus.

material immunoreacted for enkephalin ("woolly fibers," Haber and Nauta, ref. 11) provides a light-microscopic criterion for determining the extent of the globus pallidus. In such material the dense plexus of enkephalin-positive "woolly fibers" filling the main mass of the globus pallidus is seen to continue without interruption ventrally into the infracommissural region where it extends rostrally over a wide area bordering the ventral side of the striatum and bed nucleus of the stria terminalis (11,32). Interestingly, such material also shows that this infracommissural plexus extends around the lateral border of the nucleus of the diagonal band into the deep, fibrocellular layer of the olfactory tubercle, in agreement with an earlier suggestion, made by Heimer (12) on cytoarchitectural grounds, that the tubercle is a striato-pallidal complex, as well as with the description by Ribak and Fallon (27) of large cells associated with the islands of Calleja and electronmicroscopically indistin-guishable from pallidal neurons.

Since the density of the enkephalin-positive intrapallidal fiber plexus varies little throughout its extent, it cannot serve to delineate the ventral pallidum from the main, supra-, and retrocommissural mass of the globus pallidus. Such a delineation is, however, possible in sections processed for substance P-like immunoreactivity. Such material reveals a dense plexus of substance P-positive "woolly fibers" that, with minor exceptions, is coextensive with the infracommissural enkephalin-positive plexus. But, unlike the latter, it extends over only a short distance into the main pallidal mass, then abruptly declines in density and only very sparsely extends through the large remainder of the globus pallidus. The curved line along which this decline in density of the substance P-positive "woolly-fiber" plexus occurs suggests itself as the border between the ventral pallidum (vp) and the remaining part of the globus pallidus, here for purposes of contrast to be referred to as *dorsal pallidum* (dp) (ref. 10; see also Fig. 2 in which the extent of the substance P-positive plexus is indicated by a stipple pattern).

In summary, the ventral pallidum is here defined as the largely infracommissural region massively pervaded by enkephalin-positive and substance P-positive (and probably additional) striatofugal fibers terminating in the peridendritic manner characteristic of the striatopallidal projection.

DIFFERENTIAL PROJECTIONS FROM DORSAL AND VENTRAL PALLIDUM

The evidence that the subdivision of the striatum into a limbic-afferented and a "nonlimbic" district is mirrored in a ventral versus dorsal dualism in the intrapal-lidal distribution of the striatopallidal projection raises the question whether the separateness of the two striatal exit lines might not extend even beyond the globus pallidus. To investigate this question, a small deposit of tritiated leucine was placed in either the dorsal or the ventral pallidum in a large number of rats; the distributions of fibers radioactively labeled by each of these isotope placements were then registered autoradiographically, carefully charted, and compared.

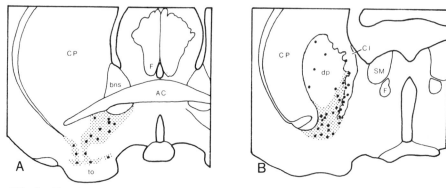

FIG. 2. Drawings of two frontal sections, respectively, at the level of the anterior commissure **(A)** and a short distance behind it **(B)**. The substance P-positive plexus, coextensive with the ventral pallidum, is indicated by stippling (cf. Haber and Nauta, ref. 11). Coarser black dots represent strongly acetylcholinesterase-positive intrapallidal neurons. Note that such cells are much more numerous in the ventral pallidum (stippled area) than in the dorsal pallidum (dp in **B**). Omitted in this illustration are the many further cholinergic neurons that are found in the nucleus of the diagonal band and other basal forebrain structures at these same transverse levels. For abbreviations, see legend to Fig. 1.

The results of these experiments showed pronounced differences between the exit lines from the dorsal and ventral pallidum, respectively. The findings are illustrated by Fig. 3 and can be summarized as follows.

1. The efferent connections of the dorsal pallidum (Fig. 3B) compose the classical projection from the external pallidal segment and involve primarily the subthalamic nucleus and substantia nigra. This pallidal exit line appears to extend the striato-pallidal projection arising from the "nonlimbic" dorsolateral striatal sector (heavy arrow in 3B), the striatal region, which in turn receives its main telencephalic input from the sensorimotor cortex (3A).

2. The ventral pallidum projects, like the dorsal pallidum, to the subthalamic nucleus and substantia nigra, but it has further projections to several structures implicated in the circuitry of the limbic system, particularly the amygdala, the lateral habenular nucleus, and the mediodorsal nucleus of the thalamus (Fig. 3C). It projects more sparsely to the hypothalamus, to the ventral tegmental area, and to more caudal regions of the midbrain tegmentum, including the region of the pedunculopontine nucleus. Of some special interest are those projections of the ventral pallidum that ascend to the anteromedial cortex and an adjoining region of the sensorimotor cortex: There is evidence suggesting that this projection, as well as the one to the amygdala, originates largely, at least, from the cholinergic cells

FIG. 3. Two partly segregated striatofugal conduction lines described in the text. **A:** "limbic" *(shaded)* and "nonlimbic" striatal subdivisions and their respective main telencephalic afferents. **B:** the conventionally described striatofugal line leading from the motor cortex-innervated "nonlimbic" striatal subdivision to the dorsal pallidum *(heavy arrow)*, which in turn projects to the subthalamic nucleus and substantia nigra; **C:** the line leading from the limbic-afferented striatal subdivision to the ventral pallidum *(heavy arrow)* and from there not only to subthalamic nucleus and substantia nigra but also to the frontocingulate and medial sensorimotor cortex, lateral habenular and mediodorsal thalamic nucleus, amygdala, hypothalamus, ventral tegmental area, and more caudal and dorsal tegmental regions. For abbreviations, see legend to Fig. 1.

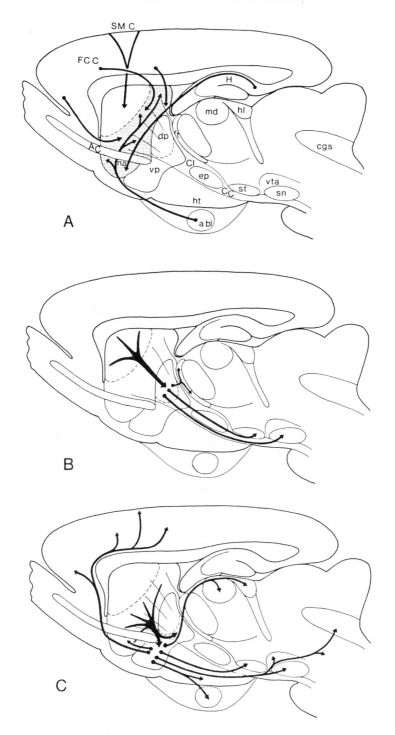

of the so-called magnocellular basal nucleus that lie embedded in the ventral pallidum (8). All these exit lines from the ventral pallidum, however, appear to lie in the transsynaptic extension of that component of the striatopallidal projection (heavy arrow in 3C) which originates from the limbic-afferented striatum, that is to say, the large striatal region innervated by a remarkable variety of afferents from within the circuitry of the limbic system (the shaded region in Fig. 3A).

DISCUSSION

The findings discussed in the foregoing account further document the pallidal nature of the infracommissural region designated ventral pallidum (VP). The region shares several features of its cytology, histochemistry, and afferent connectivity, with the main, retrocommissural mass of the globus pallidus (dorsal pallidum; DP), and the combination of its efferent connections with the subthalamic nucleus and substantia nigra is likewise characteristically pallidal. That the VP must none-theless be viewed as a distinctive part of the globus pallidus is indicated by (a) its dense plexus of substance P-positive striatopallidal fibers, which is not shared by the DP, (b) its selective innervation by the anteroventromedial, limbic-afferented striatal quadrant, and (c) the evidence that its projections involve not only the subthalamic nucleus and substantia nigra, but also various limbic system-associated structures.

More in general, the outcome of the experiments described above indicates that the limbic versus nonlimbic dichotomy in the innervation of the striatum reflects itself in the existence of two partly segregated striatofugal conduction lines. The current evidence of this continued dualism is schematically illustrated by Fig. 3 and can be summarized as follows. A dorsolateral sector of the anterior striatum, receiving only sparse afferents of limbic origin but, instead, heavily innervated by the sensorimotor cortex (17), projects to an anterodorsolateral region of the main, supra- and retrocommissural (i.e., conventionally recognized) mass of the globus pallidus. This pallidal region ("dorsal pallidum") in turn gives rise to a projection that forms the classical pallidofugal pathway descending to the subthalamic nucleus and substantia nigra (Fig. 3B). By contrast, the heavily limbic-innervated antero-ventromedial striatal region (shaded in Fig. 3A) projects to the largely infracom-missural, but partly also supra- and retrocommissural ventral pallidum. From the pallidum, in turn, efferents pass not only to the subthalamic nucleus and substantia nigra but also to various limbic system-associated structures, in particular the amygdala, frontocingulate (and adjoining sensorimotor) cortex, mediodorsal tha-lamic nucleus, lateral habenular nucleus, hypothalamus, ventral tegmental area, and more caudal and dorsal regions of the midbrain tegmentum (Fig. 3C).

As thus defined, the two striatopallidofugal lines share the subthalamic nucleus and substantia nigra as common distribution targets. If it is assumed that both these target structures, first and foremost, are components of the somatic-motor system, the present findings suggest both as sites where central skeletomuscular mechanisms are accessible to striatopallidal output of limbic antecedents, conveyed by the line leading from the limbic-afferented ventromedial striatum over the ventral pallidum. It is possible that further sites of such access lie farther caudally in the midbrain. In the experiments described in the foregoing account, isotope injections in the ventral pallidum (but not dorsal pallidum) were found to label rather sparse fibers distributed over wide regions of the midbrain tegmentum, including the dorsal area containing the nucleus tegmenti pedunculopontinus. It is of interest to note that fibers of very similar tegmental distribution have been traced from the nucleus accumbens in both rat (6,24) and cat, and it would thus seem that the system in question contains striatal as well as pallidal efferents. The available auto-radiographic material provided no evidence that either of these fiber categories actually terminates in the region of the pedunculopontine nucleus (rather than merely passing through it to the adjacent central grey substance), but recent studies with the aid of the anterograde marker PHA-L, have shown that some efferents from the region here called ventral pallidum indeed terminate in and about the pedunculopontine nucleus (7,30). Swanson et al. (30) interpret this as suggesting a limbic innervation of the "mesencephalic locomotor region" of Grillner and Shik (5).

A third route by which the limbic system could be thought to have access to central somatic-motor mechanisms could lead from the limbic-innervated striatum over the strongly acetylcholinesterase-positive cells embedded in the ventral pallidum. The present anterograde evidence, suggesting that at least some of these cells project to the sensorimotor cortex, only confirms earlier findings in retrograde-labeling experiments (20,29).

Even more difficult to interpret from a functional point of view are the limbico-striatopallidofugal lines leading to various limbic and limbic system-associated structures, summarized in Fig. 3C. From one vantage point, these connections could be viewed collectively as a differentiated "return loop," enabling the limbic system to monitor the effect of its outputs to the striatum (and thus possibly acting as an aid in adjusting the organism's motivational set to the output efficacy of the central somatic-motor system). But other possibilities must be considered. The question arises, for example, if one significance of the much interrupted limbico-striatopallido-limbic circuit here proposed may not lie in the fact that the striatum is the site of an unusually wide variety of intricately interspersed neurotransmitters and neuromodulators (cf. ref. 4), particular combinations of which might be required for optimal functioning of limbic and cortical mechanisms, no less stringently than the same or other combinations are required for optimal somatic-motor function. The possibility of such a general functional role of the corpus striatum suggests itself from a remarkable parallel between the "limbic" and "nonlimbic" trans-striatal conduction lines: both prominently include channels over which part of their impulse flow can be led back to the domain of its origin in the cerebral hemisphere. To be more explicit, the familiar "extrapyramidal motor circuit," motor cortex→striatum→pallidum→thalamic VA-VL complex→premotor cortex→motor cortex (Fig. 4A) appears to have limbic counterparts in the sequences: limbic system→striatum→ventral pallidum→amygdala, and, limbic system→

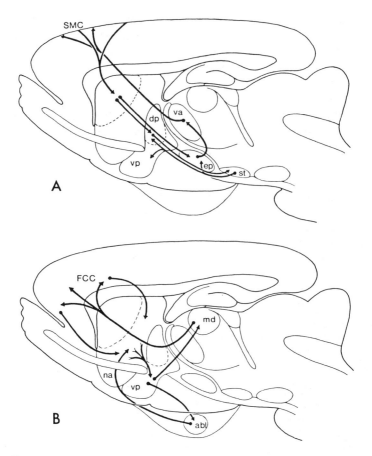

FIG. 4. The extrapyramidal circuit of the motor cortex **(A)** compared with analogous trans-striatal circuits involving the amygdala and frontocingulate cortex **(B)**. To avoid excessive complexity of the diagrams, no attempt has been made to include possible cross-roads between **A** and **B**, such as the one suggested by the reciprocal connection of the ventral pallidum with the subthalamic nucleus. For abbreviations, see legend to Fig. 1.

striatum→ventral pallidum→thalamic mediodorsal nucleus→frontal and anterior limbic cortex (Fig. 4B). If it is considered likely, on the basis of long-known anatomical connections, that the function of the striatum expresses itself, in part, through a major circuit affecting the mechanisms of the motor cortex, the more recent anatomical data here reviewed make it appear no less likely that the striatum, through an analogous though less massive circuit, can affect the mechanisms of the prefrontal cortex and thus a class of functions that seem more likely to be cognitive than primarily skeletomuscular.

ACKNOWLEDGMENTS

The foregoing account is based in large part on studies made possible by NSF Grant BNS-8306284 and PHS Grants RO1 NS19945 and PO1 MH 31154.

REFERENCES

1. Carman, J. B., Cowan, W. M., Powell, T. P. S., and Webster, K. E. (1965): A bilateral cortico-striate projection. *J. Neurol. Neurosurg. Psychiatry*, 28:71–77.
2. Fallon, J. H., and Ribak, C. E. (1980): Multiple neurotransmitter studies in the islands of Calleja complex of the basal forebrain. III. Connections, correlations and reservations. *Soc. Neurosci.*, 6:114. *(Abstract)*.
3. Fox, C. A., Andrade, H. N., LuQui, I., and Rafols, J. A. (1974): The primate globus pallidus. A Golgi and electron microscope study. *J. Hirnforsch.*, 15:75–93.
4. Graybiel, A. M., and Ragsdale, C. W. (1983): Biochemical anatomy of the striatum. In: *Chemical Neuroanatomy*, edited by P. C. Emson, pp. 427–504. Raven Press, New York.
5. Grillner, S., and Shik, M. T. (1973): On the descending control of lumbosacral spinal cord from the "mesencephalic locomotor region". *Acta Physiol. Scand.*, 87:320–333.
6. Groenewegen, H. J., and Russchen, F. T. (1984): Organization of the efferent projections of the nucleus accumbens to pallidal, hypothalamic, and mesencephalic structures: a tracing and immunohistochemical study in the cat. *J. Comp. Neurol.*, 223:347–367.
7. Groenewegen, H. J., and van Dijk, C. A. (1984): Efferent projections of the ventral pallidum in the rat as studied with the anterograde transport of Phaseolus vulgaris leucoagglutinin (PHA-L). *Neurosci. Lett.*, [*Suppl*.18:]58. *(Abstract)*.
8. Grove, E. A., Haber, S. N., Domesick, V. B., and Nauta, W. J. H. (1983): Differential projections from AChE-positive and AChE-negative ventral-pallidum cells in the rat. *Soc. Neurosci.*, 9:16. *(Abstract)*.
9. Haber, S. N., Groenewegen, H. J., Grove, E. A., and Nauta, W. J. H. (1985): Efferent connections of the ventral pallidum in the rat. Evidence of a dual striato-pallidofugal pathway. *J. Comp. Neurol.*, 235:322–335.
10. Haber, S. N., and Nauta, W. J. H. (1981): Substance P, but not enkephalin, immunoreactivity distinguishes ventral from dorsal pallidum. *Soc. Neurosci.*, 7:916. *(Abstract)*.
11. Haber, S. N., and Nauta, W. J. H. (1983): Ramifications of the globus pallidus in the rat as indicated by patterns of immunohistochemistry. *Neuroscience*, 9:245–260.
12. Heimer, L. (1978): The olfactory cortex and the ventral striatum. In: *Limbic Mechanisms, the Continuing Evolution of the Limbic System Concept*, edited by K. E. Livingston and O. Hornykiewicz. pp. 95–187. Plenum Press, New York.
13. Heimer, L., and Wilson, R. D. (1975): The subcortical projections of the allocortex: similarities in the neural associations of the hippocampus, the piriform cortex, and the neocortex. In: *Golgi Centennial Symposium*, edited by M. Santini. pp. 177–193. Raven Press, New York.
14. Hill, J. M., and Switzer, R. C. (1984): The regional distribution and cellular localization of iron in the rat brain. *Neuroscience*, 11:595–603.
15. Jacobson, S., and Trojanowski, J. Q. (1975): Amygdaloid projections to prefrontal granular cortex in Rhesus monkey demonstrated with horseradish peroxidase. *Brain Res.*, 100:132–139.
16. Jones, E. G., and Powell, T. P. S. (1970): An anatomical study of converging sensory pathways within the cerebral cortex of the monkey. *Brain*, 93:793–820.
17. Kelley, A. E., Domesick, V. B., and Nauta, W. J. H. (1982): The amygdalostriatal projection in the rat—an anatomical study by anterograde and retrograde tracing methods. *Neuroscience*, 7:615–630.
18. Kemp, J. M., and Powell, T. P. S. (1970): The cortico-striate projection in the monkey. *Brain*, 93:525–546.
19. Krettek, J. E., and Price, J. H. (1974): A direct input from the amygdala to the thalamus and the cerebral cortex. *Brain Res.*, 67:169–174.
20. McKinney, M., Coyle, J. T., and Hedreen, J. C. (1983): Topographic analysis of the innervation of the rat neocortex and hippocampus by the basal forebrain cholinergic system. *J. Comp. Neurol.*, 217:103–121.
21. Nauta, W. J. H. (1961): Fiber degeneration following lesions of the amygdaloid complex in the monkey. *J. Anat. (Lond.)*, 95:515–531.
22. Nauta, W. J. H., and Domesick, V. B. (1981): Ramifications of the limbic system. In: *Psychiatry and the Biology of the Human Brain*, edited by S. Matthysse. pp. 165–188. Elsevier, New York.
23. Nauta, W. J. H., and Domesick, V. B. (1984): Afferent and efferent relationships of the basal ganglia. In: *Functions of the Basal Ganglia*. (Ciba Foundation symposium 107), pp. 3–29. Pitman, London.
24. Nauta, W. J. H., Smith, G. P., Faull, R. L. M., and Domesick, V. B. (1978): Efferent connections and nigral afferents of the nucleus accumbens in the rat. *Neuroscience*, 3:385–401.

25. Porrino, L. J., and Goldman, P. S. (1979): Selective distribution of projections from amygdala to prefrontal cortex in Rhesus monkey. *Soc. Neurosci.*, 5:280. *(Abstract).*
26. Powell, T. P. S. (1973): Sensory convergence in the cerebral cortex. In: *Surgical Approaches in Psychiatry*, edited by L. V. Laitinen and K. E. Livingston. pp. 266–281. Medical and Technical Publishing Co. Ltd., Lancaster, UK.
27. Ribak, C. E., and Fallon, J. H. (1983): The islands of Calleja complex of rat basal forebrain. I. Light and electron microscopic observations. *J. Comp. Neurol.*, 205:207–218.
28. Ricardo, J. (1980): Efferent connections of the subthalamic region in the rat. I. The subthalamic nucleus of Luys. *Brain Res.*, 202:257–271.
29. Saper, C. B. (1984): Organization of cerebral cortical afferent systems in the rat. II. Magnocellular basal nucleus. *J. Comp. Neurol.*, 222:313–342.
30. Swanson, L. W., Mogenson, C. J., Gerfen, C. R., and Robinson, P. (1984): Evidence for a projection from the lateral preoptic area and substantia innominata to the 'mesencephalic locomotor region' in the rat. *Brain Res.*, 295:161–178.
31. Switzer, R. C., and Hill, J. (1979): Globus pallidus component in the olfactory tubercle: evidence based on iron distribution. *Soc. Neurosci.*, 5:79. *(Abstract).*
32. Switzer, R. C., Hill, J., and Heimer, L. (1982): The globus pallidus and its rostroventral extension into the olfactory tubercle of the rat: a cyto- and chemoarchitectural study. *Neuroscience*, 7:1891–1904.
33. Van Hoesen, G. W., and Pandya, D. N. (1975): Some connections of the entorhinal (area 28) and perirhinal (area 35) cortices of the Rhesus monkey. I. Temporal lobe afferents. *Brain Res.*, 95:1–24.
34. Van Hoesen, G. W., Pandya, D. N., and Butters, N. (1975): Some connections of the entorhinal (area 28) and perirhinal (area 35) cortices of the Rhesus monkey. II. Frontal lobe afferents. *Brain Res.*, 95:25–38.
35. Webster, K. E. (1961): Cortico-striate interrelations in the albino rat. *J. Anat. (Lond.)*, 95:532–545.
36. Webster, K. E. (1965): The cortico-striatal projection in the cat. *J. Anat. (Lond.)*, 99:329–337.
37. Williams, D. J., Crossman, A. R., and Slater, P. (1977): The efferent projections of the nucleus accumbens in the rat. *Brain Res.*, 130:217–227.
38. Wilson, R. D. (1972): Efferent connections of the nucleus accumbens in the rat. Master's Thesis, Massachusetts Institute of Technology.

The Limbic System: Functional Organization and
Clinical Disorders, edited by B. K. Doane and
K. E. Livingston. Raven Press, New York © 1986.

Biochemical Patterns in Limbic System Circuitry: Biochemical–Electrophysiological Interactions Displayed by Chemitrode Techniques

M. Girgis

Faculty of Medicine, University of Sydney, Australia 2006

Descriptive associations between limbic epilepsy and mental disorders are very old and are found throughout the literature. Recent investigations have shown that dysfunction of the limbic system of the brain underlies many disturbances of emotion and may result in some psychotic manifestations. The interseizure symptomatology of some patients with psychomotor (limbic) epilepsy may be indistinguishable from that of paranoid schizophrenia (19,25). Irritative lesions in or near the limbic cortex give rise to epileptic discharges accompanied by emotional feelings of terror, fear, strangeness, unreality, sadness, wanting to be alone, and feelings of paranoid nature (21). There may be also distortions of perception, again reminding one of the endogenous toxic psychosis (6,15,17,20,24). Maclean believes that of all the clinical entities, there is perhaps none that has a greater potentiality for shedding light on mechanisms underlying psychic functions in man than psychomotor or limbic epilepsy.

Mark and Ervin (22) found that 81% of 42 patients with EEG foci in the temporal lobes had a diagnosis of schizophrenia, whether or not there was an associated epilepsy. Personality disorder is the most frequent diagnosis (3). Depression is next, followed by the diagnosis of inadequate personality and psychosis. The behavioral consequence of a focal lesion must depend on whether it is an ablative lesion or a stimulatory lesion. Most clinical situations involve a lesion that is mixed ablative-stimulatory. Goddard (16) believes that the *kindling model* provides an example of pure stimulatory lesion, whereas surgical removal usually produces a pure ablative lesion. Thus, theoretically, separate examination of the two components of the more clinically relevant mixed lesion should be possible. The argument in favor of a stimulatory lesion in the vicinity of the amygdala being capable of triggering rage or *dyscontrol* (22) has come from experiments using direct electrical stimulation through depth electrodes.

REGIONAL DISTRIBUTION OF NEUROTRANSMITTERS
WITHIN THE LIMBIC SYSTEM

One of the greatest advances in neuroscience of the last decade, and one that has extremely far-reaching implications, has been the localization in the mammalian brain of neuronal systems using specific and identifiable substances as transmitters of nervous activity across synaptic junctions. Electron microscopy has shown that nerve fibers in the brain contain in their terminals synaptic vesicles similar to those seen in nerve endings in the peripheral nervous system. Moreover, the peripheral transmitter acetylcholine (ACh) and norepinephrine (NE) are present in the brain, and the activity of central neurons can be shown to be modified when these substances are brought into contact with them, e.g., the method of microiontophoresis.

Cholinergic Limbic System

Studies of the mammalian cholinergic system have lagged substantially behind those of the catecholaminergic system. One major contributing factor to explain this phenomenon has been the lack, until recently, of good sensitive and specific chemical methods for the assay of choline and ACh. Within the past two decades and, especially within the past few years, several chemical methods for assaying tissue choline and ACh have been developed which seriously rival the best bioassay methods; they all exhibit properties and reproducibility and chemical specificity. The idea of my monograph on limbic epilepsy (11) was spurred by the recent marked upsurge in the study of the metabolism and function of ACh in the limbic system. This is most evident from the steady and consistent increase in the number of papers on topics related to cholinergic mechanisms and limbic epilepsy.

Acetylcholinesterase enzyme (AChE), which is responsible for hydrolizing ACh, is strongly bound to membranes and very stable. It can be detected histochemically in serial frozen sections of brain prepared for light microscopy as well as with the electron microscope. This technique can be used as a reliable means of detecting central cholinergic neurons. On the whole, it could be inferred from our own investigations that AChE-bearing neurons in general are better developed in phylogenetically older parts of the brain. The concentration of AChE exists in the whole "limbic system" and in some nuclei which have fairly direct connections with it (11). It is not yet quite clear why the limbic structures are so rich in AChE. "Perhaps it has a protective function, preventing the development of bizarre sensitivity in susceptible cells" (13). The prevalence of available AChE may ensure that the sensitivity of ACh is maintained within a limited safe range.

Monoaminergic Pathways

The monoamines (MA), which are known to act as transmitter substances in the brain, can be studied more directly than the cholinergic system, since the transmitters themselves can be converted to fluorescent isoquinoline compounds by exposure to formaldehyde vapor and so can be visualised *in situ* with the light microscope. The intensity of fluorescence produced by the Falck technique gives an indication of the concentration of transmitter substance in a monoaminergic neuron. The disposition of the MA systems of the brain, as revealed by the Swedish workers, is as follows. The cell bodies of NE neurons are located in the medulla and the pons. The largest group forms the nucleus ceruleus, all the cells of which are NE neurons. Ascending NE fibers form a ventral system supplying the midbrain reticular formation, central grey and the nuclei of the hypothalamus, and a dorsal system arising from the nucleus ceruleus that supplies the thalamus, hippocampus, and cerebral cortex. Other fibers from the nucleus ceruleus enter the cerebellum.

The cell bodies of 5-hydroxytryptamine (5-HT) neurons are located in midline or raphe nuclei in the medulla, pons, and midbrain and have similar course to that of the NE system. The dopamine (DA) neurons have their cell bodies in the zona compacta of the substantia nigra, in the ventral tegmentum of the midbrain (VTA), and in the hypothalamus. The well-known nigroneostrial dopaminergic pathway is related to movement disorders. The VTA connections with the nucleus accumbens have recently been implicated in schizophrenic psychoses.

SYNERGY OF MESOLIMBIC CHOLINERGIC- MONOAMINERGIC MECHANISMS

The cell bodies of MA neurons occupy different situations in the brain from those of cholinergic neurons, but the course and distribution of their fibers are, to some extent, similar. Both are largely ascending in the upper brainstem. Ascending cholinergic and most MA fibers travel in the medial forebrain bundle (MFB). The neostriatum, nucleus accumbens, olfactory tubercle and some amygdaloid nuclei, receive a heavy cholinergic and DA innervation. The two systems operate in close synergy. Dopamine in particular has been implicated as an inhibitory transmitter in the amygdala. The apparent presence of *cholinergic* and *monoaminergic* neurons in the limbic system suggests a certain parallel with the peripheral autonomic nervous system. In the hippocampus, for example, histochemical stains have indicated that its main afferent pathways are cholinergic in type. On the other hand, autoradiography and fluorescent studies have detected a notable concentration of NE in the hippocampus. Serotonin studies have indicated a relatively high concentration in the grey matter of the hippocampus.

These findings are of special interest in view of the evidence that tranquilizing and psychotropic drugs known to affect the metabolism of serotonin and NE, appear to have some predilection of action on hippocampal function as revealed by changes in the EEG (21). MacLean also points out that the limbic system seems not only to exert powerful influences on the autonomic and neuroendocrine centers, but may also be the reacting organ to double antagonistic (and probably synergistic) innervation, which is similar in many respects to the autonomic innervation of the peripheral organs. Finally, there is a difference between the central cholinergic and MA systems that recalls a distinction between the parasympathetic and sympathetic innervation of the periphery, and which may well have functional implications: the cell bodies of MA neurons tend to be further removed from their target areas. In some regions of the brain, e.g., the superior colliculus and the olfactory tubercle, and also the neostriatum, the cholinergic innervation appears to be largely an intrinsic one. This suggests that the MA systems are more divergent than the cholinergic systems and may be expected to produce more generalized effects.

KINDLING MODEL OF LIMBIC EPILEPSY

Adamec et al. (1) presented evidence on lasting behavioral after-effects of repeated amygdaloid stimulation. Their data show that predatory behavior in the cat can be altered following daily repeated amygdaloid stimulation. They did not stimulate the cats to the point of behavioral convulsions, but repeated the stimulus a few times to lower the after-discharge threshold. This was done bilaterally. The rat-killing behavior of these cats was studied before and after the threshold reduction. Of central importance to the current argument (kindling model of limbic epilepsy) are the data of these investigators showing marked alteration of evoked potentials following kindling in the amygdala. Potentials evoked in secondary sites by test pulses applied to the primary (kindled) focus are increased in amplitude following kindling. All components of potentials evoked in the hippocampus, preoptic area, ventromedial nucleus of the hypothalamus and frontal pole by amygdaloid stimulation, were increased in amplitude following amygdaloid kindling.

Electrical Versus Cholinergic Kindling

The changes in brain function produced by repeated electrical stimulation are numerous, easily detectable, and appear to be permanent. Several lines of evidence demonstrate that when the amygdala is stimulated, long-lasting changes occur somewhere in the brain. Most of this work has been done on amygdaloid kindling, which probably serves as a good model for most limbic kindling. Although the kindling effect can be obtained by stimulating areas outside the amygdala, responsive areas are largely restricted to the limbic system and related structures. Within the limbic system, the amygdala has been found to be particularly responsive (20,23). There is also a suggestion that the responsiveness of particular areas is related directly to the extent of their connections with the amygdala. Limbic system epileptiform after-discharge develop as the experiment progresses.

Several experiments have shown that the changes in neural response underlying many of these developments are not restricted to the primary (stimulated) focus. After completion of amygdaloid kindling, for example, fewer stimulations are required in secondary limbic sites to develop generalized seizures, even after removal of the "kindled" primary focus. These "transfer" experiments established that transsynaptic changes in neural response were developing as a result of the kindling treatment. There are a number of features of the kindling effect which are consistent with the hypothesis that synaptic transmission is permanently facilitated between neural structures as a result of kindling. It has not yet been determined, however, that the kindling effect is a result of changes at the synaptic level. Nevertheless, in view of the fact that many examples of synaptic plasticity have been demonstrated, it seems reasonable at this stage to concentrate on the synapse and in neurotransmitters in our investigation of the kindling phenomenon.

LIMBIC CHOLINERGIC HYPERSENSITIVITY

It was explained above that there are some data that support the hypothesis that synaptic transmission is permanently facilitated between neural structures as a result of the kindling effect. We will now concentrate on the possible neurotransmitter mechanisms underlying limbic epilepsy. The changes in neural response underlying the kindling processes are not restricted to the primary focus. Several lines of evidence demonstrate that when the amygdala is stimulated, either electrically or chemically, long-lasting changes occur somewhere in the limbic brain. These changes may be irreversible. The effect can be related to seizure activity present at the time of stimulation.

In my own studies with low doses of physostigmine injected into the basal amygdaloid nucleus of the monkey, I observed similar changes (7). Two hours after intracerebral injection of 5 μl of physostigmine, the animal became restless and then rhythmic licking and chewing movements appeared. Bursts of high-voltage spike- and wave-discharges developed immediately afterward. In all cases these discharges occurred first and remained maximal in the area of injection, i.e., the basal amygdaloid nucleus. The paroxysmal discharges (spike, sharp wave, polyspike, and wave) were always observed in the amygdala after a latency of 2 hours, and they continued for several days or sometimes weeks after a single injection of physostigmine. In the postictal stage, spikes occurred in records taken 3 weeks afterward, and they showed high-amplitude slow-wave patterns. One pattern was characterized by high-voltage waves appearing at a frequency of 8 to 10 cps. A second pattern was characterized by polyspikes of 10 to 12 cps frequency (Fig. 1).

During these amygdaloid paroxysmal discharges, which appeared after the injection of physostigmine, we noticed a series of complex behavioral phenomena: myoclonus localized in the ipsilateral muscles of facial expression. Protrusion of the tongue and rhythmic licking and chewing movements followed this initial manifestation and were always associated with excessive salivation. Occasionally, an expression of anger occurred. However, real rage became more apparent if the animal was approached a few hours after the end of the manifestations mentioned.

These manifestations lasted 2 to 3 min and were followed by postictal generalized loss of tone and a brief period of confusion during which time the animal was unresponsive, looking around aimlessly. After regaining the usual alertness, the animal became aggressive and remained so throughout the period of experimentation. During the first few weeks after physostigmine injection, the aggressive reaction was unprovoked. The animals would attack any person approaching the cage. No overt epileptic convulsions were seen in these animals.

During the first few weeks, when unprovoked aggression was the most characteristic feature, the EEG recording showed continuous high amplitude activity. This

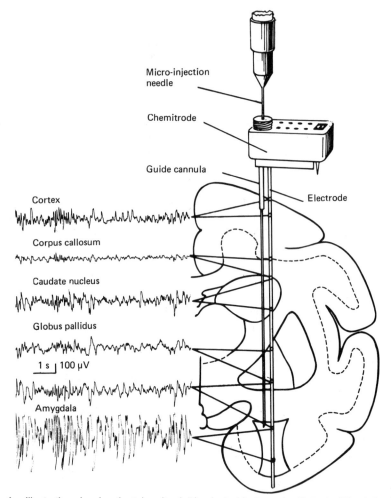

FIG. 1. Illustration showing the "chemitrode" implanted in the animal's brain. Microinjection of physostigmine was injected by means of a Hamilton microsyringe. The EEG record shows the hyperactivity at the site of injection (basal amygdala).

was temporarily antagonized by an injection of atropine, to reappear the next day. However, after repeated injections of atropine, the EEG recordings gradually reverted to normal appearance. In some animals the abnormal EEG activity lasted up to 7 weeks (for further details see ref. 7). Unlike the electrographic changes, the behavioral changes never regained normal status. As already mentioned, the clinical picture changed in degree from "unprovoked" to "provoked" aggression. Currently, we are using scopolamine instead of atropine because it is more effective in blocking the behavioral and EEG changes. The effects of this anticholinergic drug are reported to exceed those of atropine more than 10 times, and its specific central action has also been emphasized.

In my investigations referred to above, an attempt was made to study the relationship between the cholinergic system of the amygdala and epileptiform discharges. Human psychomotor epilepsy is characterized by intermittent ictal and interictal seizure activity. Few experimental models are available for the study of the underlying physiopathology. I was motivated in my investigation by the possibility of obtaining EEG and possibly behavioral patterns in the monkey, comparable to those of limbic epilepsy in man. The physostigmine injections were made in the basal amygdala, an area which shows very high AChE activity in the brains of all the primates examined using histochemical procedures. The amygdala has one of the lowest thresholds for EEG seizures and overt convulsions following electrical stimulation. In the chemical investigations mentioned above, I have found that the amygdala and other related limbic structures have a marked cholinergic hypersensitivity.

PARTICIPATION OF MUSCARINIC CHOLINERGIC RECEPTORS IN KINDLING

During recent years there has been increasing evidence of the involvement of cholinergic mechanisms in the cortical mediation of desynchronized activation of the EEG which characterizes the "arousal" response. It has been shown that the rate of liberation of ACh from the surface of the neostigmized cortex in the cat may increase two to four times during desynchronized cortical activations with arousal, as compared with that obtained during slow wave and spindle sleep. Furthermore, studies of chronically isolated cortex, which have been reported to show spontaneous epileptiform discharges, show increased sensitivity to topically applied ACh. Increased reactivity of the isolated cortex to ACh suggests that supersensitivity to endogenous ACh may be a factor in cortical epileptogenesis.

Partial or total isolation of the cerebral cortex was offered recently as a model for the study of focal epilepsy by several investigators (5,18). The authors investigated the implications of denervation (or "disuse") supersensitivity to putative transmitter. It was indicated that after weeks or months, the isolated cortex showed spontaneous epileptiform discharges and increased sensitivity to topically applied ACh. Isolated cortex may sustain prolonged epileptiform after-discharges. This is one measure of supersensitivity.

A causal relationship between supersensitivity and an alteration in the cholinergic system has been suggested, based on the observations that there is a decrease in AChE activity in isolated cortex, and a *decrease in AChE activity parallels the increase in supersensitivity.* Increased reactivity of the isolated cortex to ACh suggests that supersensitivity to endogenous ACh may be a factor in cortical epileptogenesis. All my histochemical studies in mammalian brains (referred to above) point to the fact that some of the highest (AChE) activity in the whole brain is to be found in limbic structures, particularly the basal amygdala. Studies on the effect of cortical under-cutting and long-term electrical stimulation on synaptic AChE showed that a decrease in AChE activity parallels the increase in supersensitivity. A decrease in the activity of AChE and the supersensitivity in under-cut cortex are likely to be the consequences of the loss of cholinergic innervation and of synaptic "disuse" following denervation.

It has been suggested that the phenomenon of supersensitivity of the neuronally isolated cortex may be explained by an increased sensitivity of subsynaptic and possible nonsynaptic membranes as a consequence of denervation. This is analogous to the supersensitivity observed in denervated muscle. Cannon suggested that abnormality of cortical cells in epilepsy might be the result of loss of innervation of cells—another example of increased sensitivity in denervated structures. The increased excitability has been likened to the degeneration supersensitivity that develops in peripheral structures after interruption of their neural input.

It is not yet clear if the neural changes that underlie amygdaloid kindling take place within cholinergic circuits or if these circuits simply play a supportive role in seizure development. The possibility that cholinergic circuits are involved in the kindling process is indicated by the fact that atropine retards amygdaloid kindling (2). This and other aspects of cholinergic hypersensitivity have recently been discussed by Vosu and Wise (26) and Wasterlain (28), who found that ACh was the only neurotransmitter for which they could demonstrate a relationship to kindling phenomena. Vosu and Wise found that repeated cholinergic stimulation (carbachol) produced behavioral seizures after several applications, similar to those seen with electrical stimulation, suggesting an important role for cholinergic circuitry in subcortical propagation of epileptiform activity. Similar results were presented by Wasterlain et al. (28) who further showed that mixing the injected carbachol with the muscarinic cholinergic antagonist atropine reduced seizure. It has recently been reported (9) that only a few electrical kindling stimuli are needed to produce prolonged supersensitivity to intracerebrally injected physostigmine. This supersensitivity is correlated with further progression of kindling. Scopolamine, given intramuscularly in doses of 120 µg/kg suppresses these kindling-induced seizures.

Our own findings and those mentioned above show that cholinergic kindling sensitivity of limbic structures parallel electrical kindling sensitivity (10). This fits best with the hypothesis that it is cholinergic circuits at the site of stimulation that mediate both *electrically* and *chemically* induced kindling and that are involved in the retardation of seizure development by anticholinergic drugs.

RESERPINE DRAMATICALLY FACILITATES THE KINDLING PROCESS

There have been reports in the literature that reserpine facilitates the kindling process (2). These authors used intraperitoneal injections of reserpine. In our laboratory we developed a technique by which reserpine could be delivered intracerebrally in a steady-state flow by means of an osmotic minipump (Fig. 2). Reserpine was injected at a rate of 1 µl/hr for a week (taken from a solution of 2.5 mg/ml). On the seventh day, electrical kindling stimuli (of the amygdala) were

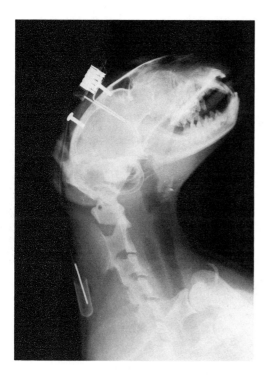

FIG. 2. X-ray study of the cat skull showing the implantation of the chemitrode (target: nucleus accumbens septi). The self-powered osmotic minipump, containing reserpine, is implanted subcutaneously and is connected to the needle via a catheter. The chemical is delivered at the rate of 1 μl/hr (2.5 mg/ml reserpine solution) for a week. On about the sixth day of implantation, electrical kindling stimuli were started. It was found that reserpine dramatically facilitates the kindling process (see Fig. 5 for summary).

FIG. 3. EEG record showing AD in limbic structures after four electrical kindling stimuli of the reserpinized basal amygdala (the *top* tracing is central amygdala-globus pallidus; the second is central amygdala-basal; the third and fourth are within the basal amygdala; the fifth tracing is within the hippocampus).

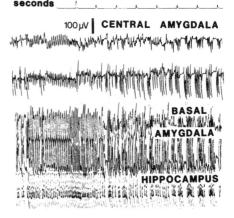

started, resulting in full-blown seizure after the sixth day (see Fig. 3 and histogram for summary). Chronic intracerebral microperfusion of reserpine was found to dramatically facilitate the kindling process in all areas tested (such as amygdala, hippocampus, and nucleus accumbens septi) (Fig. 4). Other than the locomotor retardation that these animals had, all showed signs that indicate a possible "cholinomimetic" action of reserpine. Ipsilateral constriction of the pupil and diarrhea

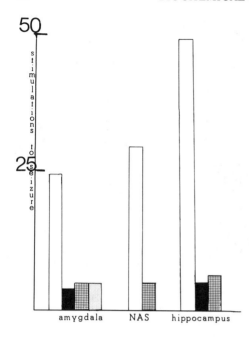

FIG. 4. Seizure development in three groups of experiments following electrical stimulation ☐ of the amygdala, nucleus accumbens septi (NAS), and hippocampus. Physostigmine ■, reserpine ▦, and 6-hydroxy-dopamine ▨ dramatically facilitate the kindling process when given before the electrical kindling stimuli. The clear column represents the results of the control experiments (electrical kindling stimuli only); the following is a representative kindling parameter: 600 μA, 2 sec trains of biphasic pulses, 60 Hz frequency. Saline injections prior to electrical stimulations do not facilitate the kindling process.

TABLE 1. *Comparison of the effects of intracerebrally injected physostigmine (PHYS), reserpine (RES), and 6-hydroxydopamine (6-OHDA)*[a]

	PHYS	RES	6-OHDA
Kindling facilitation	+	+	+
EEG hyperactivity	+	+	
Locomotor retardation	+	+	
Pupillary constriction	+	+	
Diarrhea	+	+	
Salivation	+		

[a]The results indicate that reserpine appears to have more actions in common with the known cholinomimetic drug (physostigmine) than can be explained by its catecholaminolytic effect alone. This is also further confirmed by the comparison with the well-known catecholaminolytic drug shown in the table. This is indirect evidence for the cholinomimetic effect of reserpine.

were common. Reserpine was, for a long time, thought to have only monoaminolytic effects (see Table 1 for details).

Currently, we are testing the effects of glutamic acid on the kindling process. In another series of experiments we are aso using kainic acid in minimal doses prior to the glutamate minipump. This catalyzing the reaction acted as a primer in the production of the original (pathological) locus found in the human limbic epilepsy. As stimulation of ACh receptors results in sustained seizure activity which damages the brain by unknown mechanisms, and as endogenous glutamate has possible excitotoxic action, it seems likely that glutamate may have a role in the brain damage associated with sustained limbic seizures. All these findings are reported in detail elsewhere (12).

REFERENCES

1. Adamec, R. E., Stark-Adamec, C., Perrin, R., and Livingston, K. E. (1980): In: *Limbic Epilepsy and the Dyscontrol Syndrome*, edited by M. Girgis and L. G. Kiloh, pp. 117–132. Elsevier; Amsterdam.
2. Arnold, P. S., Racine, R. J., and Wise, R. A. (1973): *Exp. Neurol.*, 40:457–470.
3. Bingley, T. (1958): *Acta Psychiatr. Neurol.*, 33:[*Suppl.*120].
4. DeJong, R. N. (1957): *Neurology*, 1:1–14.
5. Ferguson, J. H., and Jasper, H. H. (1971): *EEG Clin. Neurophysiol.*, 30:377–390.
6. Gastaut, H. (1953): *Epilepsia*, 2:59–96.
7. Girgis, M. (1978): *Epilepsia*, 19:521–530.
8. Girgis, M. (1980): *"Limbic Epilepsy and the Dyscontrol Syndrome*, edited by M. Girgis and L. G. Kiloh, pp. 149–160. Elsevier, Amsterdam.
9. Girgis, M. (1981): *Brain Res.*, 208:379–386.
10. Girgis, M. (1981): *EEG Clin. Neurophysiol.*, 51:417–425.
11. Girgis, M. (1981): *Neural Substrates of Limbic Epilepsy*, Warren H. Green Inc., St. Louis.
12. Girgis, M., Harris, K.: *Neuroscience. (in press)*.
13. Girgis, M., Hofstatter, L. (1979): In: *Modern concepts in Psychiatric Surgery*, edited by E. R. Hitchcock, H. T. Ballantine, Jr., and B. A. Meyerson. pp. 151–160. Elsevier, Amsterdam.
14. Girgis, M., Kent, J., Kohlhardt, S., Rasko, J., and Stobo, P. (1981): *Br. Res. Bull.*, 7:719–723.
15. Gloor, P. (1960): In: *Handbook of Physiology*, edited by J. Field, H. W. Magoun, and V. E. Hall. Am. Phys. Soc., Washington D.C., pp. 1395–1425.
16. Goddard, G. (1980): In: *Limbic Epilepsy and the Dyscontrol Syndrome*, edited by M. Girgis and L. G. Kiloh, pp. 107–116. Elsevier, Amsterdam.
17. Jackson, J. H. (1899): *Lancet*, 1:79.
18. Jasper, H. H. (1969): In: *The Physiogenesis of the Epilepsies*, edited by Gastaut. Thomas, Springfield.
19. Kiloh, L. G. (1980): In: *Limbic Epilepsy and the Dyscontrol Syndrome*, edited by M. Girgis and L. G. Kiloh, pp. 231–238. Elsevier, Amsterdam.
20. Kreindler, A., and Steriade, M. (1964): *Arch. Ital. Biol.*, 102:576–586.
21. MacLean, P. D. (1962): *J. Nerv. Ment. Dis.*, 135:289–301.
22. Mark, V. H., and F. R. Ervin (1970): *Violence and the Brain.* Harper & Row, New York.
23. Olds, J. (1958): In: *Reticular Formation of the Brain*, edited by H. H. Jasper, pp. 20–42. Little Brown & Co., Boston.
24. Penfield, W., and Jasper, H. (1954): *Epilepsy and Functional Anatomy of the Human Brain.* Little Brown & Co., Boston.
25. Smith, J. S., and Kiloh, L. G. (1977): In: *Psychosurgery and Society*, p. 70, Pergamon Press, London.
26. Vosu, H., and Wise, R. A. (1975): *Behav. Biol.*, 13:491–495.
27. Wada, J. A. (1980): In: *Limbic Epilepsy and the Dyscontrol Syndrome*, edited by M. Girgis and L. G. Kiloh, pp. 133–148. Elsevier, Amsterdam.
28. Wasterlain, C. G., Jonec, V., and Holm, S. G. (1978): *Neurology (Minneap.)*, 28:346–352.

The Limbic System: Functional Organization and
Clinical Disorders, edited by B. K. Doane and
K. E. Livingston. Raven Press, New York © 1986.

A Simplified Perspective on the Basal Ganglia and Their Relation to the Limbic System

Haring J. W. Nauta

*Division of Neurosurgery, The University of Texas Medical Branch,
Galveston, Texas 77550*

The complexity of forebrain circuitry is quickly evident to anyone choosing to study the subject. The challenge, to many, has been the exposition of that complexity to the fullest extent possible while at the same time not losing sight of any ordering principles that could allow both a simplified understanding and a vantage point suggesting further experimentation. The new tract-tracing methods available in the past decade have allowed progress in both categories of endeavor: They have provided many new anatomical details exposing further complexity, while, at the same time, they have provided evidence that principles of order may exist which actually appear simpler than previously recognized.

This chapter briefly summarizes the results of some tract-tracing experiments applied to the basal ganglia in cat and monkey. The experiments have been documented more comprehensively elsewhere (12,14,15). Although at first the results seem only to complicate the understanding of forebrain circuitry by adding yet more projections to already swollen lists, the detail they provide, when seen together with data from many other sources, suggests some principles of order applicable to much of the forebrain and encompassing parts of both the motor system and the limbic system. If the reader will first bear with some of these details, the principles of order may be seen to follow from them.

EXPERIMENTS: THEIR EXPECTED AND UNEXPECTED FINDINGS

The experiments themselves are straightforward "tract tracing" studies based on the autoradiographic anterograde method applied separately to several of the recognized components of the corpus striatum in cat and to the subthalamic nucleus in cat and monkey. Many of the findings were anticipated by earlier studies based on degeneration techniques. For example, the autoradiographic studies confirmed the known projection of caudate nucleus and putamen to the external and internal pallidal segments and to the substantia nigra (17,26); the external pallidal segment showed the expected evidence of a massive projection to the subthalamic nucleus; the internal pallidal segment was found to project to the thalamic nuclei ventralis lateralis, ventralis anterior, and centrum medianum and to the midbrain nucleus tegmenti pedunculopontinus pars compacta (17); and, finally, the subthalamic nucleus did indeed show evidence of a massive projection to the internal pallidal segment (1).

However, in addition to the anticipated projections enumerated above, the experiments also showed clear evidence of several pathways whose presence or extent could not have been predicted with confidence from earlier degeneration studies. Although it must be admitted that evidence of these additional pathways was occasionally noted in the degeneration studies, such evidence was usually attributed to damaged fibers of passage and therefore considered artifactual. Because so little confidence could be placed in their existence, few conceptual schemes took the projections seriously into account. However, with the evidence from the autoradiographic tracing method, the existence of these pathways appeared on firmer ground.

These newly characterized pathways can be summarized as follows. The external pallidal segment now appears to project prominently, not only to the subthalamic nucleus, but also to the thalamic reticular nucleus, and in lesser density to the caudate nucleus, putamen, cortex, and substantia nigra. The efferent projections of the internal pallidal segment likewise appear more extensive than previously suspected. Evidence of efferent projections were found not only to the ventralis lateralis-ventralis anterior (VL-VA) nuclei complex and centrum medianum of the thalamus and to the midbrain reticular formation, but also there was clear evidence of a prominent projection to the lateral habenular nucleus (12). Likewise, the efferent projections of the subthalamic nucleus appeared more extensive than previously recognized. The subthalamic nucleus of both cat and monkey could be determined to project not only to the internal pallidal segment as previously reported, but also massively to the external pallidal segment and to the nondopaminergic part of the substantia nigra (15). In addition, there was evidence of sparse projections to the caudate nucleus and putamen and to the midbrain nucleus tegmenti pedunculopontinus, pars compacta (TPC).

TWO CONCLUSIONS BASED ON THESE DATA

For the purpose of the following discussion, the findings of these autoradiographic tracing studies can be summarized by two general statements. First, the efferent projections of the pallidal complex appear to be more extensive than previously appreciated and include projections not only to structures obviously identified with the motor system, but also to structures whose functional associations are either poorly characterized, or, in the case of the lateral habenular nucleus, traditionally identified as part of the limbic system. Second, the main efferent projections of the subthalamic nucleus are distributed to the external pallidal segment, the internal pallidal segment, and the nondopaminergic part of the substantia nigra.

HOW THESE TWO CONCLUSIONS SUGGEST A SIMPLIFIED SCHEME OF BASAL GANGLIA ORGANIZATION

First Conclusion

The first conclusion, that the efferent projections of the basal ganglia are more extensive than appreciated earlier, undermines the tacit assumption of earlier schemes that the basal ganglia outflow is directed exclusively to the motor system. To remain within such a concept it would be necessary to redefine the lateral habenular nucleus as part of the motor system or to specifically exclude the pallido-habenular projecting cells from inclusion in the basal ganglia. Although this remains an alternative interpretation, it now seems more economical to view the basal ganglia as part of a telencephalic outflow system afferented by many functional subdivisions (as they can be identified in the cerebral cortex) and directed, in turn, to several diencephalic and mesencephalic cell groups (Figs. 1 and 2). This basal ganglia outflow system is characterized by two conspicuous features that distinguish it from a more direct telencephalic outflow system typified by the internal capsule and cerebral peduncle. First, whereas the latter outflow links directly with the thalamus or other subcortical structures, the basal ganglia outflow system has two interposed neurons, one in the striatum and another in the pallidum or nigra. Second, whereas the direct outflow system may extend caudally to pontine, medullary, or even spinal cord levels, the basal ganglia system does not extend caudally beyond the midbrain (Fig. 1). Both outflow systems can be viewed as lying on the effector side of an imaginary watershed between sensory and motor systems, but there is no necessity to consider either system as exclusively related to movement. Just as the corticospinal and corticobulbar tract form only part of the internal capsule system, the classical ansa lenticularis, directed at the ventral anterior thalamic complex, forms only part of the basal ganglia outflow system. This perspective—that obvious motor system affiliation is not a prerequisite for a structure to be considered part of the basal ganglia—provides part of the impetus to look for a new scheme of basal ganglia organization. It leads to the impression that we may have been excluding some telencephalic cell territories from inclusion in the basal ganglia because of known connections with, for example, the limbic system. This prompts the question, "Just what are the boundaries of the basal ganglia cell groups, and what criteria should be applied to choosing such boundaries?"

Second Conclusion

The second conclusion suggested by the anatomical data—that the main projections of the subthalamic nucleus are to the external pallidal segment, the internal pallidal segment, and the nondopaminergic part of the substantia nigra—provides another impetus to look for a new scheme of basal ganglia organization. The confluence of the subthalamic outflow with that of the striatum appears remarkable and all the more so since the confluence occurs in a cell territory divided by the

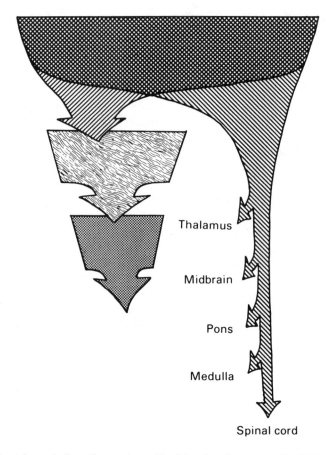

Thalamus

Midbrain

Pons

Medulla

Spinal cord

FIG. 1. Two telencephalic outflow systems. The "direct" outflow system (typified by the internal capsule-cerebral peduncle) is on the right; the basal ganglia outflow system, on the left. Note that the basal ganglia outflow system is polysynaptic with links in the striatum and pallidum. Note also that while the "direct" outflow system may extend caudally to pontine, medullary, or even spinal levels, the basal ganglia outflow system does not extend caudally beyond the midbrain. ▨ cortex; ⟍ striatum; ▨ pallidum and nondopaminergic substantia nigra; ◹ internal capsule system; ⟋ cortico-striate pathway.

internal capsule system. The two parts of the globus pallidus on one side of the internal capsule, and the nondopaminergic substantia nigra on the other, each receive dense projections from both the subthalamic nucleus and the striatum. This coincidence in their major sources of input suggested that other similarities between them might exist as well and that their separation by the internal capsule system might be fortuitous (13). Again, the boundaries of the basal ganglia cell groups are called into question, this time by the impression that we may have been considering as separate two cell groups really belonging to one and the same neuronal aggregate.

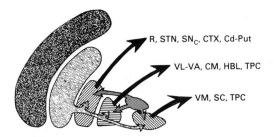

R, STN, SN$_C$, CTX, Cd-Put

VL-VA, CM, HBL, TPC

VM, SC, TPC

FIG. 2. Afferent and efferent projections of the tier III structures (pallidum and nigra). Note the confluence of afferents from the striatum and subthalamus in these tier III structures. The collective distribution of efferents from the tier III structures is fairly widespread. Abbreviations: CM, centrum medianum; Cd-Put, caudate nucleus and putamen; CTX, cortex; HBL, lateral habenular nucleus; R, nucleus reticularis thalami; SC, superior colliculus; SNc, substantia nigra, pars compacta; STN, subthalamic nucleus; TPC, nucleus tegmenti pedunculo-pontinus, pars compacta; VL-VA, ventralis lateralis and ventralis anterior nuclei of the thalamus; VM, nucleus ventralis medialis of the thalamus. ▨ cortex; ▨ striatum; ▨ external pallidum; ▬ internal pallidum; ▨ subthalamic nucleus; ▨ nondopaminergic substantia nigra.

A PROPOSED SIMPLIFIED SCHEME OF BASAL
GANGLIA ORGANIZATION

From the foregoing it may be instructive to envision what the telencephalon and basal ganglia would look like if one ignored any divisions imposed by the great white matter bundles and by current concepts of functional association. One would then be left to base the grouping of cell territories on such criteria as a common histological organization, similar input/output relations, and similar transmitter chemistry. The basal ganglia could then be seen as part of a three-tiered telencephalic organization, as shown in Fig. 3. This organization has been described in more detail earlier (13), and only its main features will be described here (see Fig. 3).

The uppermost tier (tier I) represents an aggregate of the cortical structures: the neocortex and the allocortex, of which the hippocampal formation is a part. The second tier (tier II) is composed of the striatum, as already understood to include the caudate nucleus and putamen, and, in addition, the territories of the nucleus accumbens septi and parts of the olfactory tubercle given the collective term "ventral striatum" by Heimer and Wilson (10). These authors have long emphasized the close association or continuity of the traditional striatum with the ventral striatum. The third tier (tier III) is composed of two pallidal segments, the non-dopaminergic part of the substantia nigra and also parts of the substantia innominata.

A major feature of this scheme concerns the projections between the three tiers and the number of neurons present in each of the tiers. There are massive projections from tier I to tier II, and from tier II to tier III. It is also apparent that the volume of each tier and the number of neurons in each tier appear to diminish progressively when proceeding radially from tier I to tier II to tier III (22,24,25). Although at the time considering only the striatum and pallidal complex, Papez (18) compared

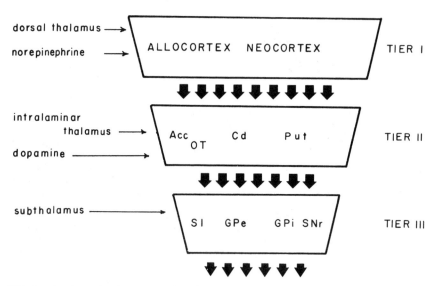

FIG. 3. A schematized representation of some major connections in the basal ganglia. Abbreviations: Acc, nucleus accumbens septi; Cd-Put, caudate nucleus and putamen; GPe, external pallidal segment; GPi, internal pallidal segment; OT, olfactory tubercle; SI, substantia innominata; SNr, nondopaminergic substantia nigra.

this aspect of basal ganglia circuitry with spokes of a wheel. Later when the prominence of the cortical projections to the striatum was appreciated (11,23,27), the impression arose of a funnel-like convergent conduction from the cortex through the basal ganglia to the motor thalamus. With the more broadly defined cell groupings proposed here, it still appears reasonable to continue with the notion that the basal ganglia (tier II and tier III) provide the substrate for a funnel-like, polysynaptic efferent conduction channel from the cortex, but now the efferent target appears to be a variety of structures in the diencephalon and mesencephalon, not just the motor thalamus.

EVIDENCE THAT THESE EXPANDED GROUPINGS ARE LEGITIMATE ORGANIZATIONAL UNITS

The evidence that these expanded groupings—tiers I, II, and III—form legitimate coherent cell aggregates comes from several independent sources, as described below.

Evidence from Histological Studies

There are some characteristic features of histological organization that remain constant throughout each of the tiers. The cortical tier (tier I) is characterized by an abundance of pyramidal cells having roughly conical or cylindrical dendritic domains each oriented with its long axis normal to the cortical surface and thereby suggesting a columnar organization. In contrast, the histology of the striatal tier

(tier II) is characterized by cells having roughly spherical or oblong dendritic domains, highly arborized and extending only a short distance from the cell body. Instead of a columnar organization, as seen in cortex, the striatal cells appear to form clustered groupings (see ref. 19 for a review). Likewise, the pallidal tier (tier III) also shows some uniformity in histological organization. Here, the neurons appear to have long, obliquely branching dendrites that, on electron microscopic examination, appear to be densely covered with afferent axon terminals (5).

Evidence from Comparative Anatomy

In all mammals the cerebral cortical structures represent a sizable population of cells requiring a fairly massive afferent and efferent conduction system. Both the afferent conduction system to the cortex and the "direct" efferent system (discussed earlier) are carried in the prominent internal capsule. To link the cortex directly with the thalamus and other brainstem structures, this major fiber system must find its way between, through, or around cell groups of the basal ganglia. As it takes a different course through the basal ganglia in different mammalian species, the internal capsule can be seen to subdivide the nuclei of the basal ganglia in different ways (Fig. 4).

Probably the best known configuration is that seen in primates where the internal capsule forms a coherent bundle separating the caudate nucleus from the putamen. The internal capsule then runs dorsal to the external and internal pallidal segments to course between the internal pallidal segment and the substantia nigra, thereby separating these latter two cell groups. In the carnivore, the internal capsule again forms a coherent bundle separating the caudate nucleus from the putamen and again runs dorsal to the external pallidal segment but, in this order of mammals, forms a brushwork as it traverses the internal pallidal segment (or "entopeduncular nucleus") before regrouping to form a coherent bundle on the ventral surface of the brainstem, the cerebral peduncle. In the rodent the configuration is again different, with the internal capsule forming a brushwork through the striatum and through the external and internal pallidal segments, and only groups to form a coherent bundle on the ventral surface of the brainstem as it becomes the cerebral peduncle, thereby respecting the territory of the substantia nigra. The cetaceans (whales and porpoises) are perhaps the only order of mammals in which "nature got it right" and respected the entire territory of the tier III grouping. In this order of mammals the cephalic flexure appears to draw the basal ganglia rostroventrally and, in so doing, leaves the internal capsule to course dorsal to the entire complex formed by the external pallidal segment, internal pallidal segment, and substantia nigra (tier III) (21).

From this comparative anatomical viewpoint, it appears that the course of the internal capsule through the basal ganglia is extremely variable and therefore is unlikely to provide a fundamental criterion for deciding the boundaries of basal ganglia component cell groups.

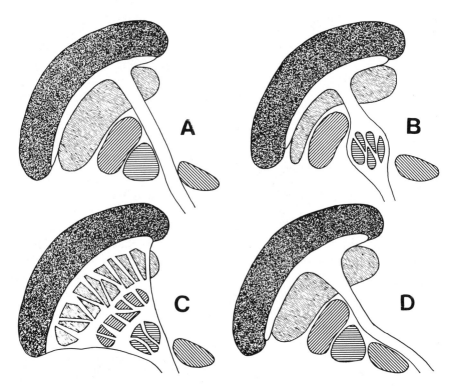

FIG. 4. The comparative anatomical aspects of the relationship between the internal capsule and the basal ganglia structures as discussed in the text. Note that the course of the internal capsule is quite variable in different mammalian orders. As the internal capsule traverses the territory of the tier III structures (pallidum and nigra), it may either course between the internal pallidal segment and substantia nigra (as in primates, *A*); penetrate one (carnivore, *B*) or both (rodent, *C*) pallidal segments; or course around the entire pallidum-nigra complex (as in whales, *D*).

Evidence from Neurochemistry

Also in support of the present scheme are data showing similar patterns of transmitter chemical usage throughout each tier. In tier I, a major afferent and efferent transmitter appears to be glutamate and/or aspartate (4). Norepinephrine afferents also appear to be distributed throughout the structures of tier I (6), setting it apart from tiers II and III in which norepinephrine afferents appear sparse or absent. The territories comprising tier II are perhaps most easily characterized by their dense dopamine innervation (6) and by their patch-like dense staining for acetylcholinesterase (8). Common to the components of tier III are prominent γ-aminobutyric acid (GABAergic) inputs from the striatum (3,9,20) and perhaps also the subthalamic nucleus (16).

Evidence from Single-Unit Recordings

Recent physiological evidence also suggests a coherence of at least the pallidal complex with the nondopaminergic substantia nigra. Based on single-unit recordings in awake behaving monkeys, DeLong and Georgopoulos (2) discovered movement-related units in a somatopic organization straddling the internal capsule to involve both pallidal segments and the nondopaminergic substantia nigra. Neurons in the internal pallidal segment and nondopaminergic substantia nigra showed similar patterns of spontaneous activity. Furthermore, units related to orofacial movements were found in the lateral parts of the substantia nigra in a distribution suggesting a continuation with the orofacial representation in the adjacent internal pallidal segment.

Important to the notion that the basal ganglia may form a telencephalic outflow system subserving more than just movement is the observation (7) that large parts of the pallidal complex contain units showing no evident relation to movement.

IMPLICATIONS FOR LIMBIC SYSTEM CONCEPTS

The finding that the outflow of the basal ganglia is directed to more than just the motor system and the finding that only some of the basal ganglia neurons can be shown to change their discharge patterns in relation to movement (7) raises many questions about the organization and functions of the basal ganglia and their relation to the limbic system. The perspective presented here emphasizes that the basal ganglia appear to form only one of two telencephalic outflow systems and that both outflow systems appear to subserve each major subdivision recognized in the cerebral and limbic cortex. It appears likely that as the motor cortex uses both the basal ganglia outflow system and a direct outflow system (the internal capsule), the limbic or allocortex similarly uses both outflow systems. The hippocampal formation has long been known to give rise to the fornix, which projects to a part of the striatum, the nucleus accumbens septi (5a), and to a part of the diencephalon, the hypothalamus. The precommisural fornix is distributed to the nucleus accumbens whereas the postcommisural fornix continues beyond to link directly with the hypothalamus. In other words, the precommisural fornix links with the basal ganglia outflow system, and the postcommisural fornix behaves like the direct outflow system.

It goes without saying that the basal ganglia are involved with the organization and execution of movements. The question remains, however, what else are they involved with? One interpretation is that the movement-related parts of the basal ganglia form only an isolated, if major, subset of the basal ganglia outflow system. Other parts of the basal ganglia would be seen then as forming an isolated, but parallel, organization subserving other functional subsystems, such as the limbic system. Another point of view is that the limbic system may actually provide an input to the motor system via the basal ganglia outflow system and that the unexplained or "nonmotor" output simply represents a feedback to these nonmotor sources of afferents. Which point of view comes closer to the truth will depend on a better understanding of the opportunities for circumferential interactions among the predominantly radially oriented circuits within the basal ganglia. Assuming that parts of both interpretations may be correct, it may be reasonable to suggest that the basal ganglia reflect the continuum of motor-related parts of the brain, beginning with simple movements and increasing in complexity through more complicated sequences of movements to patterns so complex that they can only be called behaviors. Just as there may be a predominantly motor part of the cortex and a motor part of the striatum and a motor part of the globus pallidus and substantia nigra, so too there may be a predominantly limbic part of the cortex, a limbic part of the striatum, and a limbic part of the pallidum. From this perspective one might expect that a single pathological process affecting different foci within a given tier could lead to vastly different clinical manifestations, just as focal lesions within different parts of the internal capsule can produce vastly different clinical manifestations. Perhaps neurological illnesses which today appear very dissimilar, such as movement disorders and behavior disorders, may some day be shown to have similar pathological mechanisms.

REFERENCES

1. Carpenter, M. B., and Strominger, N. L. (1967): Efferent fiber projections of the subthalamic nucleus in the rhesus monkey. A comparison of the efferent projections of the subthalamic nucleus, substantia nigra and globus pallidus. *Am. J. Anat.*, 121:41–72.
2. DeLong, M. R., and Georgopoulos, A. P. (1979): Motor function of the basal ganglia as revealed by studies of single cell activity in the behaving primate. *Acta Neurol.*, 24:131–140.
3. Fonnum, F., Grofova, I., Rinvick, E., Storm-Mathisen, J., and Walberg, F. (1974): Origin and distribution of glutamate decarboxylase in substantia nigra in cat. *Brain Res.*, 71:77–92.
4. Fonnum, F., Søreide, A., Kvale, I., Walker, J., and Walaas, I. (1981): Glutamate in cortical fibers. In: *Glutamate as a Neurotransmitter*, edited by G. DiChiara and E. L. Gessa, pp. 29–42, Raven Press, New York.
5. Fox, C. A., Andrade, A. N., LuQui, I. J., and Rafols, J. A. (1974): The primate globus pallidus: A Golgi and electron microscope study. *J. Hirnforsch.*, 15:75–93.
5a. Fox, C. A. (1943): The stria terminalis, longitudinal association bundle and precommissural fornix fibers in the cat. *J. Comp. Neurol.*, 79:277–295.
6. Fuxe, K. (1965): Evidence for the existence of monoamine neurons in the central nervous system— IV. Distribution of monoamine nerve terminals in the central nervous system. *Acta Physiol. Scand.*, 64[Suppl.247]:37–85.
7. Georgopoulos, A. P., DeLong, M. R. (1978): The globus pallidus of the monkey: Neuronal activity in relation to movement. *Soc. Neurosci.*, 4,43. *(Abstract).*
8. Graybiel, A. M., and Ragsdale, C. W., Jr. (1978): Histochemically distinct compartments in the striatum of human, monkey, and cat demonstrated by acetythiocholinesterase staining. *Proc. Natl. Acad. Sci. USA*, 75:5723–5726.
9. Hattori, T., McGeer, P. L., Fibiger, H. C., and McGeer, E. (1973): On the source of the GABA-containing terminals in the substantia nigra. Electron microscopic autoradiographic and biochemical studies. *Brain Res.*, 54:103–114.
10. Heimer, L., and Wilson, R. D. (1975): The subcortical projections of the allocortex: Similarities in the neural associations of the hippocampus, the piriform cortex, and the neocortex. In: *Golgi Centennial Symposium*, edited by M. Santini, pp. 177–193. Raven Press, New York.
11. Kemp, J. M., and Powell, T. P. S. (1970): The cortico-striate projection in the monkey. *Brain*, 93:525–546.
12. Nauta, H. J. W. (1974): Evidence of a pallidohabenular pathway in the cat. *J. Comp. Neurol.*, 169:263–290.
13. Nauta, H. J. W. (1979): A proposed conceptual reorganization of the basal ganglia and telencephalon. *Neuroscience*, 4:1875–1881.
14. Nauta, H. J. W. (1979): Projections of the pallidal complex: an autoradiographic study in the cat. *Neroscience*, 4:1853–1873.
15. Nauta, H. J. W., and Cole, M. (1978): Efferent projections of the subthalamic nucleus: an autoradiographic study in monkey and cat. *J. Comp. Neurol.*, 180:1–16.

16. Nauta, H. J. W., and Cuenod, M. (1982): Perikaryal cell labeling in the subthalamic nucleus following the injection of ³H-γ-aminobutyric acid into the pallidal complex: an autoradiographic study in cat. *Neuroscience*, 7:2725–2734.
17. Nauta, W. J. H., and Mehler, W. R. (1966): Projections of the lentiform nucleus in the monkey. *Brain Res.*, 1:3–42.
18. Papez, J. W. (1942): A summary of fiber connections of the basal ganglia with each other and with other portions of the brain. *Res. Publ. Assoc. Res. Nerv. Ment. Dis.*, 21:21–68.
19. Pasik, P., Pasik, T., and DiFiglia, M. (1979): The internal organization of the neostriatum in mammals. In: *The Neostriatum*, edited by I. Divac and R. E. Berg, pp. 5–36. Pergamon Press, Oxford, England.
20. Precht, W., and Yoshida, M. (1971): Blockage of caudate-evoked inhibition of neurons in the substantia nigra by picrotoxin. *Brain Res.*, 32:229–233.
21. Riese, W. (1924): Zur vergleichenden Anatomie der Striofugalen Faserung. *Anat. Anz.*, 57:487–494.
22. Schroder, K. F., Hopf, A., Lange, H., and Thörner, G. (1975): Morphometrischstatistiche Strukturanalysen des Striatum, Pallidum, und Nucleus Subthalamicus beim Menschen—I. Striatum. *J. Hirnforsch.*, 16:333–342.
23. Szabo, J. (1962): Topical distribution of the striatal efferents in the monkey. *Exp. Neurol.*, 5:21–36.
24. Thörner, G., Lange, H., and Hopf, A. (1975): Morphometrisch-statistische Strukturanalysen des Striatum, Pallidum und Nucleus Subthalamicus beim Menschen—II. Pallidum. *J. Hirnforsch.*, 16:401–413.
25. Von Bonin, G., and Shariff, G. A. (1951): Extrapyramidal nuclei among mammals: a quantitative study. *J. Comp. Neurol.*, 94:427–439.
26. Voneida, T. J. (1960): An experimental study of the course and destination of fibers arising in the head of the caudate nucleus in the cat and monkey. *J. Comp. Neurol.*, 115:75–87.
27. Webster, K. E. (1961): Cortico-striate interrelations in the albino rat. *J. Anat.*, 95:532–545.

The Limbic System: Functional Organization and
Clinical Disorders, edited by B. K. Doane and
K. E. Livingston. Raven Press, New York © 1986.

Is the Limbic System a Limbic System? Studies of Hippocampal Efferents: Their Functional and Clinical Implications

C. E. Poletti

Massachusetts General Hospital, Harvard Medical School, Boston, Massachusetts 02114

The word *limbic* means to "rim around." The limbic lobe got its name because the limbic cortex "rims around" the medial aspect of the telencephalon. Papez postulated that the limbic lobe was functionally subserved by a circuit reverberating around it and relayed through the diencephalon. MacLean later extended the concept to define a limbic system that included all principal afferent and efferent connections of the limbic lobe. Nevertheless, Papez's view prevailed for many years; namely, that the limbic lobe is a largely self-contained functional system whose principal efferent and afferent connections were relayed to and from other limbic structures.

This chapter discusses our concept of the nature and mechanisms of action of the temporal lobe limbic system by (a) reviewing the data from a series of experiments on hippocampal and amygdalar efferents done in our laboratories; (b) alluding to two new clinical therapies derived from this data—one in the field of temporal lobe epilepsy, the other in cancer pain suppression; and (c) using this data to reformulate a concept of hippocampal function in particular and of the temporal lobe limbic system in general.

HIPPOCAMPAL EFFERENTS: A SERIES OF PHYSIOLOGICAL, ANATOMICAL, AND METABOLIC STUDIES

Traditional View of Hippocampal Efferent Function

The earlier concept of hippocampal functional organization was based on four hypotheses. First, the hippocampus was thought to act as a single unit; common functions were ascribed to the portion of the hippocampus adjacent to the entorhinal cortex (anterior or ventral hippocampus) and to its more posterior and dorsal portion. Second, it was thought that the common functions of the hippocampus were subserved by common efferent projections; i.e., that virtually the entire influence of the hippocampus was conveyed via the fornix to the hypothalamus and thalamus. Concomitantly, it was the belief that the hippocampus and amygdala function independently through their respective projection systems and have common functions only to the extent that their respective efferent systems project to the same diencephalic structures. Third, hippocampal influence was thought to be almost entirely inhibitory, primarily because behavioral studies showed an arrest of behavior during hippocampal activation. Fourth, the hippocampal efferent system, the fornix, was thought to project almost exclusively to the septum and the mammillary bodies. From here its influence was believed to be relayed to the anterior thalamic nuclei, to the cingulate cortex, and finally back into the hippocampus—the limbic circuit proposed by Papez.

Hippocampal Influence on Unit Activity of the Basal Diencephalon

Questioning this concept of hippocampal functional organization, MacLean in 1968 designed a study of the influence of the anterior and posterior hippocampus on unit activity in the hypothalamus, preoptic region, and basal forebrain in the awake primate. The results of this study conflicted in several ways with the then current hypotheses of hippocampal functional organization outlined above. First, it seems now to have been an extremely insightful idea to study the efferent output of the anterior and posterior portions of the hippocampus separately, for although it was known then that these two regions receive different afferent inputs, their efferent projections were still believed to be very similar. In this study shock stimulation of the anterior hippocampus was clearly more effective in eliciting unit responses than was stimulation of the posterior hippocampus; this difference was most marked for units in the hypothalamus (Fig. 1). Second, 83% of unit responses to hippocampal stimulation were excitatory. This indicated that at the neuronal level, at least, the influence of the hippocampus is not predominantly inhibitory. Third, hippocampal stimulation elicited a relatively high percentage of responsive units not only in the region of the mammillary bodies, but throughout the hypo-

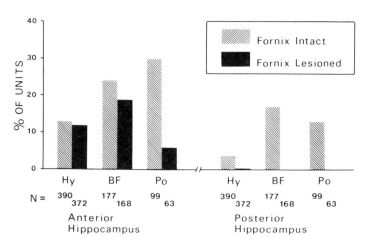

FIG. 1. Percentages of responsive units in hypothalamus, basal forebrain, and preoptic region in the intact animal and in animals with fornix lesions for anterior and posterior hippocampal stimulation; *(N)* number of units tested.

thalamus; even larger percentages of units responded in the basal forebrain and preoptic areas (Fig. 1). The four structures showing the highest percentage of responses were the diagonal band (54%), the medial preoptic region (36%), nucleus accumbens (31%), and the perifornical nucleus of the hypothalamus. This finding indicated that the primary influence of the hippocampus was distributed throughout the basal diencephalon and was by no means predominantly restricted to the mammillary bodies or even just the hypothalamus. The fourth surprising finding in this initial study was physiological evidence for direct projections of fornix fibers to a number of structures not known at the time to receive fornix afferents. Thus, not only were short latencies found in the lateral septum (11 msec) and in the mammillary bodies (13.5 msec)—structures known to receive fornix fibers—but also in the medial preoptic area (11 msec) and in the perifornical nucleus of the hypothalamus (10 msec)—structures not known at the time to receive direct hippocampal projections in the primate (8).

Fornix Projections to Basal Forebrain, Preoptic Areas, and Hypothalamus

In order to investigate the direct fornix projections suggested by these short latencies, an anatomical study of fornix system projections was also done in the squirrel monkey. Using the Voneida silver degeneration staining technique, specific fornix projections to the medial preoptic area (both pre- and postcommissural) and to the perifornical nucleus were confirmed. More important, and confirming the impressions from the preceding physiology study, the overall picture that emerged showed only a small portion of fornix fibers going to the mammillary bodies. Most of the fibers projecting below the anterior commissure distributed to structures in the basal forebrain and preoptic areas (7) (Fig. 2).

Returning to the initial physiological data, with these new anatomical findings one can appreciate at least three apparently inconsistent results.

1. In the bed nucleus of the stria terminalis (BNST), the effect of afterdischarges elicited in the hippocampus is only minimal 15 sec after the beginning of the afterdischarge; then within 28 sec more, a major recruitment of slow-wave and unit activity occurs. It thus takes many seconds for the full effect of an afterdischarge to reach the BNST, even though the anatomical study shows hippocampal fornix fibers direct to this nucleus.

2. Afterdischarges elicited in the hippocampus produce maximal slow-wave and unit activity in the midportion of the ventromedial nucleus (VMN) of the hypothalamus, but they have very little influence on either the upper or lower poles of the nucleus, even though the anatomical study shows fornix fibers distributing specifically to the superomedial rim of the VMN.

3. Shock stimulation of the anterior hippocampus, compared to the posterior hippocampus, was responsible for twice as many unit responses, even though other anatomical studies of the fornix system have shown that fornical fibers originate from the anterior and posterior hippocampus in approximately equal numbers.

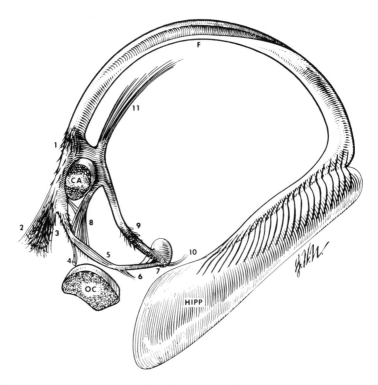

FIG. 2. Composite drawing of subcallosal hippocampal fornix projections in the squirrel monkey to basal forebrain, preoptic, hypothalamic, and thalamic structures. *(1)* Medial and lateral septal projections. *(2)* Basal forebrain projections including nucleus of the diagonal band, nucleus accumbens, gyrus rectus, olfactory tubercle, and putamen. *(3)* Medial and lateral preoptic precommissural fibers. *(4)* Diagonal band projections toward the amygdala. *(5)* Projections via MFB through lateral hypothalamus. *(6)* "Lateral corticohypothalamic tract," precommissural fibers turning medially to tuberal region. *(7)* Precommissural fibers entering the lateral and caudal aspect of the medial mammillary nucleus adjacent to the entrance of the descending fornix column. *(8)* "Medial corticohypothalamic tract" (postcommissural) projections to medial preoptic and anterior hypothalamic areas. *(9)* Medial and lateral perifornical area. *(10)* Prerubral area. *(11)* Thalamic projection including nucleus reuniens, paraventricularis, anterior-ventral, and lateral dorsal.

To explain these and several other apparent discrepancies in the data, the present author in 1970 hypothesized, for the first time, that a significant portion of the hippocampal influence on the basal diencephalon is exerted independently on the fornix system and originates primarily from the anterior hippocampus.

Hippocampal Influence on Basal Diencephalic Unit Activity in Primates with Complete Lesions of the Fornix System

Therefore, to test the possibility of a major nonfornix anterior hippocampal influence, the first physiological study was repeated, but this time in squirrel monkeys with complete bilateral lesions of the fornix system. As hypothesized, whereas the influence of the posterior hippocampus was virtually abolished by sectioning the fornix system, shock stimulation of the anterior hippocampus still produced a major influence on the basal diencephalon (Fig. 1). Furthermore, whereas the influence of the anterior hippocampus on the preoptic region was markedly decreased by sectioning the fornices, the influence of the anterior hippocampus on the basal forebrain was only slightly diminished, and on the hypothalamus the effect was diminished even less. (Fig. 1). From these studies one can also conclude that most of the hippocampal influence on the hypothalamus in the intact animal comes in fact from the anterior hippocampus and is exerted by nonfornix pathway(s) (12,13).

The next step was to determine how this nonfornix anterior hippocampal influence is exerted on the basal diencephalon. Further analysis of the combined data revealed two sets of interesting observations:

1. With the fornix lesioned, the three structures showing the greatest percentage of responses were the BNST, nucleus accumbens, and the VMN (Fig. 3).

2. In the fornix-lesioned animals, hippocampal shock stimulation affected 19% (18/95) of VMN units in the lesioned animals compared to 4% (4/99) in the intact

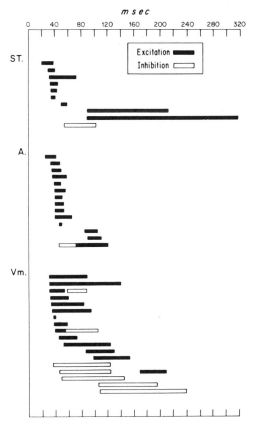

FIG. 3. Graphic display of responses in the three structures with the highest percentage of responses: bed nucleus stria terminalis, nucleus accumbens, and ventromedial nucleus of hypothalamus. For each structure, responses arranged with initially excited units above initially inhibited units in the order of increasing latency.

animal. The VMN was the only structure found to have a greater hippocampal influence with the fornix sectioned.. Furthermore, in the intact animal in the center of the nucleus there were no unit responses but a very large positive inhibitory slow wave. Once the fornix was sectioned, this inhibitory slow wave disappeared, and many units in the midportion of the nucleus then showed an effect from hippocampal stimulation. This effect was both excitatory and inhibitory (Fig. 3).

The first of these observations called to mind the anatomical studies showing amygdalar projections to the BNST, nucleus accumbens, and the VMN. The second set of observations, in particular, called to mind the beautiful and extensive series of physiological experiments by Gloor and his colleagues (2) on the efferent influence of the amygdala on the hypothalamus. In the VMN they had found dual opposing influences of the amygdala: an excitatory influence on units in the core of the VMN, mediated by the ventralamygdalofugal pathway; and an inhibitory influence on units in the poles of the nucleus, mediated by the stria terminalis. These observations and considerations clearly raised the hypothesis that the major nonfornix anterior hippocampal influence on the hypothalamus and basal forebrain was being conveyed via the amygdala.

Anterior Hippocampal Influence on Amygdala Unit Activity

In order to test for the possibility that the physiological influence from the anterior hippocampus passes first directly to the amygdala, the next study in this series investigated the influence of the hippocampus on unit activity in the amygdala, again in the awake intact squirrel monkey.

Following shock stimulation to the anterior hippocampus, 20% of units throughout the amygdala were affected. In sharp contrast, only 2% of units were affected by stimulation of the posterior hippocampus. From the anterior hippocampus short latency unit responses, many driven by single shocks of low intensity, were found especially in the central and basomedial nuclei. These were short enough (12 msec) to permit relay to the hypothalamus and basal forebrain, where unit responses to anterior hippocampal stimulation in the fornix-lesioned animal were found at appropriately longer latencies (22–28 msec). Furthermore, whereas the influence of the anterior hippocampus on units in the central nucleus is predominantly excitatory, the hippocampal influence on basomedial unit activity is predominantly inhibitory (5).

Anterior Hippocampal Influence Mediated to the Hypothalamus and Basal Forebrain via the Stria Terminalis and Ventralamygdalofugal Pathway

The last link in this story of nonfornix anterior hippocampal efferents was to test whether the influence of the anterior hippocampus on the amygdala is then in turn relayed to the hypothalamus and basal forebrain via the two efferent pathways of the amygdala: the stria terminalis and the ventralamygdalofugal pathway.

To test this hypothesis, we used Sokoloff's 2-desoxyglucose technique. The results were quite striking. One of the considerations for calling the limbic system a unified system is based on the belief that afterdischarges tend to spread throughout the system in a nonrestricted distribution. The findings of this study, in contrast, showed that the spread of afterdischarges elicited in the hippocampus follows specific patterns as a function of the site of origin of the afterdischarge. Thus, when the afterdischarge is elicited in the posterior hippocampus, there is propagation of the afterdischarge only within the hippocampus on either side, with some increased metabolic activity in the septum. When, however, the afterdischarge is elicited in the anterior hippocampus with activation of the subiculum, then the hippocampal afterdischarges spread ipsilaterally to the entorhinal cortex, the amygdala, the hypothalamus, the preoptic areas, and to the basal forebrain (3) (Fig. 4).

Using this model, the final part of the study was to see if the propagation of these afterdischarges from the anterior subicular region of the hippocampus to the basal diencephalon was being mediated, at least in part, via the stria terminalis. Accordingly, the above study was repeated in animals with lesions of the fornix system and in animals with lesions of both the fornix system and the stria terminalis. With the fornix lesioned, the VMN and adjacent areas of the hypothalamus, for instance, showed a little less metabolic activity than in the intact animal. However, lesioning the stria terminalis in addition virtually eliminates the nonfornix influence of the anterior hippocampus on the hypothalamus. Yet, even in the animals with the fornix and stria terminalis lesioned, there is still increased metabolic activity— though less intense—in the lateral preoptic region and throughout the basal forebrain. Since these areas are known to receive extensive direct projections of the ventralamygdalofugal pathway (VAF), it seems likely that part of the nonfornix spread of activity of the anterior hippocampus to the basal diencephalon is also mediated by the VAF (9).

Clinical Implications of Nonfornix Anterior Hippocampal Influence on the Basal Diencephalon

Of some interest is the fact that these basic science findings now have had some clinical therapeutic benefits in the field of temporal lobe epilepsy. Most patients with temporal lobe epilepsy treated with temporal lobectomy are found to have a focus of pathology in the anterior hippocampal region. Based on the above discoveries in animals, it was therefore proposed that in some patients suffering from temporal lobe epilepsy the seizure may originate in the anterior hippocampus and spread to the amygdala before reaching the diencephalon. Accordingly, instead of initially treating these patients surgically with a temporal lobectomy, it was further proposed that satisfactory results might be obtained by a much smaller stereotactic lesion, interrupting the pathway from the anterior hippocampus to the amygdala. Recently, a patient has been identified in whom such a lesion gave very satisfactory long-term results (10). Since such a lesion might be tolerated bilaterally, without any memory deficit, this new treatment might offer for the first time hope of surgical therapy for patients suffering from bilateral foci.

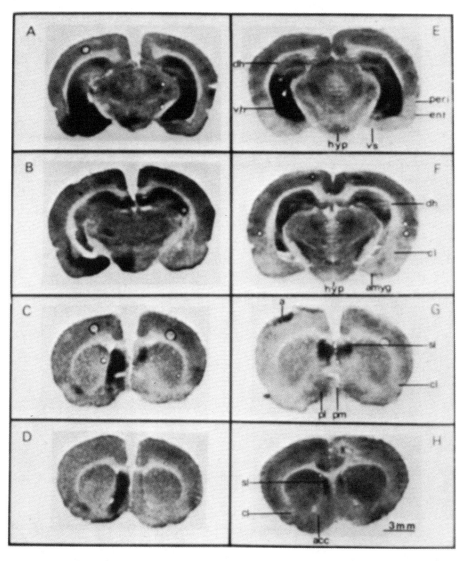

FIG. 4. Deoxyglucose autoradiographs of coronal brain sections comparing the pattern of activity, at four different levels, in a rat with afterdischarges initiated in the ventral subicular cortex **(A–D)** and in a rat with afterdischarges initiated in the ventral hippocampus **(E–H)**. Note the bilateral increases in activity throughout the ventral hippocampus *(vh)* **(A, E)** and the dorsal hippocampus *(dh)* **(B, F)**. Only direct activation of the ventral subicular cortex resulted in increased activity in the ventral subicular *(vs)* and entorhinal *(ent)* cortex, and the deep layers of the perirhinal *(peri)* cortex **(A)**. Additional structures affected by ventral subicular activation were the ipsilateral amygdala *(amyg)* **(B)**, claustrum *(cl)* **(B–D)**, hypothalamus *(hyp)* **(A, B)**, medial *(pm)* and lateral *(pl)* preoptic nuclei **(C)**, nucleus accumbens *(acc)* **(D)**, and the entire extent of the lateral septum *(sl)* **(C, D)**. Outside the hippocampal formation, only the dorsal aspect of the lateral septum showed increased activity bilaterally in both groups of animals **(C, D, G, H)**. Note the lesion at the electrode tip in **E**. The increased density at *a* is an artifact due to a fold in the cortex.

Reformulated View of Hippocampal Efferent Function

This series of experiments has helped modify our traditional view of hippocampal efferent function. We now know that

1. Although hippocampal influence at the behavioral level appears inhibitory, at the neuronal level in the basal diencephalon at least, its influence is predominantly excitatory.

2. Hippocampal influence is not focused on the region of the mammillary bodies but is distributed throughout the hypothalamus. Furthermore, the influence of the hippocampus on the preoptic areas and basal forebrain may be even greater than its influence on the hypothalamus. Similarly, the fornix system in the primate projects only a relatively small portion of fibers to the mammillary region, with other projections throughout the hypothalamus, and comparably prominent direct projections to both the medial and lateral preoptic areas, as well as throughout the basal forebrain.

3. A major portion of hippocampal influence on the basal diencephalon is not mediated via the fornix system.

4. The anterior and posterior portions of the hippocampus have different anatomical and physiological functional projections: The posterior hippocampus influences the basal diencephalon exclusively via the fornix system with major inputs to the basal forebrain, the preoptic region, and with less prominent inputs to the hypothalamus. In contrast, the major influence of the anterior hippocampus on the hypothalamus and basal forebrain is exerted via the amygdala, whereas the major influence of the anterior hippocampus on the preoptic region appears to be mediated via the fornix system. Accordingly, the hippocampus and the amygdala now are shown not to act as separate structures within the temporal lobe. The hippocampus has a prominent direct effect on amygdala unit activity and the amygdala in turn integrates and exerts a major portion of the anterior hippocampal influence on the hypothalamus and basal forebrain.

5. The anterior hippocampus, as is the case with the amygdala, exerts a dual excitatory and inhibitory influence on the ventromedial nucleus of the hypothalamus: an inhibitory effect via the fornix system and an excitatory effect via the amygdala.

FUNCTIONAL IMPLICATIONS OF OUR CURRENT VIEW OF HIPPOCAMPAL EFFERENTS; REFORMULATION OF THE PAPEZ HYPOTHESIS; DIRECT LIMBIC INFLUENCE ON LOWER BRAINSTEM AND SPINAL CORD; THE LIMBIC SYSTEM AS A NONLIMBIC SYSTEM

Hippocampal Formation Structured for Opposing Functions

Past reports have detailed that cutting only the fornix does not in itself alter memory. This finding now makes more sense given the knowledge that a major portion of hippocampal influence is not mediated via the fornix. Paralleling the above physiological distinctions between the influences of the anterior and posterior hippocampus are now many functional studies showing different and often opposing functions of the anterior and posterior portions of the hippocampus. These studies now include endocrine and autonomic functions in addition to behavioral.

We now know that the anterior hippocampus exerts a major influence on the hypothalamus and basal forebrain via the amygdala. This new concept can be looked at in two ways: We can think of the functional influence of the anterior hippocampus as being merely relayed via the amygdala; or we can look at it the other way and say that one of the functions of the amygdala is to integrate and modulate the influence of the anterior hippocampus. This latter formulation is probably the most correct. It is most consistent, for instance, with Mishkin's recent study (4) showing that both the anterior hippocampus and the amygdala are involved in memory function together and that a lesion of either one alone does not significantly alter memory. Since we have shown that the anterior hippocampus exerts a direct effect on most of the nuclei in the amygdala, we can then conclude that the functions primarily associated with the anterior hippocampus modulate those functions associated specifically with the amygdala.

Let us say a few speculative words on opposing temporal lobe limbic functions. Gloor and his colleagues have shown opposing influences of different parts of the amygdala on the basal diencephalon. Similarly for the hippocampus, on the basis of functional studies and now the above-mentioned physiological studies, we know that the anterior and posterior hippocampus also have opposing influences. Furthermore, it appears now that even the anterior hippocampus (at least in the case of the ventromedial nucleus of the hypothalamus) itself has opposing influences. So this gives us a picture of the temporal lobe limbic system as inherently organized and structured with subsystems for opposing autonomic, endocrine, vegetative, and behavioral functions. Is this a strange way for the limbic system to act? From what we already know and think about the limbic system, I would judge that this picture is exactly what we would expect. We know that the limbic system plays a major role in affective behavior. As MacLean has formulated, it is involved primarily in behavior related to survival of the self and survival of the species. What involves more feeling than behavior related to survival of the self and survival of the species? Isn't it this survival behavior that encompasses opposing functions and behavioral acts and thoughts? Is not this survival behavior full of opposing and conflicting courses of action, feeling, and thoughts? There are many examples that we can think of in our own lives: It is clear that as children we love our parents more than anybody, but on another level we occasionally feel instead that we hate them the most also. In sexual love, how rapidly love can turn to hate; in passion, from killing one's loved one to killing oneself instead; in war, from standing at the bridge sacrificing oneself to hold off the enemy to save one's fellow man to turning and fleeing to save one's own skin. If the limbic system is especially active in survival behavior, then is it not mandatory that it should have subsystems intimately juxtaposed for rapidly exerting opposing influences and subserving opposing behaviors?

Evaluation of the Papez Hypothesis: Is the Principal Influence of the Hippocampus Directed into the Papez Circuit?

Up to this point, the studies of hippocampal influence cited have focused on efferent projections to the basal diencephalon: in particular, the hypothalamus, the preoptic areas, and the basal forebrain. The next question that can be asked is, Where does this hippocampal influence on the basal diencephalon go? Is Papez's theory correct that hippocampal influence on the diencephalon is relayed primarily to the cingulate cortex and then back to the hippocampus to complete the Papez circuit? From the foregoing data, we have seen that only a relatively small proportion of hippocampal influence is projected to the mammillary region or to other basal diencephalic structures with potential synaptic relays to the cingulate cortex. The possibility remains, however, that a major proportion of hippocampal influence is exerted directly on the anterior thalamic nuclei with a relay to the cingulate cortex.

Is the Papez theory then in fact correct? Surprisingly, a search of the literature revealed no satisfactory experimental tests of the Papez theory. Therefore the next experiment in this series was an evaluation of the influence of the hippocampus on the cingulate cortex. In order to compare this influence with that already found in the preceding studies, the same experimental design was used; i.e., a study of the influence of anterior and posterior hippocampal shock stimulation and the influence of propagating afterdischarges elicited in the hippocampus. Unit activity was studied in the cingulate cortex.

The results of this study indicated that the hippocampus has a relatively very small influence on cingulate cortex unit activity. Using extracellular techniques in the intact awake monkey, 412 units were studied during hippocampal shock stimulation; of these, only 2% (9) showed any hippocampal influence. Similarly, unit activity and the elicitation of slow-wave activity during propagating hippocampal afterdischarges appeared to be relatively minor compared to that seen in the basal diencephalon (1) (Fig. 5).

Comparing the results of this study with the preceding studies, we had to conclude that the primary influence of the hippocampus is not projected on the cingulate cortex, but in all likelihood on the basal diencephalon. To examine this conclusion let us return to the study of the propagation of hippocampal afterdischarges using the 2-desoxyglucose technique. In this study there was extensive spread of the afterdischarges, as evidenced by increased metabolic activity throughout both hippocampi, and ipsilaterally in the subiculum, amygdala, hypothalamus, preoptic areas, and basal forebrain. However, there was no perceptible alteration of metabolic activity in the cingulate cortex. This study therefore confirmed the preceding conclusion.

From this data it appears that the first half of the functional circuit proposed by Papez (projection of the hippocampal influence to the cingulate cortex) represents only a very small proportion of the efferent influence of the hippocampus. The

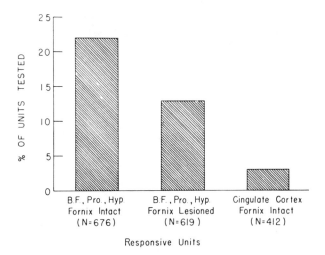

FIG. 5. Percentage of units responsive to hippocampal volleys in cingulate cortex (2%) compared with hypothalamic, preoptic, and basal forebrain regions also in the intact primate (22%) and after lesions of the fornix system (13%).

overwhelming influence of the hippocampus appears to be exerted on the diencephalon. The functional implication is that the primary role of the hippocampus is not to participate in a functional limbic circuit contained within the limbic lobe but instead that the hippocampus exerts its role by influencing the functions associated with structures downstream, especially the basal diencephalon.

Direct Limbic Influence on Lower Brainstem and Spinal Cord

If we then postulate that the primary orientation of the efferent influence of the temporal lobe limbic system is downstream, then the final question to be asked is, Does the temporal lobe limbic system have a direct major influence on the brainstem and/or the spinal cord?

To initially evaluate this hypothesis, two additional studies have recently been completed. The first, again a physiological study in the awake monkey, evaluated hippocampal and amygdalar influence on the periaqueductal grey nucleus (PAG) in the midbrain. PAG has recently been found to participate in the descending analgesic system (DAS): PAG neurons project to the nucleus raphe magnus, which in turn projects down the dorsolateral funiculus of the spinal cord to inhibit the response of dorsal horn nociceptive neurons to peripheral noxious stimulus. That PAG similarly might be modulated by higher structures seemed likely, and the limbic system appeared particularly implicated. Let us assume, as postulated by MacLean, that one of the principal group of functions of the temporal lobe limbic system is preservation of the self and preservation of the species. What role then does the limbic system play in the perception of pain? Perceiving pain, in the traditional view, is certainly important for survival. Yet, one can imagine that suppression of pain may at times be equally important for survival—both of the self and of the species. For example, if a male monkey is fighting with an intruder, his life would seem to be placed in increased jeopardy if at the first hint of any injury he retreated. Boxers must suppress pain during their fights. World War II soldiers, as documented by Beecher, usually felt no pain from even severe wounds until they were safely away from the enemy. Similarly, pain suppression must be important for survival of the species in those cases where the individual is fighting to protect other members of his group. Furthermore, propagation of the species would not be encouraged, for instance, if every time a male monkey in amorous pursuit of his chosen mate stopped in his tracks whenever he stepped on a sharp twig.

Accordingly, it seemed reasonable as part of the working conceptual hypothesis to determine whether the temporal lobe limbic system exerted a major influence on PAG with potential activation of the descending pain-suppressing system. Of 67 units studied throughout the rostrocaudal extent of the PAG, 51% of units (34/ 67) showed significantly altered firing in response to hippocampal or amygdalar stimulation. The influence of the amygdala, especially that of the corticomedial and basolateral nuclei, was particularly prominent. A number of the responses in PAG showed a latency short enough to be consistent with direct projections from the amygdala to PAG (17). These physiological data complement several anatomical studies showing amygdalar neurons projecting directly to PAG.

Clinical Implications

Of incidental note, these basic science findings again proved to have clinical ramifications: By drawing attention to limbic modulation of the descending analgesic system, this study indirectly led to the first use (now a worldwide procedure) of the chronic focal spinal application of morphine to suppress nociceptive transmission in the dorsal horn of patients suffering from cancer pain (6) (Fig. 6).

The final question, May the temporal lobe limbic structures exert a direct influence even below the brainstem?, was investigated using a new technique for retrograde tracing (microlatex beads). This most recent study showed amygdalar neurons, especially in nucleus centralis, with direct projections to both the dorsal and ventral quadrants of the spinal cord (16).

THE LIMBIC SYSTEM AS A NONLIMBIC SYSTEM

In summary and conclusion, this extensive series of experiments indicates the following:

1. The hippocampus has a major dual influence exerted throughout the basal diencephalon. This dual influence, with opposing effects on the ventromedial nucleus of the hypothalamus, is mediated directly via the fornix and through the amygdala.

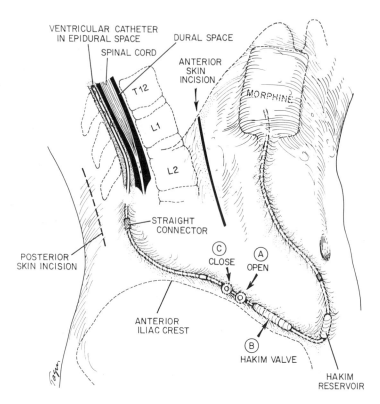

FIG. 6. Focal spinal morphine for cancer pain suppression. Completely indwelling catheter system consisting of a morphine reservoir, one-way valves in tandem permitting pumping by intermittent compression of intervalvular tubing, and an on-off valve for long-term administration of morphine into the epidural space. For operation the on-off valve is opened **(A)**, the Hakim valve is pumped 20 times **(B)** delivering 2 ml of morphine, and the on-off valve is then closed **(C)**.

2. The influence of the hippocampus on the cingulate cortex and its inferred participation in the limbic circuit postulated by Papez appears to be comparatively minor.

3. In contrast, the temporal lobe limbic system has a major influence in the brain stem on the PAG and direct projections to the spinal cord.

Based on this extensive physiological and anatomical data, we propose that the limbic system is not functioning as a limbic system; i.e., it does not function as a reverberating circuit rimming the telencephalon. Instead, one has to conclude, we believe, that the temporal lobe limbic structures exert their functional role primarily by a direct influence on structures downstream in the neuraxis: the diencephalon, the midbrain, and even on the spinal cord. This concept infers that the temporal lobe limbic system plays a significant, direct role in most of the functions associated with the basal diencephalon and on some specific functions of the brainstem and spinal cord.

The working hypothesis thus formulated is that the temporal lobe limbic system modulates virtually all the functions of the brainstem, including behavioral responses to fight and flight, pain suppression, sexual maturation, and autonomic and endocrine activity. In this view, the temporal lobe limbic system is functioning as the next evolutionary stage above the hypothalamus and basal forebrain. Just as the evolution of the hypothalamus represented an amplification and refinement of functions subserved until then by the lower brainstem, so we believe the evolution of the limbic system represented, in turn, an amplification and refinement of hypothalamic control and function. We should not forget that the limbic system was very well developed at a time when the neocortex was just developing. The author does not personally believe, as postulated by MacLean, that the brainstem, when it developed, inculcated the behavioral patterns attributed to animals at that stage of evolution; nor that the limbic system subserves primarily those behavioral patterns associated with its stage of evolution.

It may be more fruitful for further investigation not to formulate our concept of the limbic system as a system that functions primarily in preservation of self and preservation of the species, because, after all, in the earliest stages of evolution of the nervous system was not almost the entire system devoted to survival? Even at the level of the brainstem, including the hypothalamus and the thalamus, virtually all the functions are related to survival, either of the self or the species.

Yet, with the evolutionary development of the limbic system and archicortex, we see again not only a new system for improved integration and control of preceding systems (in the brainstem and the spinal cord), but we also see, probably for the first time, the appearance of a system that subserves behavior less related merely to survival. Thus, the limbic system appears for the first time to permit some early cognitive functions and rudimentary primary emotions.

Finally, to put this view of the limbic system in perspective with the entire central nervous system, one can turn to the development of the neocortex. The development of the neocortex not only again provides a new system for improved integration and modulation of the functions associated with the brainstem and archicortex, but it completes the capacity for higher cognitive functions and refined feelings—intellectual and emotional abilities that can be used not only to further survival abilities once more but also to permit the exploration of knowledge and the enjoyment of emotional experiences virtually unrelated to the survival of man.

REFERENCES

1. Dagi, T. F., and Poletti, C. E. (1983): Reformulation of the Papez circuit: Absence of hippocampal influence on cingulate cortex unit activity in the primate. *Brain Res.*, 259:229–236.
2. Dreifuss, J. J., Murphy, J. T., and Gloor, P. (1968): Contrasting effects of two identified amygdaloid efferent pathways on single hypothalamic neurons. *J. Neurophysiol.*, 31:237–248.
3. Kliot, M., and Poletti, C. E. (1979): Hippocampal afterdischarges: Differential spread of activity shown by the [^{14}C]deoxyglucose technique. *Science*, 204:641–643.
4. Mishkin, M. (1978): Memory in monkeys severely impaired by combined but not separate removal of amygdala and hippocampus. *Nature*, 273:297–298.
5. Morrison, F., and Poletti, C. E. (1980): Hippocampal influence on amygdala unit activity in awake squirrel monkeys. *Brain Res.*, 192:353–369.

6. Poletti, C. E., Cohen, A. M., Todd, D. P., Ojemann, R. G., Sweet, W. H., and Zervas, N. T. (1981): Cancer pain relieved by long-term epidural morphine: Two case reports with permanent indwelling systems for self-administration. *J. Neurosurg.*, 55:581–584.
7. Poletti, C. E., and Creswell, G. C. (1977): Fornix system efferent projections in the squirrel monkey: An experimental degeneration study. *J. Comp. Neurol.*, 175:101–128.
8. Poletti, C. E., Kinnard, M. A., and MacLean, P. D. (1973): Hippocampal influence on unit activity of hypothalamic, preoptic, and basal forebrain structures in awake, sitting squirrel monkeys. *J. Neurophysiol.*, 36:308–324.
9. Poletti, C. E., Kliot, M., and Boytim, M. (1984): Metabolic influence of the hippocampus on hypothalamus, preoptic, and basal forebrain exerted through amygdalofugal pathways. *Neurosci. Lett.*, 5:211–216.
10. Poletti, C. E., Kliot, M., and Kjellberg, R. N. (1983): A proposed stereotactic operation for temporal lobe epilepsy. *Congr. Neurolog. Surgeons Ann. Meet., 1983.*
11. Poletti, C. E., Kliot, M., and Zervas, N. T. (1979): Hippocampal afterdischarges: Differential spread of activity shown by the [^{14}C]2-deoxyglucose technique. *Eur. Soc. Stereotactic Functional Neurosurg., 4th, France, 1979.*
12. Poletti, C. E., and Sujatanond, M. (1977): Evidence for a second hippocampal diencephalic pathway comparable to the fornix system: A unit study in the awake monkey. *Proc. Soc. Neurosci.*, 3:203.
13. Poletti, C. E., and Sujatanond, M. (1980): Evidence for a second hippocampal efferent pathway to hypothalamus and basal forebrain comparable to the fornix system: A unit study in the awake monkey. *J. Neurophysiol.*, 44:514–531.
14. Poletti, C. E., Sujatanond, M., Kinnard, M. A., Creswell, G. C., Morrison, F., Kliot, M., Kjellberg, R. N., Zervas, N. T., Sweet, W. H., and MacLean, P. D. (1977): Experimentally based proposal for modified temporal lobectomy in temporal lobe epilepsy. *Ann. Meet. Am. Acad. Neurolog. Surg., Hawaii, 1977.*
15. Poletti, C. E., Sweet, W. H., Pilon, R. N., and Schmidek, H. H. (1982): Pain control with implantable systems for the long-term infusion of intraspinal opioids in man. In: *Operative Neurosurgical Techniques: Indications and Methods.* edited by H. H. Schmidek, and W. H. Sweet, pp. 1199–1212. Grune and Stratton, Orlando.
16. Sandrew, B. B., Edwards, D. L., Poletti, C. E., Foote, W. E. (1986): Amygdalar projections to the spinal cord. *Brain Res. (in press).*
17. Sandrew, B. B., and Poletti, C. E. (1984): Limbic influence on the periaqueductal grey: A single unit study in the awake squirrel monkey.. *Brain Res.* 303:77–86.

The Limbic System: Functional Organization and
Clinical Disorders, edited by B. K. Doane and
K. E. Livingston. Raven Press, New York © 1986.

Kindling and the Forces That Oppose It

Graham V. Goddard, Michael Dragunow, Eiichi Maru, and
E. Keith Macleod

Department of Psychology, University of Otago, Dunedin, New Zealand

The relevance of the kindling effect to the topic of this volume is that it provides evidence of seizure-related changes in brain function that may have behavioral correlates. Kindling is appropriately thought of as a progressive and lasting sensitization to seizure provocation. It is induced by stimulation, or the activity during seizures, and, although it does not seem to depend on any detectable tissue damage, it is very long lasting and perhaps permanent. The changes that underlie kindling involve changes in neural connectivity that may have lasting behavioral consequences.

But the question of epilepsy-related personality or behavior change is not restricted only to long-lasting effects. There are often obvious behavioral changes during ongoing partial seizures. And there are profound effects on behavior immediately following a major convulsion. During this postictal period the patient is often confused, irrational, and may be emotionally labile or flat. Postictal effects are progressively diminishing, but may last for a considerable time, and will include both general features and focal features such as Todd's paralysis. Furthermore, it is generally accepted that some patients deviate from their normal disposition during the prodromal period leading up to a major convulsion. Thus, in theory, the possibilities for epilepsy-related psychological effects include both general and focal consequences of prodromata, auras, subclinical ongoing partial seizures, and the various stages of recovery from postictal depression. Thus, the question of whether an epilepsy can result in a true interictal personality change is greatly confused because at any given moment the patient is either having a seizure, or is somewhere in time between the last convulsion and the next.

Sato (55) has drawn attention to the distinction between the postictal factors that involve reduced levels of consciousness and the truly interictal factors affecting behavior. But the list of factors that can come into play at different times between one seizure and the next is much longer (Fig. 1). We are concerned here with the underlying neural mechanisms that change with various time courses during and following a seizure. Our aim is to provide a theoretical framework from which the question of behavioral effects of epilepsy can be reexamined.

We shall describe the experimental evidence for changes in brain function of short, intermediate, and long-term duration that result from seizures and are likely

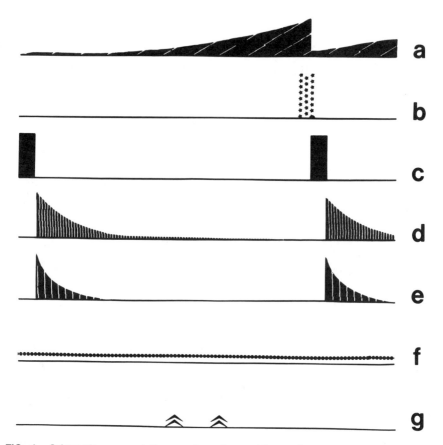

FIG. 1. Schematic representation over time of several factors that may be associated with an epilepsy. Time runs from left to right. Two seizures are represented in **c.** An aura preceding the second seizure is represented in **b.** Following each seizure are postictal factors that decay over time, some slowly, **d,** and some more rapidly, **e.** The probability of another seizure rises as time passes since the last seizure. This rising probability may be associated with increasing endogenous excitants, and these may give rise to prodromata when sufficiently strong. They are depicted in **a.** If interictal personality factors are also present, they are supposed to be present as a constant background, as in **f.** Observations of the psychological state of a patient at any moment in time are likely to be influenced by the sum of all factors **a–f** present at the time. The *arrows* in **g** indicate times at which interictal factors, if present, are least contaminated by ictal, prodromal, or postictal factors, but note that even at the times marked, the interictal factor may not be the only one active.

to have behavioral implications. Often these changes in brain function are revealed experimentally as changes in seizure susceptibility.

One of the first systematic investigations of long-term alterations in seizure susceptibility was described by Sacks and Glaser in 1941 (53). They found that convulsant doses of metrazole administered to rats on alternate days produced resistance to the metrazole so that, on average, the convulsant threshold dose was raised by one-third. After a 4-week drug-free interval, however, the tolerance had disappeared, giving way to a susceptible state in which the minimal convulsant dose was reduced to about two-thirds of the initially effective dose. Thus it appeared that two opposite effects were occurring with repeated metrazole injection: a desensitization, with a time course measured in days, and a longer lasting supersensitivity measured in weeks. The supersensitivity was investigated further by injecting metrazole at weekly intervals. With this regimen no tolerance was evident, but an increased susecptibility developed and persisted for at least 7 weeks after the final injection. Some of the supersensitive rats were then given a rest period of 3 months and challenged with an alternate-day injection of metrazole. Again tolerance developed, suggesting that these two opposing processes are independent and additive: the tolerance being a transient event superimposing on the more permanent supersensitivity.

It was not clear from this pioneering study of Sacks and Glaser how much of each of the two effects were attributable to metabolic/pharmacokinetic effects, how much to toxic/necrotic effects, or how much to nondrug factors associated with the seizures themselves. It is our contention that neither the hyposensitivity nor the hypersensitivity was entirely pharmacokinetic because, as we shall show, similar effects are found with electroconvulsive shock (ECS) and focal electrical stimulation. We suggest, furthermore, that alterations in behavior are likely to accompany both processes.

Essig and his colleagues (17–19) found that repeated ECS threshold determinations that ended with convulsions in cats produced elevations in ECS thresholds when thresholds were measured once or twice daily. However, threshold measurements at intervals of 3 days or more decreased ECS thresholds. Thus the threshold elevations were transient events opposing the more durable threshold reductions. Subconvulsive electroshocks did not elevate seizure thresholds, suggesting that the seizure was causing the threshold elevations. Essig and Flanary showed that repeated ECS (four times per day for 20 days) produced a greater elevation of ECS threshold than one ECS stimulation.

Herberg and Watkins (31) showed that seizures induced by focal self-stimulation of the hypothalamus in rats produced a resistance to further hypothalamic seizures which lasted for 2 hr. To show that this inhibition of seizures was not just a focal effect, Herberg et al. (30) showed that seizures induced by septal stimulation also produced suppression lasting about 2 hr of the seizures induced by hypothalamic stimulation. Audiogenic seizures also produced a transient block of the hypothalamic seizures. Thus both Essig and Herberg have suggested that the transient suppression of seizures by antecedent seizures is a general phenomenon related to the seizure itself rather than to the method of seizure induction.

Both transient inhibitory effects and long-term facilitatory effects of seizures on subsequent seizures have been reported also in kindling.

Kindling is a change in brain function caused by repeated focal stimulation that results in a lasting predisposition to epileptiform convulsions (26). It is revealed as a progressively more generalizing focal convulsion with a progressively lowering threshold. It has been observed in reptiles, amphibians, rodents, lagomorphs, felines, canines, and primates; animals with more complex brains show the most complex and severe convulsions. The areas of the brain from which kindling may be observed include almost the entire forebrain, although some structures, especially anterior neocortex and the limbic system, are more sensitive and responsive than others. A rule of thumb is that the rate of kindling of a focus in the limbic system decreases with its synaptic distance from the amygdala (for review see ref. 25).

Goddard et al. (26) showed that kindling from the amygdala only occurred with interstimulus intervals of 20 min or greater, with an interval of 24 hr being optimal. Stimulation at 5- or 10-min intervals did not kindle major motor seizures. Evidence of seizure activity was observed but, instead of generalizing, it eventually diminished and disappeared. Racine et al. (52) also found that rats kindled from the amygdala with interstimulus intervals of 15 min did not develop bilateral clonic seizures. This minimum interstimulus interval necessary for the completion of kindling may vary with age, however, since Moshé et al. (46) report that kindling from the amygdala in weanling rats did occur with an interstimulus interval of 15 min. If the changes presumed to underlie kindling are opposed by refractory periods that follow all or some of the trials, this refractory period would appear to last longer in adult rats and less long in weanling rats. This difference in the time course of refractory periods may be related to the differential development of inhibitory mechanisms in the limbic system.

Transient suppression of kindled seizures can also be produced by ECS. Tsuru et al. (57) found that ECS delivered 2 hr and 55 min prior to amygdala stimulation retarded kindling. Handforth (29) reported that ECS delivered 24 or 22 hr prior to daily amygdala stimulation in rats retarded kindling. He also found that 11 ECSs delivered at 12-hr intervals produced elevated kindled seizure thresholds, which lasted for 48 hr. Urca and Frenk (60) also found that ECS retarded kindling but did not greatly affect afterdischarge duration.

Direct tests for refractory periods following kindled seizures have been performed by several investigators. Mucha and Pinel (47), while kindling from the amygdala in rats, found that a single afterdischarge with accompanying motor seizure produced inhibition of seizures which lasted for 90 min. Electrical stimulation that did not produce afterdischarge did not have any seizure suppressant effects. A series of 19 repeated motor seizures, spaced 1.5 hr apart, produced a longer lasting (at least 72 hr) inhibition of seizure activity. Although the ability to trigger motor seizures had recovered after 5 days, the afterdischarge duration remained attenuated for at least 9 days after this series of convulsions. Similar refractory periods have been observed when kindling from area CA1 in rats (54) and for amygdala kindling in cats (56). Refractory periods may also be measured as elevations in seizure thresholds. Handforth (29) and Freeman and Jarvis (21) found that repeated testing of seizure thresholds at 24-hr intervals in amygdala-kindled rats produced a progressive elevation of threshold.

The differential time courses of the two opposing effects, kindling and postictal refractoriness, are best seen in studies using two or more sites of stimulation.

Goddard et al. (26) implanted rats with either bilateral amygdala electrodes or ipsilateral amygdala and septal electrodes. All rats were then fully kindled from one amygdala (primary site kindling). The rats were then kindled from the contralateral amygdala or ipsilateral septum (secondary site kindling). Kindling from these secondary sites was faster than normal for these sites. McIntyre and Goddard (39) showed that this positive transfer effect was greater if there was a delay of 14 days, rather than 24 hr, between primary and secondary site kindling. Another interesting finding was that during the secondary site kindling the latency to seizure was greater than that of the primary site. This effect was more marked when secondary site kindling began 24 hr later than when it began after 14 days. These results suggest that primary site kindling produces a long-lasting facilitation that is opposed by a shorter lasting suppression. This shorter lasting suppression, as indicated by its most sensitive measure (seizure onset latency), decays over a period exceeding 14 days.

The primary site was then retested for its ability to elicit seizures. Suppression of seizures and longer latencies were observed following the secondary site kindling than would have been expected from delay alone. The time course of this interference effect that suppressed the primary amygdala kindling was maximal when the interval between secondary and primary site kindling was 1 day, was still present, although attenuated, with an interval of 7 days, and was not present after 14 days. Similar effects were found for the latency data, with increases at 1- and 7-day intervals, but not at 14 days. Furthermore, the degree of interference was related to the number of convulsions elicited during the secondary site kindling. If secondary site kindling was taken only as far as the first behavioral class 4 seizure, there was no interference effect. Burnham (9) found that suppression of primary site seizures occurred after secondary site seizures only if the secondary site was located in the amygdala. Other sites in the limbic system cause the longer lasting facilitation, but not the suppression.

Gaito (23) also investigated the interference effect and extended the number of alternations between repeated stimulation of the primary site amygdala and repeated stimulation of the secondary site contralateral amygdala. He described an oscillatory trend in seizure latency and, to some extent, in the rate of kindling. Primary site stimulation elicited shorter latencies than secondary site stimulation over 6 to 11 alternations when 24 hr elapsed between one site and the next. An interval of 14 days between alternations abolished the differences in kindling rate but not the differences in latency. But unfortunately, the electrode placements were not confirmed histologically so bilaterally symmetrical placements were not guaranteed. It would appear that Gaito's result is in agreement with the above hypothesis of long lasting facilitation effects and short lasting interference effects, although it is not clear whether his more permanent difference in latency between the two hemispheres was due to differences in electrode placement or is evidence of slower seizure spread due to competition with the primary site for access to motor areas.

Another aspect of these interference effects has been reported by Burchfiel et al. (8). Concurrent kindling of limbic foci by alternately stimulating septum and ipsilateral entorhinal cortex every 24 hr resulted in the development of clear dominance of one focus over the other. That is, kindling from one focus progressed normally, but the other focus, despite showing local afterdischarge associated with arrest and automatisms, did not continue to kindle to the more advanced stages of motor convulsion. Which focus became dominant seemed to depend upon which first established connections with the motor seizure substrate. Similar effects were observed for septum and contralateral entorhinal cortex, amygdala and ipsilateral entorhinal cortex, bilateral amygdala, and bilateral entorhinal cortex. Furthermore, a mutual antagonism, where neither site emerged as dominant and both sites continued to show incomplete seizure development, was sometimes observed.

In this review so far we have concentrated on seizure suppression as our measure of the refractory period. However, this approach cannot answer the important question of mechanism. It is unlikely that the refractory period is a passive event related to neuronal exhaustion. Cases of status epilepticus show that seizures can occur for prolonged periods despite any such hypothesized neuronal exhaustion. Furthermore, although the decrease in oxygen tension and pH and the increase in carbon dioxide tension, which result from increased metabolic rate, depress seizures, Caspers and Speckmann (11) demonstrated that rapid spontaneous seizure arrest cannot be attributed to hypoxia, although hypercapnia may be involved. A more likely explanation is that the refractory period reflects a transient activation of endogenous anticonvulsant processes that suppress further seizures. These endogenous anticonvulsant processes are probably activated by the seizure and may be responsible for spontaneous seizure arrest as well as the postictal refractory period. Two lines of evidence derived from neurochemical and neurophysiological studies support the putative activation of endogenous anticonvulsant processes.

In most neurochemical studies of kindling the brain tissue is excised hours, days, or, at most, a week after the final generalized seizure. Thus, any observed change in brain chemistry may be seizure-induced and transitory. Conclusions about the neurochemical basis of kindling are unwarranted unless the neurochemical "trace" is shown to last as long as kindling itself. However, such studies do provide data that may be relevant to an understanding of the refractory period.

Liebowitz et al. (36) kindled from the entorhinal cortex in rats. Generalized seizures were then evoked on 5 to 7 consecutive days. The rats were killed 24 hr after their final seizure and the hippocampus was excised. The total content and release of a number of amino acids was determined to reveal an elevated level of γ-aminobutyric acid (GABA) and an increase in potassium-stimulated release of GABA in kindled hippocampi compared with unstimulated controls. Since potassium-induced release of GABA is calcium-dependent, this result may indicate that depolarization-induced release of GABA is potentiated after seizures. And since agents that potentiate GABA-mediated inhibition tend to block kindled seizures (33,35,43,64; although note ref. 33 for an opposing view.), this result would support a GABA inhibition explanation of the refractory period. This hypothesis is strengthened by the observations of Green et al. (28) who found that ECS, administered to rats, raised the convulsant threshold doses of bicuculline, isopropylbicyclophosphate, and metrazole (all GABA antagonists), but not of strychnine (a glycine antagonist) or quipazine (a serotonin agonist), for at least 30 min following the ECS convulsion.

Brain levels of adenosine have been found to increase following seizure activity (63), and increased adenosine receptor numbers have been found following chronic ECS in rats (2 days following the last seizure; ref. 48), although 1 hr after metrazole-induced seizures fewer receptors were found (65). Since adenosine is an anticonvulsant (13,14,44) and may be involved in spontaneous seizure arrest (13), these receptor increases may reflect a potentiated anticonvulsant effect of adenosine following seizure activity.

It has also been hypothesized that endorphins, released during seizures, may have inhibitory effects on subsequent seizures (34), but these effects appear to be weak (32).

Dashieff et al. (12) found decreased muscarinic cholinergic receptor binding (decreased number) in the dentate gyrus, hippocampus and amygdala of amygdala-kindled rats sacrificed at different times following their first stage 5 seizure. Rats sacrificed 1 day after their first stage 5 seizure showed decreased binding in dentate, hippocampus, and amygdala. Rats sacrificed after 3 days showed decreased binding in only dentate. Rats sacrificed after 7 days did not show decreased binding. Thus the muscarinic receptor declines were maximal in the dentate, hippocampus, and amygdala 1 day following a stage 5 seizure, were still present in the dentate 3 days later, and were back to control levels after 7 days. The transient nature of these receptor declines, together with a reported failure to find receptor declines after stages 2 and 3 of kindling, suggests that they are seizure-induced. Since acetylcholine is an excitatory neurotransmitter, these receptor declines would reflect reduced excitability and a reduced tendency for seizures. Since choline uptake and acetylcholinesterase activity were not affected by the seizures, the receptor declines were not merely compensating for increased release or decreased metabolism of acetylcholine.

Burchfiel (7) investigated the effect of hippocampal afterdischarge on the responsiveness of CA1 pyramidal cells to iontophoretically applied acetylcholine. He observed that immediately after the cessation of the afterdischarge (at a time when further stimulation did not elicit afterdischarge), there was a period of decreased responsiveness to acteylcholine, whereas 40 to 60 min later there was a supersensitivity.

Paul and Skolnick (50) found that electroshock seizures in rats resulted in elevated numbers of diazepam binding sites 15 and 30 min after the end of the seizure. By 60 min, receptor number had returned to the level of nonseizing controls. Mc-Namara et al. (42) found that amygdala kindling in rats caused significant increases in hippocampal benzodiazepine receptors in tissue excised 24 hr after the first stage 5 seizure. These receptor increases appeared to be seizure-induced rather than kindling-induced for two reasons. Larger increases were found in animals subjected to more seizures, even though all animals were kindled to the same criterion of one stage 5 seizure. And ECS also produced significant increases in hippocampal benzodiazepine receptors in rats sacrificed 1 day after the last seizure.

In a subsequent study Valdes et al. (61) localized these receptor increases to the dentate granule cells. Since benzodiazepines are potent anticonvulsants in a number of seizure models including kindling, and since they potentiate GABA-mediated inhibition, these receptor increases might be interpreted as enhanced capacity for seizure suppression. Fanelli and McNamara (20) found increased benzodiazepine binding and also found that GABA-induced enhancement of benzodiazepine binding was reduced in a kindled group 24 hr after the final stage 5 seizure. This reduced efficacy of GABA on benzodiazepine binding could be due to a number of factors, the most likely being that of greater binding of endogenous GABA in the kindled group, thus reducing the effect of exogenous GABA. This hypothesis is consistent with the data of Liebowitz et al. (36) showing an enhanced release of GABA from the hippocampus of kindled rats.

Tuff et al. (59) found increased numbers of benzodiazepine receptors in the amygdala of amygdala-kindled rats using well-washed preparations. These rats were kindled to six consecutive stage 5 seizures, and brain tissue was excised 2 weeks after the final seizure. Rats kindled from the dentate after amygdala kindling also showed an increased number of benzodiazepine receptors in amygdala and hippocampus. Of particular interest is that the receptor increases were correlated with potentiated hippocampal inhibition (see later).

However, Niznik et al. (49) found that kindling from the amygdala in rats produced reduced numbers of benzodiazepine receptors in the ipsilateral cortex and hypothalamus in unwashed tissue excised 2 weeks following the sixth stage 5 seizure. No differences were found in amygdala-pyriform cortex, hippocampus, striatum, and contralateral cortex and hypothalamus. These different results may be due to the washing procedure, as the unwashed preparations may have contained endogenous ligand in a higher concentration in kindled brain.

Despite this last inconsistent result, it would appear that kindled seizures (and seizures produced by ECS) produce neurochemical changes that have an anticonvulsant effect. These results support the hypothesis that the postictal refractory period reflects a strengthening of endogenous anticonvulsant processes that may include up-regulation of inhibitory processes (e.g., GABA, benzodiazepine receptors, adenosine) and a down-regulation of excitatory ones (e.g., cholinergic). However, findings of this sort need to be interpreted cautiously. First, with respect to the benzodiazepine receptors, we do not know if the endogenous ligand is an anticonvulsant. Second, a detected change in one neurochemical parameter implies, but does not prove, an altered biological effect. Correlative neurophysiological data, showing an altered biological response of nerve cells following seizure activity, are also required.

The second line of evidence suggesting that the refractory period is due to strengthening of endogenous anticonvulsant processes comes from single-cell recording studies and field potential studies in the hippocampus.

Fujita and Sakuranaga (22) studied membrane potential changes in the hippocampal cells of rabbits kindled from the hippocampus and found spontaneous hyperpolarizing potentials in the CA1 pyramidal cells, which were not preceded by spike bursts or depolarizations. These spontaneous hyperpolarizations were also observed in nonkindled rabbits but were of less magnitude than in the kindled rabbits. Brainstem stimulation also produced these hyperpolarizing potentials. Unfortunately, the number of seizures and the interval between the last seizure and testing were not reported. Whether the potentiation of inhibition was produced by seizure or by kindling is unclear.

The observations of Fujita and Sakuranaga presumably related the grossly recorded interictal spikes. Whether such interictal spikes reflect increased or decreased seizure susceptibility is unclear. Engel and Ackermann (16) reported that increased frequency of interictal electroencephalographic (EEG) spikes correlated with decreased seizure susceptibility in amygdala kindled rats. However, in a more extensive study, Gotman (27) found that the ongoing rate of interictal spiking did not consistently correlate with either increased or decreased seizure susceptibility. The appearance of interictal spiking in the kindled brain is an indication that kindling has occurred and that seizure susceptibility is present, but moment-to-moment rate of spiking is a poor indicator of the moment-to-moment fluctuations of seizure susceptibility.

Tuff et al. (58) found that paired pulse depression, induced by applying double pulse stimulation at the appropriate intervals to the perforant path, was potentiated after amygdala and dentate kindling. This measure of recurrent inhibition was taken 2 weeks after the completion of kindling (defined as six consecutive stage 5 seizures). Therefore, this result implies a strengthening of inhibition following kindling. Tuff et al. also found that the latency to afterdischarge onset, induced by 5 Hz stimulation of the perforant path, was increased after kindling. They interpreted this result to mean an enhanced resistance to inhibitory failure following kindling.

Goddard (24) found, when kindling from the hippocampal dentate area, that the population spike (a measure of the firing of a population of granule cells) evoked by perforant path stimulation was increased following kindling to stage 3, but decreased after kindling to stage 5 seizures. As testing was carried out 2 weeks after the final seizure, the result can be interpreted to mean a lasting decrease in excitability of the granule cells following major convulsions. Also a measure of inhibition was taken before kindling and 2 weeks after the final kindled seizure by testing the strength of the inhibitory effect of contralateral hilar stimulation on the perforant path evoked potentials. This inhibition tended to increase after kindling, although the increase was not statistically significant.

More recently, Maru and Goddard (45) have studied the time course of these changes in excitability and inhibition. Extracellular field potentials were recorded from the dentate hilus of rats before, during (20 to 23 hr after each kindling stimulation), and 1 month after the completion of kindling. Kindling potentiated the excitatory synapses (field excitatory postsynaptic potential, EPSP), and this potentiation was even more pronounced after the 1-month seizure-free interval. The input-output curve of cellular excitability was shifted to the right, particularly during late kindling trials when seizures were more intense, and the cellular discharge threshold was increased. Both of these changes indicate a reduction in excitability of the granule cells following severe convulsions that last for more than 24 hr. Interestingly, both measures had returned to prekindling baseline after 1 month without seizure. Our ongoing research indicates that this return to normal levels of excitability is a gradual process requiring more than 2 weeks to complete following a series of stage 5 convulsions. Similarly, the measure of contralateral hilar inhibition indicated that kindling produced a transient potentiation of inhibition, which, 1 month after the final seizure, also returned to baseline.

The potentiated EPSP, on the other hand, would appear to be a more durable change related to kindling, since it survived the 1-month interval without seizures and, in fact, was even more potentiated after the rest period than it had been at the end of the kindling trials. Other long-term effects of kindling have been reported. These include reductions in beta-adrenergic binding (41), raised basal levels of cyclic guanosine monophosphate (GMP) (5), and increased protein phosphorylation (62). The possible relevance of these long-term effects of kindling to human clinical epilepsy has been discussed elsewhere (25).

The various effects reviewed here, and their implications for behavior, can be summarized in reference to Fig. 1. We do not have direct evidence of the first factor—the increasing drive to seizure. In the kindling model the seizures are usually triggered by focal stimulation. However, spontaneous convulsions have been reported after prolonged kindling, and, in the case of some clinical epilepsies, it would appear that endogenous seizure-provoking factors may build up over time and contribute to the prodromata and eventually provoke the seizure. Behavioral changes and "personality factors" might be expected as part of the prodrome.

Behavioral changes during the aura and during the ictus are overt and obvious. They need no further comment here. The controversy is not over how and when seizure activity spills into motor areas to change behavior. The controversy is whether or not dramatic behavioral changes ever result from covert, or subclinical, seizure activity. We have no direct evidence concerning this matter.

Figure 1 d,e describe long- and short-lasting postictal effects. The foregoing review of evidence gives support to the notion of endogenous anticonvulsant agents that are released by the seizure. These agents presumably stop the convulsion and linger on. The rapid decaying ones ensure high resistance to seizures, not just in the same focus but generally. They would give rise to the behavioral depression and clouding of consciousness that follow major seizures. Caldecott-Hazard et al. (10) have reported short-term behavioral changes following kindled seizures in rats that might be due to rapidly decaying anticonvulsant agents. We have also cited evidence that the longer lasting postictal effects may linger for more than 2 weeks after a series of severe convulsions and involve both increased levels of inhibition and decreased levels of cellular excitability. These also can act both focally and generally. When stronger in the focus than elsewhere, they may explain Todd's palsy. It is interesting to note that an aborted focal seizure may be followed by a more striking Todd's paralysis than one that is allowed to progress and involve other areas (15).

And, finally, Fig. 1f is the more permanent behavioral change that could be called a true interictal personality factor. At the theoretical level these might be associated with kindling and the long-lasting increases in seizure susceptibility that outlive all other effects. Evidence of lasting behavioral changes resulting from kindling has been reported. McIntyre and Molino (40) and McIntyre (38) found that the ability to acquire a conditioned emotional response to an auditory stimulus was diminished in rats that had been kindled by stimulation of the amygdala but not of the anterior neocortex. Boast and McIntyre (6) observed a postkindling reduction in rats' ability to learn a passive avoidance task, but the results were bimodally distributed, with some animals severely affected and others relatively normal. Bawden and Racine (4) observed a similar but less pronounced effect on passive avoidance which did not reach statistical significance. Pinel et al. (51) report that kindling by stimulation of the amygdala, which was continued for many convulsions, produces rats that are more likely to try and avoid capture, may be difficult to handle, and sometimes very aggressive. These results have not been observed in other laboratories working with rats kindled by amygdala stimulation, perhaps because they usually discontinue stimulation after only a few bilaterally generalized convulsions.

One of the most interesting studies on this subject is that of Adamec (1) and more recently by Adamec and Stark-Adamec (2,3) (also see Adamec and Stark-Adamec, *this volume*) showing alterations in the predatory behaviour of cats. Attempts to extend these findings to rats have been unsuccessful. McIntyre (37) found no change in the mouse-killing patterns of rats postkindling, and a more extensive study by Bawden and Racine (4) found no changes in muricide, ranicide, or intraspecific aggression of their postkindled rats. Other studies of cat behavior, similar to those reported by Adamec, have not been attempted. Evidence of long-lasting increased synaptic coupling in circuits connected to the kindled focus has been observed by us and Racine and colleagues. A connectionist explanation of such personality changes, where they exist, is therefore available.

A note of caution that we wish to sound, however, is that any test of personality, or other behavioral variable, is necessarily presented at a particular moment in the patient's history. Inspection of Fig. 1 will reveal that any moment in time is likely to be influenced either by ictal events or by a concurrent combination of prodromal, postictal, and interictal factors. The severity of, and the time since, the last preceding convulsion or set of convulsions is of great theoretical importance, particularly if it was within the past 2 weeks, as is the time to the seizure which will follow the test. In some patients there may be little or no time during which interictal personality factors can be assessed in the absence of contamination by ictal, postictal, or prodromal factors.

ACKNOWLEDGMENT

This work was supported by a grant from the New Zealand Neurological Foundation.

REFERENCES

1. Adamec, R. (1976): Behavioural and epileptic determinants of predatory attack behaviour in the cat. In: *Kindling*, edited by J. A. Wada, pp. 135–154. Raven Press, New York.
2. Adamec, R. E., and Stark-Adamec, C. (1983): Partial kindling and emotional bias in the cat: Lasting aftereffects of partial kindling of the ventral hippocampus. I. Behavioural changes. *Behav. Neural. Biol.*, 38:205–222.
3. Adamec, R. E., and Stark-Adamec, C. (1983): Partial kindling and emotional bias in the cat: Lasting aftereffects of partial kindling of the ventral hippocampus. II. Physiological changes. *Behav. Neural. Biol.*, 38:223–239.
4. Bawden, H. N., and Racine, R. J. (1979): Effects of bilateral sub-threshold stimulation of the amygdala or septum on muricide, ranacide, intraspecific aggression and passive avoidance in the rat. *Physiol. Behav.*, 22:115–123.
5. Blackwood, D. H. R., Martin, M. J., Palomo, T., and McQueen, J. K. (1980): Changes in cGMP in amygdaloid kindling in rats. *Br. J. Pharmacol.* (Proc), 500P–501P.
6. Boast, C. A., and McIntyre, D. C. (1977): Bilateral kindled amygdala foci and inhibitory avoidance behaviour in rats: A functional lesion effect. *Physiol. Behav.*, 18:25–28.
7. Burchfiel, J. L. (1981): Kindling in the rat hippocampus: Studies of neurotransmitter mechanisms and transfer mechanisms. In: *Kindling 2*, edited by J. A. Wada, pp. 295–301. Raven Press, New York.
8. Burchfiel, J. L., Serpa, K. A., and Duffy, F. M. (1982): Further studies of antagonism of seizure development between concurrently developing kindled limbic foci in the rat. *Exp. Neurol.*, 75:476–489.
9. Burnham, W. M. (1971): Epileptogenic modification of the rat forebrain by direct and trans-synaptic stimulation. Unpublished PhD Thesis, McGill University.
10. Caldecott-Hazard, S., Yamagata, N., Hedlund, J., Camacho, H., and Liebeskind, J. C. (1983): Changes in simple and complex behaviour following kindled seizures in rats: Opioid and nonopioid mediation. *Epilepsia*, 24:539–547.
11. Caspers, H., and Speckmann, E. J. (1972): Cerebral pO_2, pCO_2 and pH: Changes during convulsive activity and their significance for spontaneous arrest of seizures. *Epilepsia*, 13:699–725.
12. Dashieff, R. M., Byrne, M. C., Patrone, V., and McNamara, J. O. (1981): Biochemical evidence of decreased muscarinic cholinergic neuronal communication following amygdala-kindled seizures. *Brain Res.*, 206:233–238.
13. Dragunow, M., and Goddard, G. V. (1984): Adenosine modulation of amygdala kindling. *Exp. Neurol.*, 84:654–665.
14. Dunwiddie, T. V., and Worth, T. (1982): Sedative and anticonvulsant effects of adenosine analogs in mouse and rat. *J. Pharm. Exp. Ther.*, 220:70–76.
15. Efron, R. (1961): Post-epileptic paralysis: theoretical critique and report of a case. *Brain*, 84:381–394.
16. Engel, J., Jr., and Ackermann, R. F. (1980): Interictal EEG spikes correlate with decreased, rather than increased, epileptogenicity in amygdaloid kindled rats. *Brain Res.*, 190:543–548.
17. Essig, C. F. (1969): Frequency of repeated electroconvulsions and the acquisition rate of a tolerance-like response. *Exp. Neurol.*, 25:571–574.
18. Essig, C. F., and Flanary, H. G. (1966): The importance of the convulsion in occurrence and rate of development of electroconvulsive threshold elevation. *Exp. Neurol.*, 14:448–452.
19. Essig, C. F., Groce, M., and Williamson, E. L. (1961): Reversible elevation of electroconvulsive threshold and occurrence of spontaneous convulsions upon repeated electrical stimulation of the cat brain. *Exp. Neurol.*, 4:37–47.
20. Fanelli, R. J., and McNamara, J. O. (1983): Kindled seizures result in decreased responsiveness of benzodiazepine receptors to γ-aminobutyric acid (GABA). *J. Pharm. Exp. Ther.*, 266(1):147–150.
21. Freeman, F. G., and Jarvis, M. F. (1981): The effect of interstimulation interval on the assessment and stability of kindled seizure thresholds. *Brain. Res. Bull.*, 7:629–633.
22. Fujita, Y., and Sakuranaga, M. (1981): Spontaneous hyperpolarizations in pyramidal cells of chronically stimulated rabbit hippocampus. *Jap. J. Physiol.*, 31:879–889.
23. Gaito, J. (1980): Interference effects within the kindling paradigm. *Physiol. Psych.*, 8(1):120–125.
24. Goddard, G. V. (1982): Separate analysis of lasting alteration in excitatory synapses, inhibitory

synapses and cellular excitability in association with kindling. In: *Kyoto Symposia* (EEG Clin. Neurophysiol. Suppl No. 36), edited by P. A. Buser, W. A. Cobb, and T. Okuma. Elsevier Biomedical Press, Amsterdam.
25. Goddard, G. V. (1983): The kindling model of epilepsy. *Trends Neurosci.*, 6(7):275–279.
26. Goddard, G. V., McIntyre, D. C., and Leech, C. K. (1969): A permanent change in brain function resulting from daily electrical stimulation. *Exp. Neurol.*, 25(3):295–329.
27. Gotman, J. (1984): Relationships between triggered seizures, spontaneous seizures and interictal spiking in the kindling model of epilepsy. *Exp. Neurol.*, 84:259–273.
28. Green, A. R., Nutt, D. J., and Cowen, P. J. (1982): Increased seizure threshold following convulsion. In: *Psychopharmacology of Anticonvulsants*, edited by M. Sandler, pp. 16–26. Oxford University Press, Oxford.
29. Handforth, A. (1982): Post-seizure inhibition of kindled seizures by electroconvulsive shock. *Exp. Neurol.*, 78:483–491.
30. Herberg, L. J., Tress, K. H., and Blundell, J. E. (1969): Raising the threshold in experimental epilepsy by hypothalamic and septal stimulation and by audiogenic seizures. *Brain*, 92:313–328.
31. Herberg, L. J., and Watkins, P. J. (1966): Epileptiform seizures induced by hypothalamic stimulation in the rat: Resistance to fits following fits. *Nature*, 209(5022):515–516.
32. Jarvis, M. F., and Freeman, F. C. (1983): The effects of naloxone and interstimulation interval on post-ictal depression in kindled seizures. *Brain Res.*, 288:235–241.
33. Kalichman, M. W. (1982): Neurochemical correlates of the kindling model of epilepsy. *Neurosci. Biobehav. Rev.*, 6:165–181.
34. Kelsey, J. E., and Belluzzi, J. D. (1982): Endorphin mediation of post-ictal effects of kindled seizures in rats. *Brain Res.*, 253:337–340.
35. Le Galle La Salle, G., Kaijiona, M., and Feldblum, S. (1983): Abortive amygdaloid kindled seizures following microinjection of γ-vinyl-GABA in the vicinity of substantive nigra in rats. *Neurosci. Letts*, 36:69–74.
36. Liebowitz, N. R., Pedley, T. A., and Cutter, W. P. (1978): Release of γ-aminobutyric acid from hippocampal slices of the rat following generalized seizures induced by daily electrical stimulation of entorhinal cortex. *Brain Res.*, 138:369–373.
37. McIntyre, D. C. (1978): Amygdala kindling and muricide in rats. *Physiol. Behav.*, 21:49–56.
38. McIntyre, D. C. (1979): Effects of focal versus generalized kindled convulsions from anterior neocortex or amygdala on CER acquisition in rats. *Physiol. Behav.*, 23:855–859.
39. McIntyre, D. C., and Goddard, G. V. (1973): Transfer, interference and spontaneous recovery of convulsions kindled from the rat amygdala. *EEG Clin. Neurophysiol.*, 35:533–543.
40. McIntyre, D. C., and Molino, A. (1972): Amygdala lesions and CER learning: long term effect of kindling. *Physiol. Behav.*, 8:1055–1058.
41. McIntyre, D. C., and Roberts, D. C. S. (1983): Long-term reduction in beta-adrenergic receptor binding after amygdala kindling in rats. *Exp. Neurol.*, 82:17–24.
42. McNamara, J. O., Peper, A. M., and Patrone, V. (1980): Repeated seizures induce long-term increase in hippocampal benzodiazepine receptors. *Proc. Natl. Acad. Sci. USA*, 77(5):3029–3032.
43. McNamara, J. O., Rigsbee, L. C., and Galloway, M. T. (1983): Evidence that substantia nigra is crucial to neural network of kindled seizures. *Eur. J. Pharmacol.*, 86:485–486.
44. Maitre, M., Cielielski, L., Lehman, A., Kempf, E., and Mandel, P. (1974): Protective effect of adenosine and nicotinamide against audiogenic seizure. *Biochem. Pharmacol.*, 23:2807–2816.
45. Maru, E., and Goddard, G. V. (1983): Excitability changes of dentate granule cells following perforant path kindling. A paper presented to the Australasian Winter Conference on Brain Research, New Zealand.
46. Moshé, S. L., Albala, B. J., Ackermann, R. F., and Engel, J., Jr. (1983): Increased seizure susceptibility of the immature brain. *Dev. Brain Res.*, 7:81–815.
47. Mucha, R. F., and Pinel, J. P. J. (1977): Postseizure inhibition of kindled seizures. *Exp. Neurol.*, 54:266–282.
48. Newman, M., Zohar, J., Kalian, M., and Belmaker, R. H. (1984): The effects of chronic lithium and ECT on A_1 and A_2 adenosine receptor systems in rat brain. *Brain Res.*, 291:188–192.
49. Niznik, H. B., Kish, S. J., and Burnham, W. M. (1983): Decreased benzodiazepine receptor binding in amygdala-kindled rat brains. *Life Sci.*, 33:425–430.
50. Paul, S. M., and Skolnick, P. (1978): Rapid changes in brain benzodiazepine receptors after experimental seizures. *Science*, 202:892–895.

51. Pinel, J. P. J., Treit, D., and Rovner, L. I. (1977): Temporal lobe aggression in rats. *Science*, 197:1088–1089.

52. Racine, R. J., Burnham, W. M., Gartner, J. G., and Levitan, D. (1973): Rates of motor seizure development in rats subjected to electrical brain stimulation: Strain and interstimulation interval effects. *EEG Clin. Neurophysiol.*, 35:553–556.

53. Sacks, J., and Glaser, N. M. (1941): Changes in susceptibility to the convulsant action of metrazol. *J. Pharmacol. Exp. Ther.*, 73:289–295.

54. Sainsbury, R. S., Bland, B. H., and Buchan, D. H. (1978): Electrically induced seizure activity in the hippocampus: Time course for post seizure inhibition of subsequent kindled seizures. *Behav. Biol.*, 22:479–488.

55. Sato, M. (1983): Biological aspects of interictal mental disorders in epilepsy. *Neurosciences*, 9:197–207.

56. Stock, G., Klimpel, L., Sturm, V., and Schlör, K. H. (1980): Resistance to tonic-clonic seizures after amygdaloid kindling in cats. *Exp. Neurol.*, 69:239–246.

57. Tsuru, N., Nimomuza, H., Fukuoka, H., and Nakahama, D. (1981): Alterations of amygdaloid kindling phenomenon following repeated electroconvulsive shocks in rats. *Folia Psychiatrica et Neurologica Japonica*, 35(2):167–174.

58. Tuff, L. P., Racine, R. J., and Adamec, R. (1983): The effects of kindling on GABA-mediated inhibition in the dentate gyrus of the rat: I. Paired pulse depression. *Brain Res.*, 277:79–90.

59. Tuff, L. P., Racine, R. J., and Mishra, R. K. (1983): The effects of kindling on GABA-mediated inhibition in the dentate gyrus of the Rat. II. Receptor binding. *Brain Res.*, 277:91–98.

60. Urca, G., and Frenk, H. (1982): Electroconvulsive shock disrupts amygdaloid kindling: Dissociation between behavioural and electrographic events. *Exp. Neurol.*, 78:492–502.

61. Valdes, F., Dashieff, R. M., Birmingham, F., Crutcher, K. A., and McNamara, J. O. (1982): Benzodiazepine receptor increases following repeated seizures: Evidence for localization to dentate granule cells. *Proc. Natl. Acad. Sci. USA*, 79:193–197.

62. Wasterlain, C. G., and Farber, D. B. (1982): A lasting change in protein phosphorylation associated with septal kindling. *Brain Res.*, 247:191–194.

63. Winn, H. R., Welsh, J. E., Bryner, C., Rubio, R., and Berne, R. M. (1979): Brain adenosine production during the initial 60 seconds of bicuculline seizures in rats. *Acta Neurol. Scand.*, [Suppl. 72] 60:536–537.

64. Wise, R. A., and Chinermain, J. (1974): Effects of diazepam and phenobarbital on electrically-induced amygdaloid seizures and seizure development. *Exp. Neurol.*, 45:355–363.

65. Wybenga, M. P., Murphy, M. G., and Robertson, H. A. (1981): Rapid changes in cerebellar adenosine receptors following experimental seizures. *Eur. J. Pharmacol.* 75:79–80.

The Limbic System: Functional Organization and
Clinical Disorders, edited by B. K. Doane and
K. E. Livingston. Raven Press, New York © 1986.

Mechanisms of Kindling: A Current View

*R. J. Racine and †D. McIntyre

*Department of Psychology, McMaster University, Hamilton, Ontario, Canada L8S 4K1
and †Department of Psychology, Carleton University, Ottawa, Ontario, Canada

Kindling is a permanent increase in epileptogenicity produced by spaced, re-peated electrical or chemical stimulation of the brain. Our objective in this chapter is to review some of the major hypotheses concerning the mechanisms underlying the kindling phenomenon, particularly those from our own laboratories. Many of these hypotheses have been discarded following the research they generated, but that research has nevertheless advanced our understanding of brain function. The chapter concludes with an outline of current working hypotheses. For more complete reviews of the kindling literature see Racine (46); McNamara et al. (36); Kalichman (25), and Peterson and Albertson (43).

THE SYNAPTIC POTENTIATION HYPOTHESES

One of the most striking characteristics of the kindling phenomenon is the growth in the strength of the electroencephalographic epileptiform afterdischarge (AD). The ictal spikes that are triggered within the stimulation site generally start out quite large. Spikes recorded from secondary sites are initially small and clearly evoked. Although the primary site spikes increase in amplitude as kindling pro-gresses, the most dramatic changes occur in secondary sites. In some of these, the spikes more than double in size while still appearing to be evoked. The animal shown in Fig. 1 was kindled in the amygdala and recordings were taken from several brain sites. During the first 5 or 10 sec, the secondary site AD spikes increased in amplitude but continued to be evoked even after the animal had become fully kindled (Fig. 1, AD No. 8). Although there are a number of possible expla-nations for these developments, we initially hypothesized an increase in the strength of excitatory synaptic connections between the primary and secondary sites (45,48).

We now know that kindling does produce a long-term potentiation effect in activated pathways. If stimulation pulses are applied to the amygdala before and after the completion of kindling, the responses evoked in target sites will be increased in amplitude (18,48,53,57,58). We also know that prior application of stimulation trains that are below threshold for the triggering of AD activity, but above threshold for the development of long-term potentiation (LTP), will facilitate subsequent kindling (53). Together, these results were quite encouraging. More recent results, however, suggest that LTP is not likely to be a primary mechanism

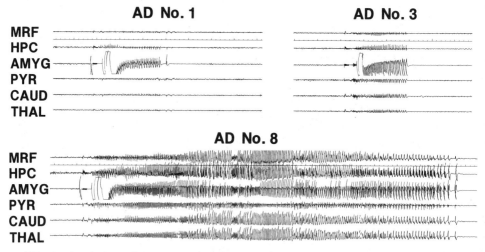

FIG. 1. A typical growth in the strength of the epileptiform afterdischarge is shown for an animal kindled in the amygdala (AMYG). The first discharge (AD No. 1) is relatively brief, and the propagation to secondary sites is weak. The third AD (AD No. 3) is still brief but propagation to secondary sites has already increased. By the eighth AD (AD No. 8), this animal is showing a full strength ictal discharge which was accompanied by a stage 5 convulsion. MRF, mesencephalic reticular formation; HPC, hippocampus; PYR, pyriform cortex; CAUD, caudate nucleus; THAL, thalamus. The second line in each set of traces is from a 1-sec timer.

of kindling, although it undoubtedly plays a role in the increase in the propagation of the discharge.

One of the first clues that kindling was based on more than LTP was that the kindling-induced potentiation effect was often unpredictable. In many cases the potentiation produced by kindling appeared to be much greater than that produced during LTP experiments (53). Our initial conclusion was that kindling resulted in very strong LTP effects, possibly owing to the increased levels of activation achieved during ictal discharges. In other cases, however, the amount of potentiation was about the same, or even less, than was seen during LTP experiments (52). In addition, the level of potentiation seen after kindling appeared to be dependent on the behavioral state to a much greater degree than after an LTP experiment. For example, the very large responses were generally only seen when the animal was in a relaxed state. We apparently had been confusing two different effects during these observations. The very large "potentiated" responses turned out to be evoked epileptiform spikes of the interictal type (22,49). It was shown that these spikes were morphologically similar to spontaneous spikes (49). Finally, drugs like diazepam, which blocked the spontaneous spikes, also blocked the evoked spikes while leaving the potentiated primary evoked response intact (ref. 51; Racine and Milgram, *unpublished observations*).

We have recently mapped various types of potentiation effects in the rat limbic forebrain, and these experiments have revealed further differences between kindling and long-term potentiation (52). Those structures which show the strongest LTP effects tend to kindle more slowly than structures showing weak LTP effects. For example, pathways into and out of the hippocampus generally support large LTP effects. Those same pathways, or their target structures, kindle quite slowly (that is, they require a large number of stimulations to develop stage 5 generalized convulsions). The lateral olfactory tract, on the other hand, kindles very rapidly but produces little or no potentiation effects in its target sites (52).

A comparison of the time course for both LTP and kindling phenomena also argues against a causal relationship. LTP can peak, or reach saturation, after a small number of trains. Kindling requires a minimum, in the most sensitive sites, of 5 or 6 epileptogenic stimulation trains to develop the stage 5 response. Most structures or pathways require between 10 and 100 stimulation trains. LTP, in our hands, decays with time constants between 4 and 15 days (52), whereas kindling appears to be permanent (45,46).

The epileptiform discharges triggered by kindling stimulations appear to recruit activity in several other structures. It was possible that the LTP effects produced by kindling were amplified because they were produced in multiple sites. We attempted to test this hypothesis by applying LTP-inducing trains in several different pathways. The expectation was that animals treated with multiple trains would show a greater facilitation of subsequent kindling than animals exposed to trains at only one site. There was, however, no difference between the groups (53).

Drugs that block kindling (e.g., diazepam) do not appear to block LTP effects (Racine and Milgram, *unpublished observations*). Drugs that facilitate kindling [e.g., reserpine, 6-hydroxydopamine (6-OHDA)] have either no effect on LTP (12,56) or may even interfere with LTP (5). Outbred rat strains that kindle rapidly do not differ in their expression of LTP effects from strains that kindle slowly (M. Steingart and R. Racine, *in preparation*).

Taken together, these observations provide convincing evidence that LTP cannot be the primary mechanism underlying the kindling phenomenon. It remains to be seen whether LTP contributes to the kindling effect. It may, for example, facilitate the development of discharge propagation. The partial facilitation of kindling by prior LTP-treatment suggests such an effect. It must be pointed out, however, that effects other than LTP may be produced during the application of potentiating trains, and it might be these effects that facilitate subsequent kindling.

THE DISINHIBITION HYPOTHESES

Epileptiform responses typically involve high levels of activation at the neuronal level. This activation takes the form of rapid discharge rates at the cellular level and a high degree of synchrony of discharge at the circuit level (11,44). The level of activation could be raised by an increase in the efficacy of excitatory synapses, but it might also be caused by a reduction of inhibition. The inhibition could be synaptic [mediated, for example, by gamma aminobutyric acid (GABA)], or it could be a voltage or ion-mediated inhibition (such as the CA^+-dependent after-hyperpolarization seen in certain pyramidal cells, e.g., ref. 40).

GABA Systems

One of the most effective means of triggering epileptiform discharge pharmacologically is by the application of drugs that interfere with GABA-mediated inhibition. At least some of these epileptic responses are similar in appearance to kindled responses (24). In addition, one of the most effective ways of blocking kindled responses is by the application of diazepam, a drug that is believed to activate GABA systems (50). There is also some evidence that GABA systems may be hypofunctional in some types of clinical epilepsy (55).

For these reasons, one of the disinhibition hypotheses that we entertained was that kindling is based on a reduction in GABA-mediated inhibition. The system that we tested was the perforant path input to the granule cells of the dentate gyrus. This pathway arises from the entorhinal cortex and produces a predominantly excitatory effect in the dentate gyrus granule cells. The excitation is followed by a powerful recurrent inhibitory effect that is believed to be mediated by GABA. GABA produces its inhibitory effect by activating chloride channels (13). The GABA inhibition lasts for about 100 msec and peaks at about 10 to 15 msec (59). In addition to the recurrent inhibition effects, there is a long-lasting afterhyperpolarization of granule cells which peaks at about 150 msec and has a half decay time of about 250 msec and which may be mediated by a voltage-dependent and/ or CA^{2+}-dependent activation of K^+ channels (40,59). This system, then, allows us to examine both types of inhibitory effect. Furthermore, because of the uniform orientation of granule cells, and because the perforant path activates many granule cells simultaneously, it was possible to use field potential recording techniques to monitor the levels of inhibition (28). This is, of course, a less direct test of inhibition than would be provided by intracellular recording, but it has the advantage that we can run chronic experiments covering a period of several weeks.

We tested inhibitory effects in the dentate gyrus by application of paired pulses (60). The first pulse triggered cell discharge (measured in the population response as a population spike, ref. 28), whereas the amplitude of the second component was affected, in part, by the strength of inhibition. By varying the interval between stimulation pulses, we could measure both strength and duration of the paired pulse depression effect. We assumed that the early component of depression (particularly around 20 msec) was dominated by GABA-mediated recurrent inhibition effects, and that the late component of inhibition (200 msec and beyond) was dominated by the late afterhyperpolarization effects. These assumptions appeared to be supported by the effects of GABA drugs (e.g., picrotoxin, muscimol, etc.), which affected primarily the early component of depression (60).

Our experiment involved the measurement of paired pulse depression effects before and after kindling. Rather than producing a disinhibition effect, kindling resulted in an increased inhibition. Both the early and the late components were affected by kindling, but the early components appeared to be affected more consistently. The effect of kindling, in fact, was very similar to the effect of diazepam, which also increases both the early and the late components of depression. In the same series of experiments we assayed for both GABA and benzodiazepine receptor binding. Kindling produced a significant increase in the number of benzodiazepine but not GABA receptors (61).

J. Miller and co-workers (42) at the University of British Columbia have also been looking at the effects of kindling on inhibition in the hippocampus. They kindled the hippocampal commissure and looked at IPSPs recorded intracellularly from both granule cells and pyramidal cells. They too found an increase in inhibition in granule cells (but not pyramidal cells). This granule cell inhibition appeared not to be Cl-mediated, and it lasted for a long period of time ($>$ 10 sec) in kindled slices, suggesting that the effect was primarily on the late afterhyperpolarization.

G. King and R. Dingledine *(personal communication)* have also looked at paired pulse effects in the hippocampal slice (using field potential techniques), and they found an increase in the depression effects similar to ours in the intact preparation. They also found evidence for some decrease of inhibition in area CA1. Additional evidence for a kindling-induced increase in inhibition, at least in the hippocampus, has been provided by Goddard (17), Maru et al. (29), and Adamec and Stark-Adamec (1). In previous single-cell recording experiments (54) we had found an increase in both the excitatory and the recurrent inhibitory responses in cells beneath the tip of an amygdala kindling electrode.

Taken together, these results do not provide much support for the hypothesis that kindling is based on a reduction of recurrent inhibition (particularly not GABA-mediated inhibition) or on a reduction in the late afterhyperpolarization. More areas must be sampled, however, before we can confidently exclude these possibilities.

Noradrenergic Systems

The other major inhibitory system to receive attention from kindling researchers is the noradrenergic system. Although the reports have been mixed, the predominant effect of norepinephrine (NE) in the forebrain (at least at α-receptors) appears to be inhibitory (27,39). Interest in the catecholamine systems increased after a report by Arnold et al. (4) that both reserpine and 6-OHDA greatly facilitated amygdala kindling. This effect was replicated and extended by Corcoran et al. (9).

Although most of the other putative transmitter systems have been investigated over the years, manipulation of the noradrenergic systems has yielded the most consistent results. Much of the recent work on noradrenergic systems and kindling has come from the laboratories of M. Corcoran of the University of Victoria and D. McIntyre of Carleton University. McIntyre et al. (33) found that a combination of 6-OHDA and desmethylimipramine (which should protect NE but not dopamine terminals) was much less effective for producing a seizure-prone animal than was 6-OHDA by itself. This result suggests that the NE system is more important for the modulation of the kindling rate than is the dopamine (DA) system (31,33). This conclusion is supported by the finding that neither pimozide (a DA antagonist) nor apomorphine (a DA agonist) had an effect on kindling rates when administered before each kindling stimulation (8), whereas propranolol (a β-adrenergic antagonist) and disulfiram (a dopamine-β-hydroxylase inhibitor) facilitated kindling.

6-OHDA lesions restricted to the ascending NE pathways have been shown to facilitate both amygdala kindling (10) and neocortical kindling (3). Ehlers et al. (14) found that knife cuts restricted to ascending NE pathways resulted in faster kindling. McIntyre (30) showed that a relatively restricted NE reduction (without DA reduction) in the pyriform-amygdala region also resulted in more rapid kindling.

NE reduction clearly facilitates kindling. It is less clear whether kindling affects the function of NE systems. If kindling is based on a noradrenergic disinhibition mechanism, then the NE system should be found to be hypofunctional. A number of assay experiments have tested postkindling levels of transmitters, enzymes, receptors, and so on, but the results are inconclusive (25,43). It would appear that the NE system is more consistently implicated than are other transmitter or neuromodulatory systems.

Fargo and Blackwood (15) reported decreases in tyrosine hydroxylase activity in the stimulated amygdala 1 month after completion of kindling, suggesting a reduced catecholamine production. Gallaghan and Schwark (8) found that NE, but not DA, content was reduced in several brain sites after kindling. McNamara (35) reported a decrease in the number of β-adrenergic receptor sites 3 days after the last kindling stimulation, and McIntyre and Roberts (32) found a similar reduction 23 days after completion of kindling. Reduction has also been reported for the α_2-adrenergic receptors following kindling (19).

Animals that have naturally low levels of monoamines also appear to be more sensitive to epileptogenic treatment. Genetically epilepsy-prone rats, for example, have been shown to have low levels of both NE and 5-hydroxytryptamine (5-HT)(21) and low turnover rates of NE (20). R. Racine and M. Steingart have bred kindling-prone and kindling-resistant rat strains at McMaster University. The kindling-prone strains showed significantly lower levels of NE but not DA in the pyriform lobe (Racine, Burnham, and Steingart, *in preparation*).

Although the evidence indicates that kindling can produce abnormalities in various transmitter systems (particularly the NE system), it remains to be seen whether these changes underlie the increased epileptogenesis in kindled animals. It is also not yet clear what abnormalities the various measures reflect. Although there have been several reports of decreased NE levels, there have also been reports of increased levels (6). In addition, turnover rates of NE have been reported to be unaffected by kindling (62), as has spontaneous and potassium-stimulated release of NE from several brain regions (26). This area is likely to remain controversial for some years to come, but the weight of evidence, such as it is, appears to point more strongly toward an involvement of NE systems than of other transmitter systems thus far tested.

THE "BURST RESPONSE" HYPOTHESES

The previously described hypotheses focused on changes at the synapse. The hypotheses considered in this section hold that the increased epileptogenesis seen in kindled animals may be due to a change in the response characteristics of the affected cells. This change could, of course, come about as a result of a reduction in tonic inhibition. In that case the mechanisms might be similar to those described in the previous section. A change in the response characteristics of the cells could also result from changes within the cell itself (e.g., a change in ion pump mechanisms, the gating characteristics of ion channels, the ability of the cell to regulate internal free ion levels, the voltage- or CA^{2+}-activated increases in K^+ conductances, etc.). Epileptiform responses can be induced in single cells, for example, by intracellular injections of scorpion venom, which alters the gating mechanism of sodium channels (2).

To investigate possible changes in response properties, it was necessary to determine more precisely which cells were affected by the kindling process. There seems to be an implicit assumption in much of the kindling literature that the stimulation site is somehow equivalent to a "primary focus," which is not necessarily true. Kindling can be accomplished by stimulation of fiber pathways, for example, and few would argue that a fiber pathway can serve as a focus.

Racine et al. (49) began a series of experiments that were designed, in part, to localize the affected cells more precisely. The working assumption was that the cells that served as the focus for spontaneous interictal activity in kindled animals were also the cells that contributed most strongly to the development of seizure susceptibility in those animals. An additional hypothesis was that area CA3 in the hippocampus might serve as the primary generator for interictal activity in kindled animals. This was based on the demonstration that area CA3 is the burst generator for penicillin-induced epileptiform responses (37,63). The development of interictal spikes was monitored in several brain areas during kindling. The main finding was that an area, or areas, in the pyriform lobe appeared to be the generator for interictal discharge, regardless of which brain area was kindled (22). These findings have subsequently been extended to additional areas, so that we now know that interictal discharge appears first in the pyriform/entorhinal/amygdala region even though the kindling stimulation may have been applied to the hippocampus, septal area, fornix/fimbria, perforant path, amygdala, or lateral olfactory tract (ref. 22; Kairiss and Smith, *in preparation*). The other structures recorded included the caudate nucleus, thalamus, and mesencephalic reticular formation. Figure 2 shows both spontaneous and evoked epileptiform spikes from an amygdala-kindled animal. Both interictal and postictal spikes are shown.

Before it became clear that the hippocampus was not the best candidate for a generator of interictal discharge, we examined the responses of hippocampal slices taken from animals kindled in the hippocampus and other areas (22,23). We looked at both field responses and intracellular responses in these slice preparations. We tested the slices in normal bathing medium and in medium containing high concentrations of K^+. We had expected more epileptogenic activity in slices from kindled animals, at least in high K^+ medium. Most of the slices did not appear to differ from control slices on any of the measures taken. There were, however, a small number of slices from kindled animals that showed increased epileptogenic

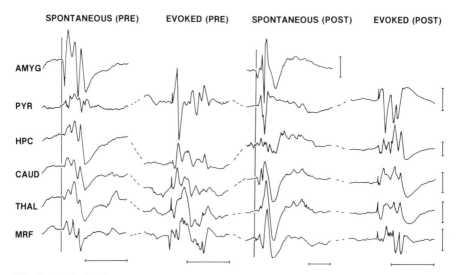

FIG. 2. Typical epileptiform spikes are shown for an animal kindled in the amygdala (AMYG). Both spontaneous and evoked spikes are shown either 48 hr after the 10th and just preceding (PRE) the 11th discharge or within 1 min after (POST) the 11th discharge. The vertical line through the spontaneous spikes indicates the spike onset, which appears to lead in the amygdala. PYR, pyriform cortex; HPC, hippocampus; CAUD, caudate nucleus; THAL, thalamus; MRF, mesencephalic reticular formation. Calibration: 75 msec; 1,500 μV.

activity in the field responses (22). The intracellular measures showed a similar indication of minor alterations in hippocampal tissue. Again, most cells did not appear to differ from control cells. Even those cells that did differ were the same on most of the measures (resting membrane potential, membrane time constants, excitatory postsynaptic potential (EPSP) amplitudes, etc.). When depolarizing pulses were applied directly to the cell, however, some of the cells from kindled slices showed strong burst responses. These depolarizing pulses bypass the usual synaptic activation and raise the possibility that the response properties, particularly the action potential generating properties, are altered. Oliver et al. (41) and King and Dingledine *(personal communication)* have also found an increased probability of epileptiform activity in hippocampal slices taken from kindled animals.

If the cells in the pyriform lobe, however, are *more* susceptible to the development of chronic epileptogenesis than are other cells, then it would be of considerable interest to look at cell responses within that area. Racine and Zaide (54) recorded, extracellularly, from single cells beneath the tip of the amygdala kindling electrode. These cells, and cells in the contralateral amygdala, were found to generate strong bursts of cell discharge. These bursts were not seen in control tissue. Fujita and Sakuranaga (16), in contrast, recorded only hyperpolarizations from hippocampal cells during interictal spikes.

Kairiss et al. (22) attempted to record from pyriform slices taken from kindled animals, without much success. These slices were taken in a roughly horizontal plane so that the lateral olfactory tract could be included. McIntyre, Wong, and

Miles (ref. 34 and *in preparation*) recently had considerable success with slices taken in a coronal plane. These slices included both amygdala and pyriform cortex, and they reliably showed epileptiform responses to directly applied electrical pulses. The epileptiform responses could be recorded from both amygdala and pyriform tissue. Intracellular recordings revealed strong burst discharges in both cell types. Slices taken from kindled animals showed reliably stronger epileptiform responses than those from control animals (Fig. 3).

In both intact preparations and slice preparations, then, the cells in the pyriform lobe appeared to be more prone to the development of chronic epileptogenicity than cells in the hippocampus. Now that the optimal regions have been determined, the way is clear for the application of neurophysiological techniques that will increase our understanding of the mechanisms underlying chronic epileptogenesis.

CURRENT HYPOTHESES

Racine and Burnham outlined a series of hypotheses about the mechanisms underlying kindling phenomena. Of interest here is their view of the mechanisms of the development of epileptogenicity in the kindled preparation. The electro-physiological experiments described above indicate that the cells that are most

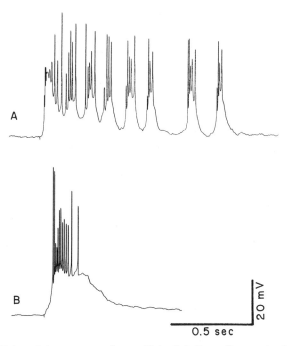

FIG. 3. Typical intracellular response of pyramidal cells in the pyriform cortex *in vitro* to synaptic input following an electrical pulse to the amygdala. **A:** Burst response with afterdischarges in tissue from a kindled rat. **B:** Burst response from a control rat. Note that the full magnitude of the action potentials has been diminished in the slow-timed *X – Y* plots.

prone to the triggering of epileptiform discharge in the acute preparation (e.g., hippocampal CA3 cells) are not the same as those that develop chronic epileptogenic properties (e.g., cells in the pyriform lobe). This difference in susceptibility to the development of chronic seizure activity can be seen in other models as well. Morillo et al. (38), for example, reported that interictal spiking appeared in subcortical structures prior to their appearance in the cortex in animals with aluminum chloride lesions of the neocortex. In at least some of these animals, the amygdala appeared to be the first structure affected. Racine and Burnham (47) described a sequence of events which they believed to be critical for the occurrence of kindling. We repeat that sequence here with slight modifications based on recent data: (a) If the kindling stimulus is applied to a structure outside the pyriform lobe, reactive discharges will eventually come to be elicited from the pyriform lobe (possibly owing to potentiation effects). (b) Once discharges begin to be triggered from structures in the pyriform lobe, the response characteristics of the cells in that region are altered. (c) The mechanism by which these response properties are altered has yet to be determined, but one possibility is a decrement in tonic inhibition provided by noradrenergic systems. Another possibility is a change within the cell itself (in membrane properties or the buffering of cations, for example). (d) Whatever the mechanism, the cells become capable of generating large depolarization shifts and strong bursts of action potentials in response to apparently unaltered input. (e) The synchronous bursts that are generated within the pyriform lobe provide a strong activation and recruitment of target structures into the discharge. (f) Although cells in other regions may be less sensitive than are cells in the pyriform region, many of these cells will also begin to show altered response characteristics after sufficiently intense and prolonged continual activation. (g) When the level of activation of forebrain structures is sufficiently strong, the convergence of this activity into brainstem motor regions drives the skeletal motor response. It remains to be seen whether there are changes localized to the brainstem or if this area is passively driven by the forebrain. (h) The strength of the convulsive response is largely determined by the level of activation of the brainstem structures that drive the response.

With respect to (f) above, we now believe that the pyriform region simply contains the most sensitive cells and that cells in other regions will also be affected if sufficiently driven. One of the reasons for this belief is the finding by Kairiss, Smith, and Racine (ref. 23 and *in preparation*) that some cells in the hippocampus are affected by kindling. Also relevant is the finding by Racine, Paxinos, Kairiss, Ngan, and Smith *(in preparation)* that large, bilateral radio frequency lesions of the pyriform lobe (including amygdala and pyriform cortex) retarded, but did not block, kindling of the septal area. Cain (7) reported that amygdala lesions retarded, but did not block olfactory bulb kindling. In fact, knife cuts or lesions of a number of different sites all failed to block kindling (Racine, Paxinos, et al., *in preparation*).

We believe that the findings reported in this review reflect substantial progress in the attempt to determine the mechanisms of kindling. It is still necessary to determine more precisely which cells are affected by the kindling stimulus, but the work of McIntyre and Wong *(in preparation)* suggests that they may be rather widespread, at least within the pyriform region. Further work should indicate if there is a smaller pacemaker population and shed light on the mechanism of burst generation in those cells.

REFERENCES

1. Adamec, R. E., and Stark-Adamec, C. (1983): Partial kindling and emotional bias in the cat: Lasting aftereffects of partial kindling of the ventral hippocampus. II. Physiological changes. *Behav. Neural. Biol.*, 38:223–239.
2. Allan, N., and Woody, C. D. (1983): Epileptiform activity induced in single cells of the sensori-motor cortex of the cat by intracellularly applied Scorpion venom. *Exp. Neurol.*, 80:491–497.
3. Altman, I. M., and Corcoran, M. E. (1983): Facilitation of neocortical kindling by depletion of forebrain noradrenaline. *Brain Res.*, 270:174–177.
4. Arnold, P. S., Racine, R. J., and Wise, R. A. (1973): Effects of atropine, reserpine, 6-hydroxy-dopamine, and handling on seizure development in the rat. *Exp. Neurol.*, 40:457–470.
5. Bliss, T. V. P., Goddard, G. V., and Riives, M. (1983): Reduction of long-term potentiation in the dentate gyrus of the rat following selective depletion of monoamines. *J. Physiol.*, 334:475–491.
6. Burnham, W. M., King, G. A., and Lloyd, K. G. (1981): Extra-focal catecholamine levels in kindled rat forebrain. *Prog. Neuropsychopharmacol.*, 5:537–541.
7. Cain, D. P. (1977): Seizure development following repeated electrical stimulation of central olfactory structures. *Ann. NY Acad. Sci.*, 290:200–216.
8. Callaghan, D. A., and Schwark, W. S. (1979): Involvement of catecholamines in kindled amygdaloid convulsions in the rat. *Neuropharmacology*, 18:541–545.
9. Corcoran, M. E., Fibiger, H. C., McCaughran, J. A., and Wada, J. A. (1974): Potentiation of amygdaloid kindling and metrazol-induced seizures by 6-hydroxydopamine in rats. *Exp. Neurol.*, 45:118–133.
10. Corcoran, M. E., and Mason, S. T. (1980): Role of forebrain catecholamines in amygdala kindling. *Brain Res.*, 190:473–484.
11. Dichter, M., and Spencer, W. A. (1969): Penicillin-induced interictal discharge from the cat hippocampus. I. Characteristics and topographic features. *J. Neurophysiol.*, 32:649–662.
12. Dunwiddie, T. V., Robertson, N. L., and Worth, T. (1982): Modulation of long-term potentiation: effects of adrenergic and neuroleptic drugs. *Pharmacol. Biochem. Behav.*, 17:1257–1264.
13. Eccles, J., Nicoll, R. A., Oshima, T., and Rubia, F. J. (1977): The anionic permeability of the inhibitory postsynaptic membrane of hippocampal pyramidal cell. *Proc. Roy. Soc. B.*, 198:345–364.
14. Ehlers, C. L., Clifton, D. K., and Sawyer, C. H. (1980): Facilitation of amygdala kindling in the rat by transecting ascending noradrenergic pathways. *Brain Res.*, 189:274–278.
15. Fargo, I. B., and Blackwood, D. H. R. (1978): Reduction in tyrosine hydroxylase activity in the rat amygdala induced by kindling stimulation. *Brain Res.*, 153:423–426.
16. Fujita, Y., and Sakuranaga, M. (1981): Spontaneous hyperpolarizations in pyramidal cells of chronically stimulated rabbit hippocampus. *Jpn. J. Physiol.*, 31:879–889.
17. Goddard, G. V. (1982): Separate analysis of lasting alteration in excitatory synapses, inhibitory synapses and cellular excitability in association with kindling. *Kyoto Symposium (EEG Suppl. No. 36)*, 288–294.
18. Goddard, G. V., and Douglas, R. M. (1975): Does the engram of kindling model the engram of normal long term memory? *Can. J. Neurol. Sci.*, 2:385–394.
19. Jeffreys, J. G. R., and Stanford, S. C. (1983): Changes in A2- and B-adrenoceptor binding sites in amygdala kindled rat brain. *Neurosci. Abst.*, 9:487.
20. Jobe, P. C., Kwang, H. K., and Dailey, J. W. (1984): Abnormalities in norepinephrine turnover rate in the central nervous system of the genetically epilepsy-prone rat. *Brain Res.*, 290:357–360.
21. Jobe, P. C., Laird, H. E., Ko, K. H., Ray, T. and Daily, J. W. (1982): Abnormalities in monoamine levels in the central nervous system of the genetically epilepsy-prone rat. *Epilepsia*, 23:359–366.
22. Kairiss, E. W., Racine, R. J., and Smith, G. K. (1984): The development of the interictal spike during kindling in the rat. *Brain Res.*, 322:101–110.

23. Kairiss, E. W., Smith, G. K., and Racine, R. J. (1983): Intracellular observations in *in vitro* hippocampus of kindled rats. *Neurosci. Abst.*, 9:489.
24. Kalichman, M. W. (1982): Pharmacological investigation of convulsant γ-aminobutyric acid (GABA) antagonists in amygdala-kindled rats. *Epilepsia*, 23:163–172.
25. Kalichman, M. W. (1982): Neurochemical correlates of the kindling model of epilepsy. *Neurosci. Behav. Rev., 6:165–181.*
26. Kant, G. J., Meyerhoff, J. L., and Corcoran, M. E. (1980): Release of norepinephrine and dopamine from brain region of amygdaloid-kindled rats. *Exp. Neurol.*, 70:701–705.
27. Langmoen, I. A., Segal, M., and Andersen, P. (1981): Mechanisms of norepinephrine actions on hippocampal pyramidal cells in vitro. *Brain Res.*, 208:349–362.
28. Lomo, T. (1971): Patterns of activation in a monosynaptic cortical pathway: the perforant path input to the dentate area of the hippocampal formation. *Exp. Brain Res.*, 12:18–45.
29. Maru, E., Tatsumo, J., Okamoto, J., and Ashida, H. (1982): Development and reduction of synaptic potentiation induced by perforant path kindling. *Exp. Neurol.*, 78:409–424.
30. McIntyre, D. C. (1980): Amygdala kindling in rats. Facilitation after local amygdala norepinephrine depletion with 6-hydroxydopamine. *Exp. Neurol.*, 69:395–407.
31. McIntyre, D. C., and Edson, N. (1981): Facilitation of amygdala kindling after norepinephrine depletion with 6-hydroxydopamine in rats. *Exp. Neurol.*, 74:748–757.
32. McIntyre, D. C., and Roberts, D. C. S. (1983): Long-term reduction in beta-adrenergic receptor binding after amygdala kindling in rats. *Exp. Neurol.*, 82:17–24.
33. McIntyre, D. C., Saari, M. and Pappas, B. A. (1979): Potentiation of amygdala kindling in adult or infant rats by injection of 6-hydroxydopamine. *Exp. Neurol.*, 63:527–544.
34. McIntyre, D. C., Wong, R. K. S., and Miles, R. (1983): Effect of amygdala kindling on pyriform cortex response: intracellular studies with in vitro slice. *Neurosci. Abst.*, 9:764.
35. McNamara, J. O. (1978): Selective alterations of regional beta-adrenergic receptor binding in the kindling model of epilepsy. *Exp. Neurol.*, 61:582–591.
36. McNaramara, J., Byrne, M., Dashieff, R., and Fitz, J. (1980): The kindling model of epilepsy: A review. *Prog. Neurobiol.*, 15:139–159.
37. Mesher, R. A., and Schartzkroin, P. A. (1980): Can CA3 epileptiform discharge induce bursting in normal CA1 hippocampal neurons? *Brain Res.*, 183:472–476.
38. Morillo, L. E., Ebner, T. J., and Bloedel, J. R. (1982): The early involvement of subcortical structures during the development of a cortical seizure focus. *Epilepsia*, 23:571–585.
39. Mueller, A. L., Hoffer, B. J., and Dunwiddie, T. V. (1981): Noradrenergic responses in rat hippocampus: evidence for mediation by α and β receptors in the *in vitro* slice. *Brain Res.* 214:113–126.
40. Nicoll, R. A., and Alger, B. E. (1981): Synaptic excitation may activate a calcium dependent potassium conductance in hippocampal pyramidal cells. *Science*, 212:957–959.
41. Oliver, A. P., Hoffer, B. J., and Wyatt, R. J. (1980): Kindling induces long-lasting alterations in response of hippocampal neurons to elevated potassium levels in vitro. *Science*, 208:1264–1265.
42. Oliver, M. W., and Miller, J. J. (1983): Characteristics of inhibitory processes in the dentate gyrus following kindling-induced epilepsy. *Neurosci. Abst.*, 9:484.
43. Peterson, S. L., and Albertson, T. E. (1982): Neurotransmitter and neuromodulator function in the kindled seizure and state. *Prog. Neurobiol.*, 19:237–270.
44. Prince, D. A. (1978): Neurophysiology of epilepsy. *Ann. Rev. Neurosci.*, 1:395–415.
45. Racine, R. J. (1972): Modification of seizure activity by electrical stimulation: II. Motor seizure. *EEG Clin. Neurophysiol.*, 32:281–294.
46. Racine, R. (1978): Kindling: The first decade. *Neurosurgery*, 3:234–252.
47. Racine, R. J., and Burnham, W. M. (1984): The kindling model. In: *The electrophysiology of epilepsy*, pp. 153–171, edited by P. Schwartzkroin, and H. Wheal. Academic Press, London.
48. Racine, R. J., Gartner, J. G., and Burnham, W. M. (1972): Epileptiform activity and neural plasticity in limbic structures. *Brain Res.*, 47:262–268.
49. Racine, R., Kairiss, E., and Smith, G. (1981): Kindling mechanisms: The evolution of the burst response versus enhancement. In: *Kindling 2*, edited by J. A. Wada. pp. 15–29.
50. Racine, R., Livingston, K., and Joaquin, A. (1975): Effects of procaine hydrochloride, diazepam, and diphenylhydantoin on seizure development in cortical and subcortical structures in rats. *EEG Clin. Neurophysiol.*, 38:355–365.
51. Racine, R., and Milgram, W. N. (1980): Post-activation potentiation and epilepsy. In: *Neurophysiological mechanisms of epilepsy*, edited by V. M. Okujava. pp. 166–173. Metsniereba, Tbilisi.

52. Racine, R. J., Milgram, N. W., and Hafner, S. (1983): Long-term potentiation phenomena in the rat limbic forebrain. *Brain Res.*, 260:217–231.
53. Racine, R., Newberry, F., and Burnham, W. M. (1975): Post-activation potentiation and the kindling phenomenon. *EEG Clin. Neurophysiol.*, 39:261–271.
54. Racine, R. J., and Zaide, J. (1978): A further investigation into the mechanisms of the kindling phenomenon. In: *Limbic Mechanisms: The Continuing Evolution of the Limbic System Concept*, edited by K. Livingston, and O. Hornykiewicz. pp. 457–493. Plenum Press, New York.
55. Ribak, C. E., Harris, A. B., Vaughn, J. E., and Roberts, E. (1979): Inhibitory GABAergic nerve terminals decrease at site of focal epilepsy. *Science*, 205:211–214.
56. Robinson, G. B., and Racine, R. J. (1984): Long-term potentiation in the dentate gyrus: effects of noradrenaline depletion in the awake rat. *Brain Res.*, 325:71–78.
57. Tanaka, A. (1972): Progressive changes of behavioral and electroencephalographic responses to daily amygdaloid stimulations in rabbits. *Fukuoka Acta. Med.*, 63:152–163.
58. Tanaka, T. (1977): Modification of amygdala-cortical evoked potentials by kindling and pentetrazol-induced generalized convulsions in cats. *EEG Clin. Neurophysiol.*, 32:281–294.
59. Thalmann, R. H., and Ayala, G. F. (1982): A late increase in potassium conductance follows synaptic stimulation of granule neurons of the dentate gyrus. *Neurosci. Lett.*, 29:243–248.
60. Tuff, L. P., Racine, R. J., and Adamec, R. (1983): The effects of kindling on GABA-mediated inhibition in the dentate gyrus of the rat. I. Paired pulse depression. *Brain Res.*, 277:79–90.
61. Tuff, L. P., Racine, R. J., and Mishra, R. K. (1983): The effects of kindling on GABA-mediated inhibition in the dentate gyrus of the rat. II. Receptor binding. *Brain Res.*, 277:91–98.
62. Wilkison, D. M., and Halpern, L. M. (1979): Turnover kinetics of dopamine and norepinephrine in the forebrain after kindling in rats. *Neuropharmacology*, 18:219–222.
63. Wong, R. K. S., and Traub, R. D. (1983): Synchronized burst discharge in disinhibited hippocampal slice: I. Initiation in CA2-CA3 region. *J. Neurophysiol.*, 49:442–458.

The Limbic System: Functional Organization and Clinical Disorders, edited by B. K. Doane and K. E. Livingston. Raven Press, New York © 1986.

Biochemical Changes in the Limbic System Following Kindling: Assay Studies

W. M. Burnham, H. B. Niznik, and S. J. Kish

Department of Pharmacology, University of Toronto, Toronto, Ontario, Canada M5S 1A8

When we discuss the topic of epilepsy with medical students, we usually suggest that "seizures don't hurt the brain" and that "the brain functions in a normal fashion between attacks." This point of view, which ignores certain neurological and psychiatric studies (2,7), has seemed justified by the fact that most epileptic patients seem quite normal between seizures.

Recent data derived from the kindling model, however, suggest that our traditional teaching may be overly optimistic. In the kindling model, repeated focal seizures, triggered in the brains of experimental animals (e.g., rats), evolve into focal-generalized attacks, apparently as the result of permanent alterations in brain function (11,23). At least in kindled rats, therefore, seizures *do* cause permanent changes in the brain. It is possible that similar changes take place in the brains of epileptic patients as well (10). This possibility makes it important to investigate the kindling process and to assess kindling-related brain changes in relation to seizure development in humans and to the changes in personality and learning ability that have sometimes been reported.

The search for structural changes in kindled brains has, so far, yielded ambiguous results (23). A number of clear-cut *biochemical* changes have been reported, however, and the field of kindling biochemistry has grown into an extensive one (12). Of particular interest are the postkindling biochemical changes that, like the kindling phenomenon itself, are long lasting. Among these are the drop in calcium binding protein reported by Baimbridge and Miller (1), the reduction in tyrosine hydroxylase activity reported by Farjo and Blackwood (9), and the change in β-noradrenergic binding observed by McIntyre and co-workers (15).

This chapter summarizes recent research concerning a fourth type of long-lasting postkindling change, the change found in benzodiazepine (BZD) receptor binding. This topic is of particular interest because of the close relation of the BZDs to the γ-aminobutyric acid (GABA) system—a system thought to play a major role in seizure control. The field also illustrates some of the complexities involved in the biochemical area and indicates the possibilities for confusion if studies are not pursued in a thorough fashion.

BASIC TECHNIQUE

Before discussing experimental data, it will be useful to summarize the basic technique used in BZD binding studies. We shall concentrate on the protocol used in our own laboratory. (Details appear in refs. 4,19,20.) Other approaches are described by McNamara et al. (16) and Tuff et al. (26).

Our basic design involves a comparison of ^{3}H-flunitrazepam (^{3}H-FLU) binding in the postmortem brains of amygdala-kindled and yoked-control rats. (^{3}H-FLU is a ligand that can be used to preferentially label the "central" type of BZD binding site.) Male Royal Victoria hooded rats are implanted in the right amygdala with chronic stimulating/recording electrodes and are kindled to a criterion of six stage 4-5 (22) seizures. Kindling stimulation is given once a day and consists of a 1-sec train of 60-Hz, biphasic, square-wave pulses with a peak-to-peak intensity of 400 μA. (Yoked controls receive matched handling, but no stimulation.) Following the sixth stage 4-5 seizure, daily stimulation is discontinued and kindled and control subjects are set aside for a stimulation-free interval (2 weeks or 2 months). They are then killed by decapitation, and the brains are quickly removed and frozen (-80°C). ^{3}H-FLU receptor binding is subsequently measured using a standard filtration assay. Nonspecific binding is defined using an excess of either unlabeled diazepam (used by previous workers) or clonazepam (now preferred for its specificity). Estimates of β_{max} (maximum number of binding sites) and K_D (affinity) are made from Scatchard plots.

EXPERIMENTAL RESULTS

The first studies of postkindling BZD receptor binding were done by McNamara et al. (16). Working 24 hours after the last seizure, these workers observed a bilateral elevation of ^{3}H-diazepam binding (β_{max}) in the hippocampi of kindled rats. A subsequent series of reports confirmed and extended these original findings (e.g., ref. 27).

Since McNamara et al. killed their subjects 24 hr after the last seizure, however, the relation of their findings to the kindling phenomenon was hard to interpret. Postictal inhibitory effects are observed in the kindling model (23), and these are still present at 24 hr. The binding abnormalities observed by McNamara et al. might have related either to kindling itself or to such transitory postictal effects.

A subsequent study by Racine's group (26) clarified this issue. Tuff et al. studied ^{3}H-FLU binding in amygdala-kindled and control rats 2 weeks after the sixth generalized convulsion. Since they planned to do GABA binding as well, they utilized a "washed" brain homogenate—a preparation in which the neural membranes are repeatedly centrifuged to remove endogenous GABA. Tuff et al. found not only the bilateral hippocampal elevations in receptor density (15%) previously reported by McNamara's group, but also bilateral elevations in amygdaloid binding (20%). These results confirmed that the kindling technique causes abnormalities in BZD binding and established that these outlast the period of transitory postictal effects.

Our own experiments began with an attempt to duplicate the results of Tuff et al. Since we did not plan to include GABA binding in our experiment, we used a simpler "unwashed" homogenate preparation that omits the multiple centrifugation steps. (This proved to be a significant difference.) Otherwise, our protocol was similar to that of Tuff et al., involving the same strain of rats (Royal Victoria hooded), the same kindling technique and kindling criterion (six generalized convulsions), and sacrifice at the same postseizure interval (2 weeks). Our findings, however, were very different. As indicated by Table 1, we failed to find elevations in either hippocampal or amygdaloid BZD binding. Instead, we found reductions (β_{max}) in two other areas, the hypothalamus and the ipsilateral cortex (19). A series of follow-up experiments confirmed these reductions and indicated that they were long lasting (2 months) and confined to the "central type" of BZD receptor (4).

The results of our follow-up studies strengthened our faith in our own findings. They did nothing, however, to resolve the conflict between our own data and the results obtained by our colleagues at McMaster. A careful examination of experimental protocols suggested that the difference in homogenates might be the crucial variable. We therefore embarked on a study in which both "washed" and "unwashed" homogenates were prepared from brains of the same kindled and control animals (20). The results obtained from the "unwashed" homogenates (not shown) were very similar to our previous findings (Table 1). The results from the "washed" homogenates, however, reproduced the pattern of ³H-FLU binding abnormalities previously reported by Tuff et al: ³H-FLU binding was normal in the hypothalamus and cortex, but bilateral elevations were seen in the amygdala and hippocampus (Table 2).

GENERAL DISCUSSION

What conclusions can be drawn from these paradoxical data? For clarity it will be useful to divide the discussion into three areas: (a) biochemical nature of the changes, (b) possible functional implications, and (c) clinical implications.

TABLE 1. β_{max} for diazepam-displaceable ³H-FLU binding to unwashed homogenates of amygdala-kindled rat brain regions[a]

Region	β_{max} (% of control)	
	Right	Left
Frontal cortex	80% ± 5[c]	97% ± 3
Amygdala pyriform	95% ± 4	93% ± 4
Hippocampus	90% ± 5	91% ± 4
Striatum[b]	104% ± 1	98% ± 5
Hypothalamus	80% ± 3%[c]	

[a]N = 7.
[b]N = 6.
[c]p < .05 as determined by Student's 2-tailed t-test for independent samples.

TABLE 2. β_{max} for ^{3}H-FLU binding to extensively washed, frozen-thawed homogenates of amygdala-kindled rat brain regions[a]

	β_{max} (% of control)	
Region	Right	Left
Frontal cortex	95% ± 5	97% ± 5
Amygdala-pyriform	120% ± 4[c]	120% ± 4[c]
Hippocampus	117% ± 5[c]	118% ± 3[c]
Striatum	92% ± 6	94% ± 8
Hypothalamus[b]	104% ± 8	

[a]$N = 5$.
[b]$N = 4$.
[c]$p < .05$ as determined by Student's 2-tailed t-test for independent samples.

Biochemical Nature of the Changes

The data discussed above make it clear that the kindling technique produces long-lasting ^{3}H-FLU binding abnormalities in the hypothalamus, limbic system, and cortex. The nature of these changes, however, is not clear. It seems unlikely that they represent simple alterations in the quantity of receptor protein, since changes of that sort should be observed in both "washed" and "unwashed" homogenates. As to their actual nature, we have only hypotheses, some of which appear below. None of these hypotheses, unfortunately, explains *both* the elevations and reductions. They account for *either* the reductions or the elevations.

Reduced Binding

The reversible reductions in β_{max} of ^{3}H-FLU binding observed in unwashed homogenates may be due to (a) the presence in kindled brains of noncompetitive inhibitors of ^{3}H-FLU binding, which are removed by the washing procedure (however, see Chiu and Rosenberg, ref. 5); or (b) a loss of receptors in kindled brains, which is restricted to a subpopulation of BZD receptors which disappears during washing (e.g., type II soluble receptors, Lo et al., ref 14; see also ref. 13).

Elevated Binding

The reversible increases in β_{max} observed in washed membranes may be due to either (a) a kindling-induced alteration of membrane structure, such that a proportion of "central type" BZD receptors is protected from solubilization during the washing procedure; or (b) a conversion of super-high (8,17,18) or super-low (3) affinity conformations of the BZD receptor (5) to normal (nM) affinity states in kindled brains. The latter changes might not be detected in unwashed membranes, possibly because of the presence of endogenous ligands/modulators, GABA, or other compounds that would maintain an equilibrium in favor of the super-high or super-low conformational states. Experiments designed to test these possibilities are currently in progress.

Functional Implications

Previous authors have suggested that the binding elevations observed in washed homogenates might be related to a seizure-induced enhancement of GABA-mediated neural inhibition (16,25,27). The present data underline the speculative nature of such theorizing. Increased binding is observed only when washed homogenates are used. Decreased binding is seen in unwashed homogenates, and the nature of the abnormalities (if any) which exist *in vivo* is not yet clear.

Having stated that warning, however, let me join in some speculation. As Dr. Goddard notes in this volume, evoked potentials are potentiated after kindling. More specifically, as Dr. Racine and I reported some years ago (24), they are potentiated in some pathways but not in others. In the amygdala-kindled rat brain, potentials are regularly augmented in the hypothalamus and cortex (Racine, *personal communication*), where Niznik, Kish, and I found BZD binding reductions, but not in the hippocampus or in the amygdala, where elevations in BZD binding are found. (Hippocampal potentials actually show more inhibition after kindling. See ref 25). It is tempting to speculate that these correlations may be more than coincidental. Much more research, however, will be required to put such speculation on a scientific basis.

Clinical Implications

We still have a large number of unanswered questions concerning the binding changes induced by kindling. We do not know, for instance, which aspect of the procedure causes the changes—the electrical stimulation, the repeated focal seizures, or the generalized seizures that develop. We do not know whether the changes relate to induced damage or whether they represent an attempt by the brain to suppress seizures. We do not even know whether the *small* changes reported so far have any *functional* meaning, although the permanent development of generalization in the kindling model indicates that some sort of functional change must take place. All of these questions require further research.

Despite these unanswered questions, however, our biochemical data generally support the notion that seizures change the brain. It may be that they are not the relatively benign phenomena we have believed them to be and that we should be making much more aggressive attempts to stop them in human patients. Further investigations of the effects of seizures on the brain will be required, as well as continuing research designed to develop more effective and less toxic antiseizure drugs.

ACKNOWLEDGMENTS

This work was supported by the Grant MT 5611 from the Medical Research Council of Canada and by the Clarke Institute of Psychiatry. H. B. Niznik has a studentship from the Savoy Foundation for Epilepsy and S. J. Kish is a Career Scientist of the Ontario Ministry of Health. The authors would like to thank Hoffmann-LaRoche Ltd. (Vaudreuil, Quebec) for their generous contributions of diazepam, clonazepam, and RO5-4864.

REFERENCES

1. Baimbridge, K. G., and Miller, J. J. (1982): Immunohistochemical loss of calcium-binding protein from dentate granule cells during kindling induced epilepsy. *Soc. Neurosci. Abst.* 8:457.
2. Bear, D. M., and Fedio, P. (1977): Quantitative analysis of interictal behaviour in temporal lobe epilepsy. *Arch. Neurol.*, 43:454–467.
3. Bowling, A. C., and DeLorenzo, R. J. (1982): Micromolar affinity benzodiazepine receptors: Identification and characterization in central nervous system. *Science*, 216:1247–1250.
4. Burnham, W. M., Niznik, H. B., Okazaki, M. M., and Kish, S. J. (1983): Binding of ^{3}H-flunitrazepam and ^{3}H-RO5-4864 to crude homogenates of amygdala-kindled rat brain: two months post-seizure. *Brain Res.*, 279:359–362.
5. Chiu, T. H., and Rosenberg, H. C. (1981): Endogenous modulator of benzodiazepine binding in rat cortex. *J. Neurochem.*, 36:336–338.
6. Chiu, T. H., and Rosenberg, H. C. (1983): Multiple conformational states of benzodiazepine receptors. *Trends Pharm. Sci.*, 4:348–350.
7. Dodrill, C. B., and Troupin, A. S. (1976): Seizures and adaptive abilities. *Arch. Neurol.*, 60:604–607.
8. Ehlert, F. Y., Roeske, W. R., and Yamamura, H. I. (1981): Multiple benzodiazepine receptors and their regulation by GABA. *Life Sci.*, 29:235–248.
9. Farjo, I. B., and Blackwood, D. H. R. (1978): Reduction in tyrosine hydroxylase activity in the rat amygdala induced by kindling stimulation. *Brain Res.*, 153:423–426.
10. Goddard, G. V. (1983): The kindling model of epilepsy. *Trends Pharm. Sci.*, 6:275–279.
11. Goddard, G. V., McIntyre, D. C., and Leech, C. K. (1969): A permanent change in brain function resulting from daily electrical stimulation. *Exp. Neurol.*, 25:295–330.
12. Kalichman, M. W. (1982): Neurochemical correlates of the kindling model of epilepsy. *Neurosci. Biobehav. Rev.*, 6:165–181.
13. Korneyev, A. Y., and Factor, M. I. (1983): Change in the B_{max} and K_D for ^{3}H-flunitrazepam observed in the course of washing rat brain tissue with distilled water. *Mol. Pharmacol.*, 23:310–314.
14. Lo, M. M. S., Strittmatter, S. M., and Snyder, S. H. (1982): Physical separation and characterization of two types of benzodiazepine receptors. *Proc. Natl. Acad. Sci. USA*, 79:680–684.
15. McIntyre, D. C., Roberts, D. C. S., Milstone, D., Edson, N., and Birras, L. (1982): Long term reduction in beta-adrenergic receptor binding following amygdala-kindling. *Soc. Neurosci. Abst.*, 8:456.
16. McNamara, J. O., Peper, A. M., and Patrone, V. (1980): Repeated seizures induce long term increases in hippocampal benzodiazepine receptors. *Proc. Nat. Acad. Sci. USA*, 77:3029–3032.
17. Mizuno, S., Ogawa, N., and Mori, A. (1982): Super high affinity binding site for ^{3}H-diazepam in the presence of Co^{2+}, Ni^{2+}, Cu^{2+} or Zn^{2+}. *Neurochem. Res.*, 7:1487–1493.
18. Mizuno, S., Ogawa, N., and Mori, A. (1983): Differential effects of some transition metal cations on the binding of B-carboline-3-carboxylate and diazepam. *Neurochem. Res.*, 8:873–880.
19. Niznik, H. B., Kish, S. J., and Burnham, W. M. (1983). Decreased benzodiazepine receptor binding in amygdala kindled rat brains. *Life Sci.*, 33:425–430.
20. Niznik, H. B., Burnham, W. M., and Kish, S. J. (1984): Benzodiazepine receptor binding following amygdala-kindled convulsions: differing results in washed and unwashed brain membranes. *J. Neurochem.*, 43:1732–1736.
21. Olsen, R. W. (1981): The GABA postsynaptic membrane receptor-ionophore complex. Site of action of action of convulsant and anticonvulsant drugs. *Mol. Cell. Biochem.*, 39:261–279.
22. Racine, R. J. (1972): Modification of seizure activity by electrical stimulation: II motor seizure. *EEG Clin. Neurophysiol.*, 32:281–294.
23. Racine, R. J. (1978): Kindling: The first decade. *Neurosurgery*, 3:234–252.
24. Racine, R. J., Gartner, J. G., and Burnham, W. M. (1972): Epileptiform activity and neural plasticity in limbic structures. *Brain Res.*, 47:262–268.
25. Tuff, L. P., Racine, R. J., and Adamec, R. (1983): The effects of kindling on GABA-mediated inhibition in the dentate gyrus of the rat. I. Paired pulse depression. *Brain Res.*, 277:79–90.
26. Tuff, L. P., Racine, R. J., and Mishra, R. K. (1983): The effects of kindling on GABA-mediated inhibition in the dentate-gyrus in the rat. II. Receptor binding. *Brain Res.*, 277:91–98.
27. Valdes, F., Dasheiff, R. M., Birmingham, F., Crutcher, K. A., and McNamara, J. O. (1982): Benzodiazepine receptor increases after repeated seizures: evidence for localization to dentate granule cells. *Proc. Nat. Acad. Sci. USA*, 79:193–197.

The Limbic System: Functional Organization and
Clinical Disorders, edited by B. K. Doane and
K. E. Livingston. Raven Press, New York © 1986.

Limbic Hyperfunction, Limbic Epilepsy, and Interictal Behavior: Models and Methods of Detection

*R. E. Adamec and **C. Stark-Adamec

*Department of Psychology, Memorial University of Newfoundland, St. John's,
Newfoundland, Canada A1B 3X9; **Department of Psychology, University of Regina,
Regina, Sasketchewan, Canada S4S OA2

This chapter is concerned with neurobehavioral phenomena that may serve as a model of the impact of limbic seizures on interictal behavioral states. These phenomena stem from a series of studies which integrate three areas of animal research: (a) ethological studies of the conflict between aggression and defense in the adult animal and in a developmental time frame; (b) neurobehavioral studies of the limbic substrates of these behaviors in adult animals; (c) and limbic kindling.

DEFINITION OF KINDLING

As originally defined by Goddard et al. (28), the term kindling refers to the phenomenon whereby repeated, temporally spaced application of brief, high-frequency trains of subconvulsive electrical pulses to limbic and cortical areas in a variety of species of animals eventually come to elicit motor convulsions that outlast the stimulus train. Convulsive behavior appears suddenly, and this aspect seems to have suggested the name. The term kindling is thus an analogy to the starting of a fire, whereby application of a low heat, or subconvulsive stimulation, causes tinder, or brain tissue, to burst into flames, or convulse. The most startling aspect of this phenomenon is its longevity. Convulsive sensitization to the stimulus appears very long lasting, having now been found to persist for as long as 1 year after brain stimulation has been terminated (47). Subsequent work by Goddard and many others (reviewed in ref. 35) has altered the initial view of sudden onset and has revealed kindling to have a graded development, advancing in definable stages in stepwise fashion with respect to some parameters of the seizure (Racine, ref. 35, has described stages in the rat).

In a general sense, kindling refers to neural processes that mediate lasting changes in brain function in response to repeated, temporally spaced application of neurobehaviorally active agents. In this most general sense, kindling processes have been inferred in a number of clinical phenomena, including the development of psychoses (33,34,36) and psychopathology associated with complex partial seizures (16,30,38).

Some of the properties of kindling are summarized in Table 1. Properties 4 and 5 in the Table have been used to suggest that limbic kindling may serve as a model of limbic epilepsy (16,17). Properties 1 to 3, however, are most relevant to the issue of the impact of kindling on behavior.

BEHAVIORAL BIAS AND LIMBIC SYSTEM EXCITABILITY

This research represents an ongoing attempt to (a) determine if limbic seizures alter limbic function interictally in such a way as to impact on behavior manifested between seizures (b) determine if the preexisting status of limbic function controlling particular behavioral states interacts with seizure discharging to determine behavioral outcome; and (c) test a number of hypotheses regarding how repeated limbic seizures alter behavior in animals and possibly in humans.

Before turning to the question of how limbic seizures influence neurobehavioral functioning, the neurobehavioral system investigated, that is the conflict between aggression and defense and the limbic substrate of these behaviors, must be described. The animal under investigation is the cat. Why the cat? The reasons for choosing the cat stem from the research by John Flynn and his colleagues on the role of the limbic system in modulating various forms of electrically elicited aggressive behavior in the cat. This work revealed the presence of at least two limbic circuits controlling predatory aggression. One, involving the basomedial amygdala, functions to tonically suppress attack and at the same time facilitates defense (5,24). A second includes the ventral hippocampus and is involved in tonic attack facilitation (37).

These circuits could be described as a set of opponent tonic modulators of attack and defense. These terms may be defined with an example. Egger and Flynn showed that alternating stimulus pulses to the lateral hypothalamus and basomedial amygdala resulted in a slowing of quiet biting attack elicited hypothalamically (latency to bite a rat). Amygdala stimulation alone could also suppress attack in cats that would spontaneously attack rodents. Placing a lesion in the basomedial amygdala resulted in a quickening of hypothalamically elicited attack when stimulus

TABLE 1. *Some properties of kindling*

---

1. Kindling is not all-or-none, but involves a progressive, long-lasting lowering of threshold to evoke an AD, or electrographic seizure, without a convulsion
2. Kindling can be induced in many species, from frogs, rats, cats, and dogs to primates
3. Kindling has been associated with long-lasting, interictally maintained synaptic potentiation with limbic system circuits
4. When carried on long enough, kindling stimulation leads to spontaneous convulsions
5. Anticonvulsant control over kindled limbic foci exerted by pharmacological agents used to treat various epileptic disorders is best with agents that are most effective in treating complex partial seizure disorders in humans

parameters were kept constant. These data suggested that the basomedial amygdala exerted some tonic, or lasting, inhibitory control over hypothalamically mediated attack behavior. Similar but converse phenomena were found when the ventral hippocampus was stimulated, or lesioned.

To reiterate, tonic means lasting exertion of some behaviorally detectable action (facilitation or suppression). Modulation means not behaviorally provocative, but affecting some parameter of the behavior (e.g., latency to perform it).

THE AGGRESSIVE AND DEFENSIVE CAT PERSONALITY AND ITS LIMBIC SYSTEM SUBSTRATE

Our original work with this system revealed that domestic cats differ behaviorally along a quantitative dimension of aggressiveness and defensiveness. The more defensive the cat, the less likely it is to attack formidable prey, that is, rats. Expressions of defensiveness were generalized in that nonrat predators were more threatened than aggressive cats by humans, novel environments, rats, and conspecific threat vocalizations, in that order. Mice pose little threat to either rat predators or nonrat predators. These response dispositions remain stable over retest periods exceeding 1 year. Given the generalized nature of defensive responses and the fact that measures of defense to various stimuli are highly correlated, we proposed that cats possess a scalable defensive "personality" trait (1,5,12).

Developmental studies designed to trace the ontogeny of attack and defense subsequently revealed that the defensive personality emerges early in life. Cats that grew to be defensive as adults showed evidence of enhanced defensive responses to environmental threat between 37 and 52 days of age. Moreover, early defensiveness correlated highly ($r = .88$) with defensive response at 1 year of age. These data suggest that defensiveness, as a trait, is the result of some unknown, experientially resistant neurodevelopmental process (13–15).

Other work in adults revealed stable neural correlates of the defensive personality. These appeared in epileptic and nonepileptic measures of excitability in the opponent limbic modulators of attack and defense.

In summary, a behavioral personality trait expressed as a predisposition or bias to respond defensively to environmental threat varies directly with: (a) seizure susceptibility (afterdischarge threshold, ADT) of the basal amygdala—the more defensive the cat, the lower the ADT; (b) limbic permeability, or propagation of seizure activity from the amygdala to thalamic and hypothalamic areas which are part of the substrate of the expression of defensive behavior—the more defensive the cat, the stronger the evocation of multiple unit activity (MUA) in areas to which the amygdala projects synaptically; (c) the degree of population neural response generated in the amygdala by species relevant stimuli—the more defensive the cat, the larger and more prolonged are the increases in MUA response in the amygdala when the cat visually orients to rats (this is not the case when the cat looks at mice); (d) defensive bias also varies inversely with seizure susceptibility of the ventral hippocampus when seizures are generated by high-frequency stimulation of an input pathway (the perforant path input to the dentate area)—the more defensive the cat, the higher the ADT (2,3,5, and *unpublished observations*).

We then tested whether these limbic excitability correlates of behavioral disposition are causally related to the defensive personality using a method borrowed from the kindling paradigm—lowering of threshold to evoke an afterdischarge (AD). When ADT of the amygdalae of aggressive cats was reduced by "partial kindling," that is, without evoking motor convulsions, cats ceased killing rats and became generally more defensive. Behavioral changes were lasting, persisting up to 4 months, or as long as the cats were kept. Associated with the behavioral change was a lasting increase in limbic permeability (3,5).

In effect, when the epileptic excitability of the limbic substrate of defense of aggressive cats was experimentally changed to resemble the excitability of defensive cats, the behavior also changed from an aggressive cat personality to a defensive cat personality.

On the other hand, it was possible to block the increase in limbic permeability, but not the decrease of amygdaloid ADT, by prior stimulation to the point of AD of the ventral hippocampus. These aggressive animals became more effective killers (faster latency to kill rats) with a trend toward decreasing defensiveness toward rats.

Taken together, the behavioral data and neural data indicate that the behavioral balance of attack and defense is under the tonic control of opponent limbic circuits, which are themselves biased and in a measurable manner. The most behaviorally relevant neural parameter appears to be limbic permeability, since behavioral changes were dependent on increases in limbic permeability and not on ADT changes alone. It should be pointed out that all of the thalamic and hypothalamic areas in which permeability increased form part of a system of cells whose electrical activation suppress predatory attack and often evoke defensive responses.

Up to this point, limbic permeability has been defined as the degree of propagation of seizure activity between limbic system structures and their output fields. Yet the behavioral disposition that correlates with limbic permeability is present interictally. Furthermore, behavioral changes induced by lowering ADT persisted interictally and were not dependent on seizure discharges for their maintenance.

These observations suggest that behavioral disposition, occurring either naturally or induced epileptically, is dependent on some form of interictally maintained modulation of transmission of nonepileptic activity, possibly as some form of potentiation of synaptic transmission. In fact, it has been reported that repeated high frequency or epileptic driving of limbic circuits lastingly facilitates conduction of nonepileptic neural activity transsynaptically (22,23,35).

We are now working on this question of the relationship between interictally manifested synaptic response to single pulse stimulation and behavioral disposition. This investigation is being carried out with cats used in the developmental studies just mentioned. It is of great interest that the 37- to 52-day age period in which defensiveness grows corresponds to a time period in which Kling and Coustan (29) observed that the amygdala begins to modulate the hypothalamic substrate of defense in cats. Early differences in defensive responses may then be the behavioral signature of differences in this neural developmental process.

For this and other reasons, we are concentrating on two pathways in the cat brain: (a) the amygdalo-ventromedial hypothalamic (VMH) pathway mediated via the ventral amygdalofugal pathway (VAF); (b) the perforant-path dentate mono-synaptic pathway. The amygdalo-VMH pathway is being investigated because this is one pathway over which changes in limbic permeability associated with behav-ioral changes were detected ictally (5). Moreover, it has been demonstrated that medial amygdala stimulation produces an evoked potential of negative polarity, which represents an excitatory synaptic input from the amygdala carried over the VAF.

An example from one of our awake cats appears in Fig. 1. The poststimulus frequency histogram below the potential is from a recording of multiple cell bursts from the VMH following amygdala stimulation with single pulses of biphasic stimuli. The evoked potential and the population cell response measured this way resemble very closely the data seen with microelectrodes (32).

Our work on this pathway so far has been to compare the response of the VMH to single pulse stimulation of the amygdala in awake cats with high and low degrees of defensive predisposition. We first determine the threshold for evocation of a potential in the VMH by single pulse stimulation of the amygdala. Then a graded intensity series of stimulations is applied in six steps from 100% to 175% of threshold. A total of 32 stimulations at each intensity are applied. Evoked potential data are sampled by computer. The computer is then used to calculate the peak height of the VMH potential as depicted in Fig. 1. Peak heights are found for each stimulation over all intensities.

Peak height of potentials (in microvolts) from defensive cats were found to exceed those of aggressive cats over the entire range of intensities (from 100% to 175% of threshold, Fig. 2; ref. 11). MUA activity just after a pulse, but before the onset of the VMH potential, was examined in the amygdala (4–6 msec) as a measure of cellular excitatory response to the stimulation. MUA activity generated around the peak of the VMH potential in the VMH was also analyzed (6–22 msec) in a similar fashion. There were no differences between groups of cats in cellular response over the intensity range examined. Threshold for evocation of a VMH potential did not differ between groups of cats, either. Taken together, these data imply that the differences in the VMH field potential reflect some differential strength of synaptic drive into the VMH from the amygdala.

We also found two differences in hippocampal response to excitatory input from the entorhinal cortex mediated via the perforant path. (a) Threshold for eliciting an AD in the ventral hippocampus (VHPC) by perforant path stimulation is higher in nonaggressive cats than it is in aggressive cats (167 μA $\pm$ 59 and 505 μA $\pm$ 74; means $\pm$ SE for aggressive and defensive cats, respectively). (b) Double pulse stimulation studies suggest that recurrent inhibition is likely stronger in nonaggres-sive cats (11).

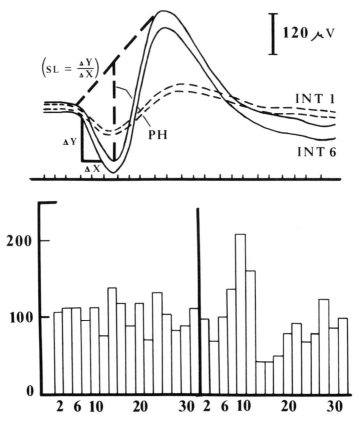

FIG. 1. The upper part of the figure contains two computer-plotted averages of potentials evoked in the ventromedial hypothalamus of an awake and freely moving cat. Double lines demark the ± 95% confidence intervals of the average. The time base below the potentials is calibrated in 1-msec intervals. Potentials were generated by single pulse stimuli to the amygdala at 100% (INT 1) and 175% (INT 6) of threshold for evocation of the VMH potential. Method of measuring slope (SL) and peak height (PH) of the potential appear in the figure superimposed on the INT 6 average. Poststimulus frequency histograms of evoked multiple unit activity (MUA) recorded simultaneously with the potential appear in the bottom part of the figure. The data are expressed as a percentage of MUA recorded just prior to the onset of stimulation. Percentage MUA represents the average of 32 samples of 30 msec at each intensity of stimulation. INT 1 histograms appear at the left, and INT 6 histograms appear at the right. Histogram counts were taken in 2-msec bins. Note that the MUA increases between 6 and 12 msec after a pulse, near the peak of the potential at INT 6. This pattern of MUA response matches quite closely published poststimulus frequency histograms recorded with microelectrodes in anesthetized cats.

When perforant path fibers from the entorhinal cortex are stimulated in awake, freely moving animals, it is possible to record a monosynaptically evoked extracellular dentate field potential (Fig. 3) consisting of at least two components: (a) a population excitatory postsynaptic potential (EPSP), which is related to the intracellularly recorded EPSP (18,31); and (b) a compound action potential that is superimposed on the EPSP and is called the population spike, representing the

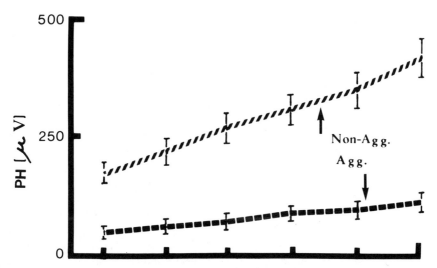

FIG. 2. Plotted in the figure are the changes in peak height (PH) of the ventromedial hypotha-lamic (VMH) potential over intensity of single pulse stimulation of the amygdala in aggressive (Agg) and nonaggressive (non-agg) cats. Means, and ± SEM over the groups of cats are plotted vs intensity of stimulation expressed as a percentage of threshold from 100% to 175% of threshold for evocation of a VMH potential by amygdaloid stimulation.

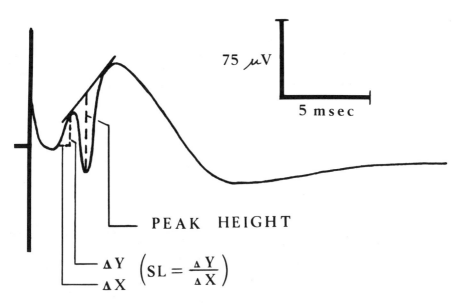

FIG. 3. Plotted in the figure is a computer average of a compound field potential evoked in the dentate area of the ventral hippocampus of an awake cat by single pulse stimulation of the per-forant path. The methods of measurement of slope (SL) of the EPSP component and peak height of the population spike are superimposed on the potential.

firing of many dentate granule cells. Field potentials remain stable for many days or weeks (21,23). It is possible, then, to draw inferences from a population field potential about cellular events.

Furthermore, the field potential may be used to indirectly measure the strength of recurrent inhibition in this system. This is done by measuring the degree of suppression of the population spike generated by the second pulse of a pulse pair to the perforant pathway. Suppression is observed when the interval between pairs (interpulse interval or IPI) falls within the time of occurrence of the recurrent IPSP. The implication is that cell firing in response to the second pulse of a pulse pair is suppressed owing to a recurrent inhibition generated by cellular firing provoked by the first pulse of the pair (7,20). We have confirmed with single cell recording in cat ventral hippocampus that suppression of the peak height of the population spike is indeed associated with a decrease in probability of firing of single cells (9).

We used the suppression of the population spike as a measure of recurrent inhibition in awake cats. Double pulse stimulation was applied to the perforant path at intensities sufficient to evoke a population spike in the dentate area (at least 150% of threshold of the dentate potential). Pulse pairs of equal amplitude and width were delivered with IPIs varying from 20 to 160 msec over four consecutive pulse pairs in a series of 20,40,80, and 160 msec. This series was repeated a total of 10 times to yield 10 paired stimulations at each IPI. Pulse pair stimulations were separated by 10 sec. Peak height of population spikes evoked by each pulse of a pair was measured, as well as the ratio of the height of the spike evoked by the second pulse of a pair divided by the height of a spike evoked by the first pulse of a pair. These ratios were averaged over the 10 stimulations at each IPI. This entire procedure was repeated four times every other day for 8 days. The results were stable over the four replications.

Data from aggressive, less defensive cats were then compared with data from less aggressive, more defensive cats. First, the peak heights of the potential evoked by the first pulse of a pair did not differ between groups of cats (Fig. 4). This is interpreted to mean that the degree of cellular activity evoked by the first pulse of a pair was equal across groups of cats and IPIs.

Groups of cats did differ with respect to the ratios of peak heights generated by the first and second pulses of a pair, however. More defensive (NA, Fig. 4) cats showed greater suppression of the second population spike than more aggressive cats (A, Fig. 4) at interpulse intervals of 20, 40, and 80 msec. Since the suppression of the second spike is taken as a measure of recurrent inhibition, these data suggest that more defensive cats show deeper and more prolonged recurrent inhibition in the ventral hippocampus than do less defensive, more aggressive cats (11).

The implication is that some tonic difference in recurrent inhibition is associated with defensive bias, which is behaviorally antithetical to aggressive disposition. The data also suggest a factor that may contribute to the higher thresholds for electrically evoked seizures in the perforant path in defensive cats.

All of these data suggest the following tentative model of functional response of the amygdala, VMH, VHPC system to excitatory input. Since the basal amygdala-

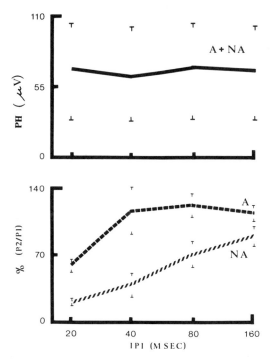

FIG. 4. Plots of peak height values of the population spikes in the ventral hippocampi of aggressive (A) and nonaggressive (NA) cats vs the interpulse interval (IPI) of pulse pairs delivered to the perforant path. The upper graph shows the peak height (PH) values obtained from potentials evoked by the first stimulus of a pulse pair. Data are averages and ± SE over both groups of cats and over 4 days of repeated testing. The lower graph shows the ratio P2/P1, where P2 is the PH of the population spike obtained from potentials evoked by the second stimulus of a pulse pair, and P1 is the PH value obtained from the potential evoked by the first stimulus of a pulse pair. Means, and ± SE over days are plotted separately for aggressive and nonaggressive cats. The ordinate of this graph is in units of a percentage of P1. The abscissas of both graphs are IPI in msec.

VMH pathway is considered to be part of the substrate of defensive biasing and suppression of aggressive behavior in the cat (4,43), limbic activity from excitatory inputs may be preferentially routed through the amygdalo-VMH pathway in more defensive cats. Little response would be expected from the ventral hippocampal system in these cats owing to its reduced excitability. In more aggressive cats, little transmission through the amygdalo-VMH pathway may occur, whereas the more excitable ventral hippocampus, a tonic faciliator of predatory aggression, may dominate limbic response.

One hypothetical extension of these findings is that in free behaving situations, differential routing of sensory evoked neural activity may determine behavioral response to that input. If complex sensory input arrives in the amygdala from neocortical analyzers (27), it is possible that the temporal neocortex is one source of species-relevant stimuli driving this system.

Our data are also consistent with the hypothesis that some form of synaptic potentiation underlies behavioral disposition (or bias) and is at least consistent with the notion that epileptically induced behavioral changes persisting interictally may be dependent on changed patterns of transmission of excitatory activity within and out of the limbic system.

EFFECTS OF REPEATED LIMBIC AD ON AGGRESSIVE AND DEFENSIVE BEHAVIOR

We are currently working on a direct test of this possibility (8,9). Cats in these studies were part of the population of defensive cats described in the developmental studies. The expression of their defensive dispositions has remained stable over retest periods of up to 3 years. The profile of evoked response in the limbic pathways described has also been found to be stable over retest periods of more than 1 week, with up to four retests of response. Moreover, evocation of two limbic ADs have been found to be without effect on these profiles.

We chose to repeatedly evoke seizure discharges in the ventral hippocampus directly, or by stimulation of the perforant path in defensive cats. Given the proposed role of the ventral hippocampus in attack facilitation, our expectation was that such a treatment would reduce defensiveness and facilitate predatory aggressiveness interictally.

To our surprise, we observed the opposite. After five to seven electrically triggered ADs (spaced 6 hr apart), which did not elicit motor convulsions, there was a lasting and pronounced increase in defensive response toward rats and conspecific threat vocalizations, a lesser change in defensive response toward mice and no change in social response to a familiar and socially rewarding human. Thus, repeated ADs seem to have heightened a preexisting, defensive predisposition. Moreover, the severity of the enhancement of defensive response was influenced by the nature of the stimulus in the case of rats, mice, and conspecific threat, and possibly by prior experience with the stimulus in the case of the familiar human.

Examination of electrophysiological changes induced by repeated ADs sheds some light on these behaviorally unexpected results. It should also be emphasized that ADs were observed to spread to the amygdala and VMH every time an AD was triggered in the VHPC system. This latter result is important for interpretation of the evoked potential results.

As mentioned, stability of evoked response had been tested and found to be stable, even after two ADs, at which time behavior had not changed. After five more ADs, and a test for behavioral change, response to control intensities of pulse pairs of amygdala and perforant stimulation were examined. The method was identical to that described for assessing naturally occurring differences between aggressive and defensive cats. These tests were always performed 1 hr after behavioral testing: (a) on the day of behavioral change (or 3 hr after the last AD), (b) 24 hr after the last AD, (c) then 1, 3, 4, and up to 8 weeks after the last AD.

We observed a lasting and stable increase in size (peak height, Fig. 5) and rate of change of the initial slope of the potential evoked in the VMH by the first pulse

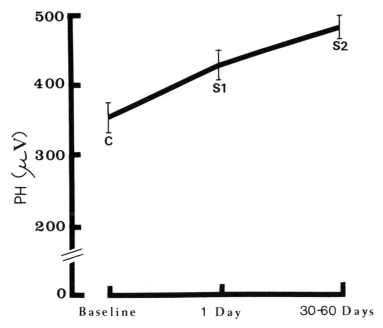

FIG. 5. The peak height (PH) of the ventromedial hypothalamic potential evoked by amygdala stimulation averaged over six cats appears in the figure. Means and SE are plotted vs three time points in the experiment: C, control prior to repeated AD; S1, one day after the last repeated AD; S2, 30–60 days after the last repeated AD. These peak heights were taken from the potential evoked by the first pulse of all paired pulse stimulations to the amygdala in each test condition.

of a pulse pair to the amygdala. No changes were noted in the ratio of the response to the second pulse of a pulse pair divided by the response to the first pulse of a pair at any IPI. Measures of population cell response in the amygdala to the stimulus pulses revealed no change in amygdaloid response to single stimuli following repeated AD. Nor were there changes noted in population cell responses evoked in the VMH at the intensities employed (9). These results suggest that some form of lasting enhancement of synaptic input in the VMH had occurred. Given that repeated ADs have been shown to enhance evoked response in limbic pathways in rats (35), it is likely that the change in VMH response was induced by the spread of ADs to the amygdala.

In a similar fashion, ADs in the perforant pathway-VHPC pathway appear to have induced a lasting potentiation of hippocampal response to input. There was a lasting enhancement (206%) of the slope of the EPSP component of the compound field potential. In contrast, there was no change in the size of the population spike evoked by the first pulse of a pair (Fig. 6A). Nor were there any changes in population cell responses in the perforant path following either pulse.

Countering this increased excitatory response to input was an equally lasting increase in suppression of the population spike evoked by the second pulse of a pulse pair at all IPIs tested (Fig. 6B; ref. 9). Given that second spike suppression

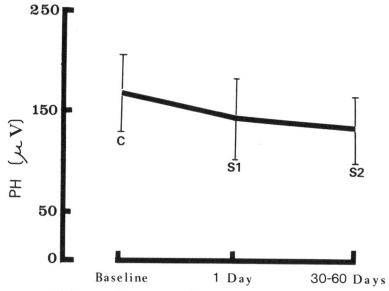

FIG. 6A. The peak height (PH) of the population spike of the ventral hippocampal potential evoked by perforant path stimulations averaged over seven cats appears in the figure. Means and SE are plotted vs three time points in the experiment: C, control prior to repeated AD; S1, one day after the last repeated AD; S2, 30–60 days after the last repeated AD. These peak heights were taken from the potential evoked by the first pulse of all paired pulse stimulations to the perforant path in each test condition.

may be used as a measure of recurrent inhibition, these data suggest that in addition to a lasting enhancement of synaptic response to input in the VMH and dentate, there was a lasting increase in recurrent inhibition in the ventral hippocampus. Similar effects of repeated limbic AD on recurrent inhibition have been reported in the rat hippocampus and have been associated with an increase in the number of benzodiazepine receptors (45,46).

Functionally, these data make sense. Facilitation of transmission of activity from the amygdala to the VMH, occurring naturally, or induced by repeated amygdaloid stimulation to AD, has been associated with enhanced defensiveness in the cat (5). Given that there was no apparent increase in population cell spiking in the VMH, the changes induced by repeated AD may have behavioral effects by increasing an excitatory modulatory input to VMH cells from the amygdala, which then interact with other sources of input to the VMH to influence behavior during actual defensive response to environmental threat. One source may be the dorsomedial tegmentum (44).

The increase in recurrent inhibition in the VHPC is also consistent with the proposed role of VHPC as an attack facilitator and defensive response suppressor. An increase in recurrent inhibition would reduce the ability of the VHPC to respond to high-frequency input and thus would attenuate transmission of activity through the hippocampus. This attenuation of function, acting perhaps like a functional

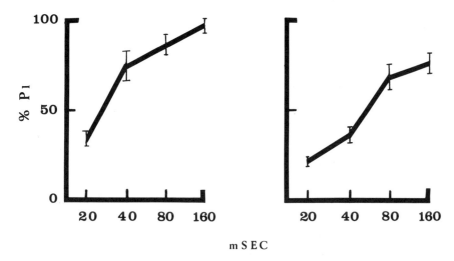

FIG. 6B. Suppression of the peak height of the population spike of the ventral hippocampal potential in response to the second pulse of a pulse pair is expressed as a percentage of the peak height of the population spike of the potential evoked by the first pulse of a pulse pair (% P1). Mean suppression and SE from seven cats are plotted vs interpulse interval of the pulse pairs in msec. Baseline data **(left)** were recorded before repeated evocation of afterdischarges (ADs) in the hippocampus. Post AD data **(right)** are the average of data observed 1 day after the last repeated AD and those recorded 30–60 days after the last AD. Note that the suppression increases at all interpulse intervals post AD.

lesion, could reduce the ability of the hippocampus to facilitate attack and attenuate defense behaviorally.

On the other hand, the enhancement of the EPSPs in the VHPC represents an increase in excitatory response to input. This change may not have any behavioral significance if cellular firing rates in the hippocampus are most relevant for modulation of behavioral response. Nevertheless, EPSP enhancement may be a contributing factor to the observed decrease in hippocampal ADT, discussed below.

To investigate the relationship between interictally manifested changes in excitability and the development of kindling, measures of latency to onset, duration, and spectral power (in the 1–70 cps band) of ADs in the amygdala, VMH, perforant pathway, and VHPC were taken. None of these were found to change following repeated AD (9). Since increase in duration and complexity of discharge is one of the hallmarks of advancing stage of kindling (35), these data suggest that little kindling was induced. The only kindling-relevant measure to change was threshold for evoking an AD in the VHPC by perforant path stimulation. These thresholds did decrease in all cats (625 ± 188 μA to 301 ± 63 μA, mean $\pm$ SE; ref. 9). These data suggest that behavioral changes may be induced by neural mechanisms, which are independent of those that mediate increases in motor convulsive response associated with kindling.

There is one intriguing discrepancy between these results and earlier studies. It has been reported by us (5) that repeated VHPC ADs induced prior to repeated amygdaloid AD in naturally aggressive cats: (a) enhance aggressiveness (b) attenuate defensiveness, and (c) block increases in transmission of epileptic activity from the amygdala to VMH when the amygdala is repeatedly stimulated. One major difference is that the cats used in the current studies are naturally defensive, having become so through some experientially resistant developmental process. As described above, the neural signatures of this process in adulthood appear as a naturally enhanced transmission of activity from the amygdala to VMH, and a naturally enhanced recurrent inhibition in the VHPC. It is possible, then, that behavioral outcome of eliciting repeated ADs in the VHPC is influenced by the naturally occurring behavioral disposition of the cat. Neurophysiologically, behavioral outcome may be determined by the naturally occurring excitability status of the limbic substrates at the time of onset of repeated AD. In the present case, repeated AD accentuated a preexisting naturally enhanced VMH response to input and a preexisting naturally enhanced recurrent inhibition in the VHPC.

CONCLUSIONS

Taken together, the data support, in part, the following hypotheses we advanced in our recent review of limbic kindling and behavior (10). These hypotheses propose that interictally maintained behavioral changes following kindling stimulation

1. Are dependent on some form of interictally maintained enhancement of transmission of neural information between limbic structures.
2. Are dependent on both increases and decreases of the ability of limbic pathways to transmit neural activity.
3. May be independent of neural mechanisms which mediate increases in motor convulsive epileptogenicity with kindling.

In addition,

4. Kindling stimulation results in enhancement of the normal behavioral functioning of some limbic areas and attenuation of function of others.
5. The behavioral outcome of repeated seizure discharges may be dependent on both (a) the behavioral disposition of the animal stimulated and (b) the brain areas stimulated.

As has been pointed out (10), an understanding of the nature of the impact of limbic seizures on behavior in animal models can only be as clear as the understanding of the neural substrate of the behavioral system examined. The data described here, and in our recent review of limbic kindling and behavior, indicate that repeated seizures induce hyperfunctional limbic and behavioral states that persist interictally in animals. By analogy, it is also possible that repeated limbic seizures in humans have interictal behavioral consequences. This analogy can only remain just an analogy until clear evidence is obtained in humans. Some support for analogous physiological changes come from Babb's (19) observations that both tetanic stimulation and ADs can induce a form of lasting potentiation of evoked potentials in human limbic system.

With respect to behavioral changes, two major and serious questions arise. First, is limbic involvement in an epileptic or an epileptic-like disorder a prerequisite for behavioral change in humans? Methods for assessing limbic involvement are still in the developmental stage, though we and others have begun to attack the problem using encephalographic power spectral analysis with promising preliminary results (6). The second question is what is the nature of behavioral change, if any? This thorny problem has a controversial and often vitriolic history (e.g., refs. 25,26,40–42). It is compounded by the complexity of the issue of adequate assessment of human behavior. Since it is indefensible to make facile generalizations from animal models to humans, the issue in humans must be approached with care taken to consider the complexity of human behavior and the complexity of sources of variation in human behavior. Both of these questions are addressed elsewhere in this volume (39).

ACKNOWLEDGMENTS

The research reported in this paper was supported by a grant to R. Adamec from the Medical Research Council of Canada (MRC grant MA 7022). The technical assistance of R. Riar, B. Vari, N. Graham, and M. Graham is gratefully acknowledged.

REFERENCES

1. Adamec, R. (1975): The behavioral bases of prolonged suppression of predatory attack in cats. *Aggress. Behav.*, 1:297–314.
2. Adamec, R. (1975): The neural basis of prolonged suppression of predatory attack. I. Naturally occurring physiological differences in the limbic systems of killer and non-killer cats. *Aggress. Behav.*, 1:315–330.
3. Adamec, R. (1975): Behavioural and epileptic determinants of predatory attack behaviour in the cat. *Can. J. Neurol. Sci.*, 457–466.
4. Adamec, R. (1976): Hypothalamic and extrahypothalamic substrates of predatory attack suppression and the influence of hunger. *Brain Res.*, 106:57–69.
5. Adamec, R. (1978): Normal and abnormal limbic system mechanisms of emotive biasing. In: *Limbic Mechanisms*, edited by K. E. Livingston and O. Hornykiewicz, pp. 405–455. Plenum Press: New York.
6. Adamec, R. (1983): Omega analysis and the discrimination of the therapeutic (psychiatric) response to Tegretol. *Perspect.* Psychiatry, 2(2):7–8.
7. Adamec, R., McNaughton, B., Racine, R., and Livingston, K. E. (1981): Effects of diazepam on hippocampal excitability in the rat: Action in the dentate area. *Epilepsia*, 22:205–215.
8. Adamec, R., and Stark-Adamec, C. (1983): Partial kindling and emotional bias in the cat: Lasting after-effects of partial kindling of ventral hippocampus. I: Behavioral Changes. Behav. *Neural Biol.*, 38:205–222.
9. Adamec, R., and Stark-Adamec, C. (1983): Partial kindling and emotional bias in the cat: Lasting after-effects of partial kindling of ventral hippocampus. II: Physiological Changes. Behav. *Neural Biol., (in press)*.
10. Adamec, R., and Stark-Adamec, C. (1983): Limbic kindling and animal behavior—Implications for human psychopathology, associated with complex partial seizures. Biol. *Psychiatry*, 18(2):269–293.
11. Adamec, R., and Stark-Adamec, C. (1984): The contribution of limbic connectivity to stable behavioral characteristics of aggressive and defensive cats. In: Modulation of Sensorimotor Activity During Altered Behavioural States. edited by R. Bandler, pp. 341–349. Alan R. Liss: New York.
12. Adamec, R., Stark-Adamec, C., and Livingston, K. E. (1983): The expression of an early

developmentally emergent defensive bias in the adult domestic cat (Felis catus) in nonpredatory situations. *J. Appl. Animal Ethol.* 10:89–108.

13. Adamec, R. E., Stark-Adamec, C., and Livingston, K. E. (1980): The development of predatory aggression and defense in the domestic cat (Felis Catus) I. Effects of early experience on adult patterns of aggression and defense. *Behav. Neural Biol.* 30:389–409.

14. Adamec, R. E., Stark-Adamec, C., and Livingston, K. E. (1980): The development of predatory aggression and defense in the domestic cat (Felis Catus). II. Development of aggression and defense in the first 164 days of life. *Behav. Neural Biol.*, 30:410–434.

15. Adamec, R. E., Stark-Adamec, C., and Livingston, K. E. (1980): The development of predatory aggression and defense in the domestic cat (Felis Catus). III. Effects on development of hunger between 180 and 365 days of age. Behav. *Neural Biol.*, 30:435–447.

16. Adamec, R. E., Stark-Adamec, C., Perrin, R., and Livingston, K. E. (1981). What is the relevance of kindling for human temporal lobe epilepsy? In: *Kindling 2,*edited by J. A. Wada, pp. 303–313. Raven Press, New York.

17. Albright, P., and Burnham, W. M. (1980): Development of a new animal seizure model: Effects of anticonvulsants on cortical and amygdala-kindled seizures. *Epilepsia*, 21:681–689.

18. Andersen, P., Bliss, T. V. P., and Skrede, K. K. (1971): Lamellar organization of hippocampal excitatory pathways. *Exp. Brain Res.*, 13:222–238.

19. Babb, T. L. (1982): Short-term and long-term modification of neurons and evoked potentials in the human hippocampal formation. *Neurosci. Res. Program Bull.*, 20(5):729–739.

20. Barnes, C. A. (1979): Memory deficits associated with senescence: a neurophysiological and behavioral study in the rat. *J. Comp. Physiol. Psychol.*, 93:74–104.

21. Barnes, C. A., McNaughton, B. L., Goddard, G. V., Douglas, R. M., and Adamec, R. (1977): Circadian rhythm of synaptic excitability in rat and monkey nervous systems. *Science*, 197:91–92.

22. Bliss, T. V. P., and Lomo, T. (1973): Long-lasting potentiation of synaptic transmission in the dentate area of the unanaesthetized rabbit following stimulation of the perforant path. *J. Physiol. (Lond.)*, 232:351–356.

23. Douglas, R. M., and Goddard, G. V. (1975): Long-term potentiation of the perforant path-granule cell synapse in the rat hippocampus. *Brain Res.* 86:205–215.

24. Egger, D. M., and Flynn, J. P. (1967): Effects of amygdaloid stimulation and ablation on hypothalamically elicited attack behavior in cats. In: W. R. Adey and T. Tokizane *Structure and Function of the Limbic System, Progress in Brain Research.* edited by W. R. Adey and T. Tokizane. Elsevier. Amsterdam.

25. Flor-Henry, P. (1976): Epilepsy and psychopathology. In: *Recent Advances in Clinical Psychiatry*, edited by K. Granville-Grossman, pp. 262–294. Churchill Livingston, New York.

26. Geschwind, N. (1977): Introduction to Psychiatric complications in the epilepsies: Current research. *McLean Hosp. J*, June, Special Issue, 6–8.

27. Gloor, P. (1972): Temporal lobe epilepsy: Its possible contribution to the understanding of the functional significance of the amygdala and of its interaction with neo-cortical-temporal mechanisms. In: *The Neurobiology of the Amygdala.* edited by B. E. Eleftheriou, pp. 723–758. Plenum Press, New York.

28. Goddard, G. V., McIntyre, D. C., and Leech, C. K. (1969): A permanent change in brain function resulting from daily electrical stimulation. *Exp. Neurol.*, 25:295–330.

29. Kling, A., and Coustan, D. (1964): Electrical stimulation of amygdala and hypothalamus in the kitten. *Exp. Neurol.*, 10:81–89.

30. Livingston, K. E. (1978): The experimental clinical interface: Kindling as a dynamic model of induced limbic system dysfunction. In: *Limbic Mechanisms*, edited by K. E. Livingston and O. Hoznykiewicz, pp. 521–534. Plenum Press. New York.

31. Lomo, T. (1971): Patterns of activation in a monosynaptic cortical pathway: The perforant path input to the dentate area of the hippocampal formation. *Exp. Brain Res.*, 12:18–45.

32. Murphy, J. T. (1972): The role of the amygdala in controlling hypothalamic output. In: *The Neurobiology of the Amygdala*, edited by B. E. Eleftheriou Plenum Press, New York.

33. Post, R. M., and Ballenger, J. C. (1981): Kindling models for the progressive development of behavioral psychopathology: sensitization to electrical, pharmacological, and psychological stimuli. In: *Handbook of Biological Psychiatry, Part IV*, edited by H. M. van Praag, M. H. Lader, O. J. Rafaelsen and E. J. Sachar. pp. 609–651. Marcel-Dekker, New York.

34. Post, R. M., Ballenger, J. C., Uhde, T. W., Putnam, F. W., and Bunney, W. E. Jr. (1981): Kindling

and drug sensitization: implications for the progressive development of psychopathology and treatment with carbamazepine. The Psychopharmacology of Anticonvulsants (The British Association for Pharmacology Monograph series), Oxford University Press: Oxford.

35. Racine, R. (1978): Kindling: The first decade. *Neurosurgery*, 3(2):234–252.
36. Sato, M., and Okamoto, M. (1981): Dopaminergic kindling and electrical kindling. In: *Kindling 2*, edited by J. A. Wada, pp. 15–29. Raven Press, New York.
37. Siegal, A., and Flynn, J. P. (1968): Differential effects of electrical stimulation and lesions of the hippocampus and adjacent regions upon attack behavior in cats. *Brain Res.*, 1:252–262.
38. Stark-Adamec, C., and Adamec, R. E. (1980): Summary of "The Integration of Applied and Experimental Psychology". *Appl. Psychol. Newslett.*, 6(1):9–12.
39. Stark-Adamec, C., and Adamec, R. E. (1984): Psychological methodology versus clinical impressions: Different perspectives on psychopathology and seizures. (This volume, Chapter 18).
40. Stevens, J. R. (1966): Psychiatric implications of psychomotor epilepsy. *Arch. Gen. Psychiatry*, 14:461–471.
41. Stevens, J. R. (1975): Interictal clinical manifestations of complex partial seizures. In: *Advances in Neurology, vol II.*, edited by J. K. Penry and D. D. Daly, pp. 85–112. Raven Press, New York.
42. Stevens, J. R. (1977): All that spikes is not fits. In: *Psychopathology and Brain Dysfunction.*, edited by C. Shagass, S. Gershorn and A. J. Friedhoff, pp. 183–198. Raven Press, New York.
43. Stokman, C. J., and Glusman, M. (1970): Amygdaloid modulation of hypothalamic flight in cats. *J. Comp. Physiol. Psychology*, 71:365–375.
44. Tsubokawa, T., and Sutin, J. (1963): Mesencephalic influence upon the hypothalamic ventromedial nucleus. *EEG Clin. Neurophysiol.*, 15:804–810.
45. Tuff, L. P., Racine, R. J., and Adamec, R. (1983): The effects of kindling on GABA-mediated inhibition in the dentate gyrus of the rat: I. Paired pulse depression. *Brain Res.*, 277:79–90.
46. Tuff, L. P., Racine, R. J., and Adamec, R. (1983): The effects of kindling on GABA-mediated inhibition in the dentate gyrus of the rat: II. Receptor binding. *Brain Res.*, 277:79–90.
47. Wada, J. A., Sato, M., and Corcoran, M. E. (1974): Persistent seizure susceptibility and recurrent spontaneous seizures in kindled cats. *Epilepsia*, 15:465–478.

The Limbic System: Functional Organization and Clinical Disorders, edited by B. K. Doane and K. E. Livingston. Raven Press, New York © 1986.

Seizure Patterns and Pharmacological Responses in the Kindling Model

Penny S. Albright, W. M. Burnham, and K. E. Livingston

Department of Pharmacology, University of Toronto, Toronto, Ontario, Canada M5S 1A8

Clinical observations have suggested that secondarily generalized seizures consist of several discrete components. A complex partial attack, for example, may begin with an aura, progress to a psychomotor state with impaired consciousness, and finally culminate in a generalized convulsion (3). The secondarily generalized seizure in humans is therefore conceptualized not as a single entity but as a series of individual attacks occurring in sequence (5).

The kindling model produces a pattern of focal onset and secondary generalization that closely resembles this clinical picture. Moreover, the various components of a kindled seizure, like those of a clinical seizure, differ in behavioral characteristics and in drug response (1,2). We have therefore come to view the kindled seizure not as a single entity but as an overlapping sequence of seizures, with focal onset followed by partial generalization and ultimately by a generalized convulsion.

Although this approach to kindled seizures has been implicit in our pharmacological work, we have seldom discussed it explicitly. We feel that it deserves further discussion and justification at the present time because of its practical implications for the growing field of kindling pharmacology.

We have therefore reviewed the anticonvulsant studies carried out in our laboratory over the past several years with reference to the concept of multiple-seizure types in the kindling model. In particular, we have concentrated on the pattern of seizure suppression observed with increasing doses of anticonvulsant drugs. We hypothesized that if the kindled seizure consists of several separate seizure subtypes, drug suppression should take place in a steplike, segmental fashion. If, on the other hand, the kindled seizure consists of a single entity, it should be suppressed in a gradual manner.

METHODS

Methods used for this work have been previously reported in detail by Albright and Burnham (1). Briefly, male Royal Victoria rats were implanted in either the anterior neocortex or the basolateral amygdala with chronic stimulating/recording electrodes. All animals were then kindled by daily stimulation with 1 sec of 60-Hz biphasic square-wave pulses administered at current levels sufficient to provoke afterdischarge (cortex, 800 μa; amygdala, 500 μa, peak-to-peak values). Daily kindled stimulation was continued until 30 generalized convulsions had been elicited. Generalized seizure threshold was then determined, and drug testing was conducted using current levels 20% above this value.

Drug testing was always preceded by 5 days of baseline testing during which vehicle effects were investigated. After baseline testing, six or seven doses of each drug were tested, a different dose being administered every 24 hr. The injection/ test interval was 30 min.

To evaluate drug effects on kindled seizures, we measured the presence or absence of afterdischarge at each drug dose as well as the presence or absence of generalized convulsive activity (stages 3, 4, and 5 by Racine's 1972 classification, ref. 4). Duration of discharge was also measured for each drug dose, and these data, not previously reported, form the basis of this chapter. For the purposes of this chapter, two drugs, carbamazepine and clonazepam, were selected for intensive review. These drugs were chosen because they represent extremes of drug action on kindled seizures. Carbamazepine, for example, is very effective in suppressing both generalized and focal activity. Furthermore, the slope of its dose–response curve is steep, indicating that small increments in dose produce large changes in response. In contrast, clonazepam's effects increase gradually over a wide range of doses, and although it is very effective in suppressing generalized seizure activity, it is not very active against focal activity.

RESULTS

Data from Individual Animals

Figures 1 and 2 illustrate the effect of carbamazepine on generalized seizures triggered from either cortex or amygdala. Representative data from single animals are presented so that the pattern of suppression may be observed. As seen in the figures, drug response is abrupt rather than gradual; that is, the kindled seizure is suppressed in a "stepwise" or segmental fashion as the dose of drug is increased. In the cortex, the seizure often disappears completely (s#433), although it may first fall back to a brief focal stage (s#434). In the amydgala, which is more drug resistant, two shortened stages (focal and intermediate) are generally seen. In both cortex and amygdala animals, the seizure disappears in segments rather than in a gradual manner.

It might be argued, however, that this abrupt pattern would appear more gradual if smaller dose intervals had been used. As mentioned previously, carbamazepine has a steep dose–response curve, and small increases in dose produce dramatic decreases in afterdischarge duration. The intervals used in this experiment may have been sufficiently large to create the appearance of abrupt suppression of seizure activity. To counteract this argument, we included clonazepam in our analysis. The anticonvulsant effects of this drug extend over a wide range of doses and thus should favor a gradual reduction in afterdischarge duration, if it occurs.

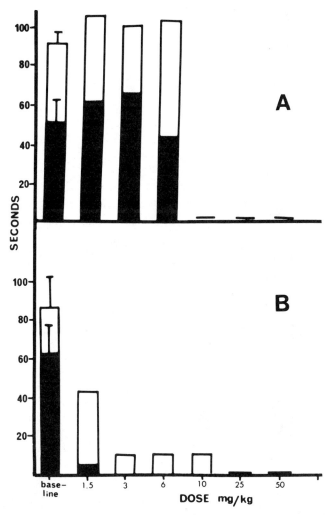

FIG. 1. Effects of increasing doses of carbamazepine on the duration of afterdischarge (□) and motor seizure (■) in individual animals. **A:** s#433 was stimulated in the cortex. **B:** s#567 received amygdala stimulation. Error bars represent standard deviations obtained from the five baseline tests.

Figures 3 and 4 show the effect of clonazepam on the generalized seizure kindled from amygdala or cortex. As seen in the figures, seizure activity also disappears segmentally with clonazepam. In the cortex, the seizure falls back to a brief focal stage (s#G9) before disappearing completely. A single intermediate stage (approximately 30 sec afterdischarge with generalized convulsive activity) is occasionally observed (s#G90). In the amygdala, an intermediate and a focal stage are again seen. (Intermediate seizures in the amygdala, in contrast to the cortex, do not involve generalized convulsive behavior). The distinct nature of these stages is well

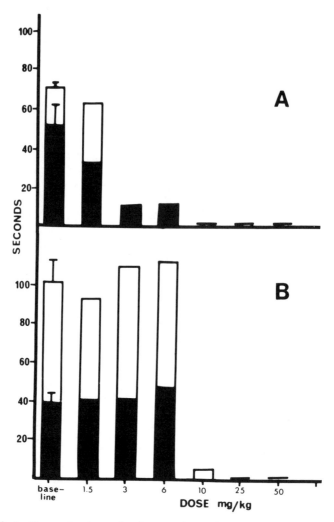

FIG. 2. Effects of increasing doses of carbamazepine on the duration of afterdischarge (□) and motor seizure (■) in individual animals. **A:** s#434 was stimulated in the cortex. **B:** s#G1 received amygdala stimulation. Error bars represent standard deviations obtained from the five baseline tests.

illustrated in Fig. 3 (s#G1), where the intermediate seizure shows little change in duration throughout a 20-fold increase in drug dose. When the dose is further increased, the siezure drops abruptly to the short focal stage.

Group Data

Figures 5 and 6 provide frequency distributions of afterdischarge duration in groups of cortex and amygdala animals receiving carbamazepine or clonazepam.

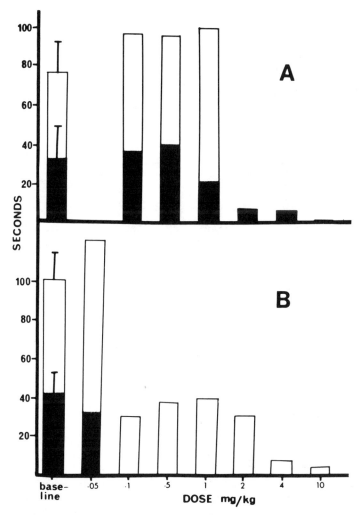

FIG. 3. Effects of increasing doses of clonazepam on the duration of afterdischarge (□) and motor seizure (■) in individual animals. **A:** s#G9 was stimulated in the cortex. **B:** s#G1 received amygdala stimulation. Error bars represent standard deviations obtained from the five baseline tests.

Afterdischarge duration is expressed as a percentage of baseline duration observed during vehicle tests. These data reflect the phenomenon observed with individual animals; that is, that long, intermediate, and focal seizures occur with few intervening stages.

Although the intermediate and focal stages are distinct in individual animals, they are difficult to separate in the group data. Typically, the focal seizure is shorter than 20 sec, whereas the intermediate seizure is longer. Some animals, however, may have relatively long focal seizures (20 sec) with a longer intermediate

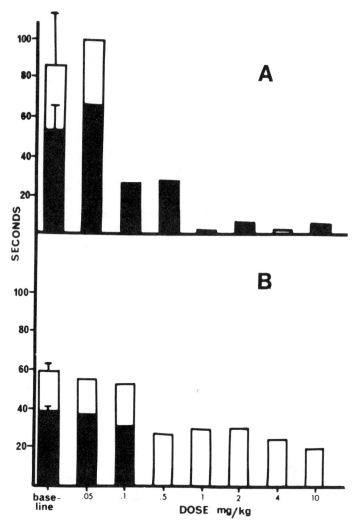

FIG. 4. Effects of increasing doses of clonazepam on the duration of afterdischarge (□) and motor seizure (■) in individual animals. **A:** s#G90 was stimulated in the cortex. **B:** s#G594 received amygdala stimulation. Error bars represent standard deviations obtained from the five baseline tests.

seizure (40 sec). Other animals may have shorter seizures of both types. This variability accounts for the apparent lack of division between these stages in the group data.

DISCUSSION

This chapter reanalyzed our previously published data on the subject of discrete seizure subtypes in the kindling model. Specifically, we have examined the pattern

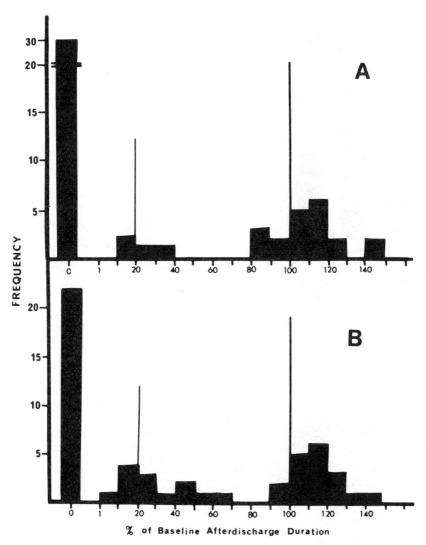

FIG. 5. Frequency distribution of afterdischarge duration in cortex **(A)** and amygdala **(B)** groups after treatment with carbamazepine. For each animal, afterdischarge duration at each dose of carbamazepine was determined as a percentage of baseline duration (baseline = 100%). On the abscissa, the line at 100% represents baseline and the line 20% represents the division between focal and intermediate stages. Baseline afterdischarge duration is approximately 100 sec ($n = 10$ cortex animals and 10 amygdala animals).

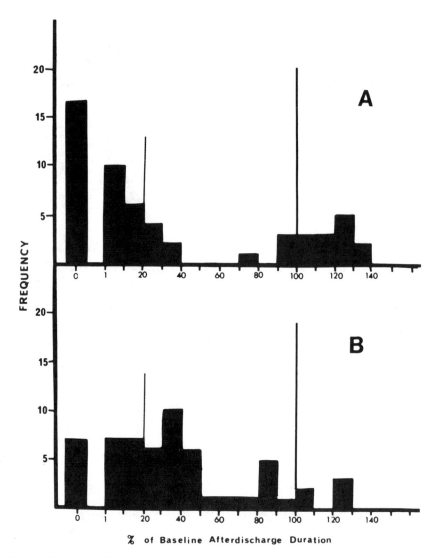

FIG. 6. Frequency distribution of afterdischarge duration in cortex **(A)** and amygdala **(B)** groups after treatment with clonazepam. For each animal, afterdischarge duration at each dose of carbamazepine was determined as a percentage of baseline duration (baseline = 100%). On the abscissa, the line at 100% represents baseline and the line 20% represents the division between focal and intermediate stages. Baseline afterdischarge duration is approximately 100 sec ($n = 10$ cortex animals and 10 amygdala animals).

of seizure suppression with increasing doses of carbamazepine and clonazepam. It was found that these drugs did not inhibit seizures gradually but instead suppressed them in an abrupt steplike fashion. Similar patterns are also observed with the other standard antiepileptic drugs tested (1). These observations are consistent with the hypothesis that the kindled seizure is not a single entity but consists of several distinct components that are differentially sensitive to therapeutic drugs. The generalized seizure is the most responsive to medication, whereas the focal discharge is the least responsive.

These findings suggest a number of interesting points. One observation is that the pattern of seizure suppression with antiepileptic drugs is a mirror image of the steplike stages seen during seizure development. For example, in the amygdala, the development of afterdischarge occurs in several sudden steplike increments (2). This pattern is analogous to the three stages seen during the drug tests described in this chapter. Similarly, in the cortex, both development and drug reversal appear to involve primarily focal and generalized stages with little intermediate activity (2). These parallels suggest that antiepileptic drugs may suppress kindled seizures by reversing the developmental process. Although the significance of this finding is still obscure, it may ultimately provide further insight into the mechanism of action of these drugs.

On the more practical level, these data suggest a particular statistical approach to kindling data. If the kindled seizure is actually composed of distinct components, antiepileptic drug ED_{50} values should not be calculated against the seizure as a whole, but rather against the individual subtypes. Furthermore, since kindled afterdischarge is not suppressed in a gradual or continuous fashion, it should be measured quantally rather than in a graded fashion. (It is more accurate to say that discharge has disappeared in half the subjects rather than to say that the mean discharge is half as long as it was.) When drug effects on kindled seizures are measured in this fashion, a clear and clinically relevant picture emerges. For example, in an earlier paper (1), we examined antiepileptic drug effects separately on cortex- and amygdala-focal and generalized seizure activity. This type of analysis facilitated our observation that the amygdala focal seizure was highly resistant to most therapeutic drugs. This factor, among others, led us to propose amygdala focal activity as a pharmacological model of complex partial seizures in man.

In addition to revealing differential sensitivity of the seizure subtypes to single drugs, this approach also reveals interesting patterns of effects when different drugs are compared. For example, Fig. 7 illustrates the anticonvulsant ED_{50} values of a variety of drugs against generalized and focal seizures kindled from the amygdala and cortex. These data allow us to divide drug effects into three distinct patterns. The first pattern is observed with the majority of the standard clinical anticonvulsants. These drugs are roughly equipotent against generalized seizures triggered from amygdala and cortex and suppress cortical focal seizures at only slightly higher doses. Much higher doses are required to suppress amygdala focal activity. The second pattern of drug effects is typical of the benzodiazepines. Generalized seizures are suppressed at low doses with slightly better suppression being seen in

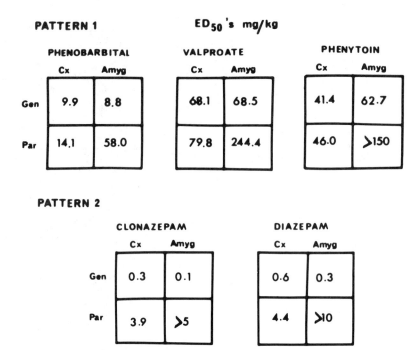

FIG. 7. ED$_{50}$ values for antiepileptic drugs against generalized and partial (focal) activity in amygdala and cortex: (Gen) generalized seizure; (Par) partial or focal seizure; (Amyg) Amygdala; (Cx) Cortex.

the case of amygdala generalized seizures. Toxic doses are required, however, to inhibit focal activity in either amygdala or cortex. The third pattern of drug effects is seen only with carbamazepine. In this case, low ED$_{50}$ values are observed for both generalized and focal seizures triggered from amygdala and cortex. Since we feel that amygdala focal activity models complex partial attacks in man (1), drugs producing this pattern would be expected to be the most effective clinically against complex partial seizures. Carbamazepine, of course, is considered by many authorities to be the drug of choice for complex partial attacks.

CONCLUSIONS

1. Like human secondarily generalized attacks, kindled seizures consist of several different seizure subtypes occurring in sequence.
2. These seizure subtypes are differently responsive to anticonvulsant drugs, with the generalized seizure being more responsive and the focal seizure being more resistant. This is also analogous to the clinical situation.
3. Anticonvulsant ED_{50} should be calculated against the different seizure types rather than against the kindled seizure as a whole. This approach provides a more accurate and statistically correct picture of drug action that more closely resembles the clinical picture. More important, however, it enables us to select drugs with special potency against amygdala focal seizures. This might ultimately lead to the development of a drug effective against complex partial attacks.

ACKNOWLEDGMENTS

The authors are indebted to Mr. Jerome Cheng for his expert technical assistance. Dr. Albright is the recipient of a postdoctoral fellowship from Medical Research Council of Canada. This research was funded by Grant No. MT-5611 from Medical Research Council of Canada.

REFERENCES

1. Albright, P. S., and Burnham, W. M. (1980): Development of a new pharmacological seizure model: Effects of anticonvulsants on cortical- and amygdala-kindled seizures in the rat. *Epilepsia*, 21:681–689.
2. Burnham, W. M. (1978): Cortical and limbic kindling: similarities and differences. In: *Limbic Mechanisms*, edited by O. Hornykiewicz and K. E. Livingston. Plenum Press, New York.
3. Daly, D. D. (1975): Ictal clinical manifestations of complex partial seizures. *Adv. Neurol.*, 11:57–83.
4. Racine, R. J. (1972): Modification of seizure activity by electrical stimulation. II Motor Seizure. *EEG Clin. Neurophysiol.*, 32:281–294.
5. Williams, D. (1965): The thalamus and epilepsy. *Brain*, 88:539–556.

The Limbic System: Functional Organization and
Clinical Disorders, edited by B. K. Doane and
K. E. Livingston. Raven Press, New York © 1986.

Role of the Human Limbic System in Perception, Memory, and Affect: Lessons from Temporal Lobe Epilepsy

P. Gloor

*Montreal Neurological Institute and the Department of Neurology and Neurosurgery,
McGill University, Montreal, Quebec, Canada H3A 2B4*

Subjectively experienced psychic phenomena are among the most striking features elicited by ictal discharge involving the human temporal lobe, as has been known since the time of Hughlings Jackson (7,8). Penfield (23,24) was the first to demonstrate that such "experiential" phenomena, as he called them (26), could be elicited by electrical stimulation of the temporal lobe in conscious man. Such experiential illusions or hallucinations frequently strike patients as being very similar to, and as vivid as, real life experiences, because they share with them a quality of experiential immediacy that frequently encompasses perceptual, mnemonic, and affective features. Sometimes one or the other of these may stand out as the predominant element or may even occur in isolation. In contrast to hallucinations experienced by psychotics, the patients do not mistake them for real life events.

Among perceptual phenomena, complex visual or auditory hallucinations (e.g., seeing a scene or a person, hearing a piece of music played, hearing someone talking) are the most common. Less frequent are gustatory and olfactory hallucinations, whereas experiential somatosensory hallucinations are curiously absent from the repertoire of subjective experiences elicited by temporal lobe discharge or stimulation. The crude cephalic or other somatic sensations, which are sometimes evoked by temporal lobe seizures or by electrical stimulation in the temporal lobe, do not have the subjective quality of experiential phenomena because they lack, in contrast to complex visual or auditory hallucinations, the close similarity to a real individual life experience. Mnemonic phenomena evoked by temporal lobe discharge often appear as memory flashbacks; i.e., the sudden reemergence in memory of a situation experienced at an earlier time in life. These evocations of a past event may be attended by the appropriate visual and auditory hallucinatory phenomena and by an appropriate affective response. Among the mnemonic phenomena one must also include the illusion of familiarity, the famous "déjà vu" sensation, for it really represents an illusion of memory, the illusion that the present is virtually identical with some situation experienced earlier. It is, in effect, the subjective experience of a memory flashback without its content. This subjective experience is a "feeling" and thus has the quality of an "affective" response. It is interesting that there apparently exists a brain mechanism that may separately encode this quasi-"affective" dimension of memory without at the same time encoding its content. Of course, such a feeling of familiarity may be associated with an appropriate visual hallucination or a true memory flashback, in which case it no longer represents a true déjà vu illusion.

The "affective" phenomena activated by temporal lobe discharge encompass the whole panoply of human emotions, although fear is by far the most common. For unexplained reasons, all other emotions are much less commonly evoked. They include emotional distress, which may be described as depression, a feeling of guilt or disgust, anger, or positive emotions, such as a feeling of elatedness, also thirst, and finally sexual emotions. The last have the subjective quality of true erotic experiences as normally evoked by actual sexual intercourse or masturbation and may sometimes culminate in orgasm (27). For unexplained reasons, erotic feelings elicited by temporal lobe discharge have almost exclusively been reported by women; they are exceedingly rare in males. The various affective responses elicited by temporal lobe discharge are usually associated with the appropriate facial expressions and visceral phenomena. In the case of fear, for example, the latter may include pupillary dilatation, pallor, and palpitations, and in the case of sexual emotions in females, they may include secretion of the vulvovaginal glands.

If one attempts to fit these observations within the framework of the known organization of temporal lobe function, one is tempted to attribute perceptual and perhaps some of the mnemonic phenomena to the activation of mechanisms represented in the temporal neocortex, whereas one would be inclined to attribute the evocation of affective states to neural activity involving limbic structures, particularly the amygdala (1–4,10,12,15–18,30). Neuroanatomical, neurophysiological, and neuropsychological evidence suggest that the main stream of information flow in the temporal lobe is directed from the neocortex toward the limbic structures (9,11,22,29), the former serving to analyze the perceptual world around us by identifying the nature and significance of external events in terms of their visual and auditory perceptual properties. The information emerging from this processing of visual and auditory sense data in the temporal neocortex is matched against past experience and then handed on to the limbic structures where, presumably in the hippocampus, memory consolidation takes place (13,14,25), while the amygdala attaches an affective connotation to the perceptual information it receives from the temporal neocortex (3,4,29). The maps of temporal lobe stimulation responses published by Penfield and Perot (26) are in remarkable accord with this concept. Not only do they demonstrate that visual and auditory perceptual and mnemonic phenomena can be elicited by temporal neocortical stimulation, they also show a certain degree of anatomical segregation of visual and auditory experiential responses elicited by temporal cortical surface stimulation in a topographical pattern that is largely congruent with the known representation of higher auditory and visual perceptual functions in monkey temporal neocortex. Thus, Penfield and

Perot (24) found the auditory responses to be clustered in the region of the first temporal convolution, whereas the visual ones had a more scattered distribution in cortical areas located more laterally, posteriorly, and inferiorly. Furthermore, Mullan and Penfield (21) reported that emotions, at least fear, were more commonly elicited from deep temporal lobe stimulation, presumably in the region of the amygdala.

It was therefore a great surprise to us, when reviewing our observations on temporal lobe seizures and electrical stimulation in 35 epileptic patients explored with stereotaxically implanted depth electrodes, that it was limbic ictal discharge or limbic stimulation, and not temporal neocortical discharge or stimulation, that elicited the whole range of experiential responses known to occur in temporal lobe epilepsy (5,6). Experiential phenomena failed to occur unless the limbic structures of the temporal lobe were involved. What was most surprising was that this was as true for complex visual or auditory perceptual hallucinations and for mnemonic phenomena as for affective ones. Furthermore, it became apparent from the analysis of the anatomical correlates of these responses that most of them were elicited from amygdaloid rather than from hippocampal or parahippocampal gyral stimulation or discharge and that, particularly in the amygdala, such responses to electrical stimulation were in more than half of the cases either not associated with an afterdischarge or only with one that remained confined to the area that had been stimulated (5). Experiential phenomena were observed in 18 (52%) of the 35 patients studied with stereotaxic exploration and occurred in 62% of the 29 patients in this series in whom the seizures were shown to arise in the temporal lobe.

Figure 1 illustrates the fact that the anatomical substrate for eliciting experiential phenomena is limbic and not neocortical. Indeed, in this 20-year-old man, right amygdaloid stimulation at 2 mA elicited an elaborate experience encompassing the complex visual hallucination of standing at noontime on a cliff by the seaside with a friend. This experience was associated with fear and represented an evocation of the memory of a past event. This was a fully integrated experience consisting of perceptual, mnemonic, and affective components, as is the case in real life. Left amygdaloid stimulation at the same intensity evoked a déjà vu illusion, and more laterally, in addition, an olfactory hallucination and the verbal expression of an affective state of exasperation. Only the experiential response induced from the right amygdala was associated with an afterdischarge, whereas those evoked from the left amygdala were not. By contrast, none of the neocortical stimulations produced any experiential responses, even though many were followed by afterdischarges.

Tables 1 to 3 document the consistency with which we found limbic structures, particularly the amygdala, rather than the temporal neocortex to be involved in the evocation of all types of experiential phenomena, be they perceptual, mnemonic, or affective. It should be emphasized that tabulating the data in this manner is somewhat artificial. As in the example just cited, an evoked experiential response may comprise perceptual, mnemonic and affective aspects. These three aspects were, however, tabulated separately, because they are not always associated with

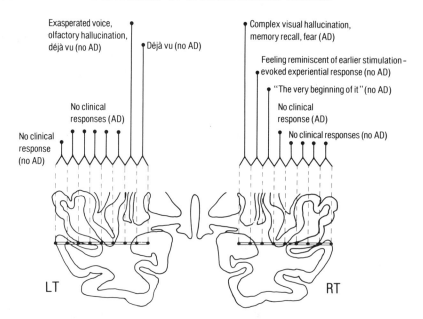

FIG. 1. Topographical distribution of responses obtained in one patient with electrical stimulations applied to adjacent pairs of contacts 5 mm apart along two horizontal depth electrode trajectories through the left and right temporal lobes. Electrode contacts 1 and 2 (most mesial) are within the amygdala; most of the others are in contact with temporal neocortical gray matter. The height of the vertical lines roughly indicates the intensity of responses elicited by electrical stimulations: (AD) afterdischarge; (LT) left; (RT) right. (From Gloor et al., ref. 6.)

TABLE 1. *Perceptual hallucinations and illusions elicited by electrical stimulation:*
Visual 23, auditory 3, olfactory 2

| | | AD | |
Stimulated structure	No AD^a or AD confined to stimulated structure	Limbic spread only	Limbic + neocortical spread
Amygdala	14	2	4
Hippocampus	1	—	4
Parahippocampal gyrus	—	—	3
Neocortex	—	—	—

^{a}AD, afterdischarge.

each other, but may occur separately or only two at the time to the exclusion of the third. Table 1 lists the perceptual hallucinations and illusions elicited by electrical stimulation. Complex visual hallucinations were by far the most common. None of these perceptual phenomena were elicited by temporal neocortical stimulation. All occurred in response to limbic stimulations, and 20 of the 28 responses were elicited by amygdaloid stimulation, 14 times without the induction of an afterdischarge or with an afterdischarge confined to the area stimulated. Table 2

TABLE 2. *Illusions of memory elicited by electrical stimulation: Déjà vu 18, memory recall 16*

Stimulated structure	No AD[a] or AD confined to stimulated structure	AD		
		Limbic spread only	Limbic + neocortical spread	Neocortical spread only
Amygdala	14	—	6	—
Hippocampus	2	—	11	—
Parahippocampal gyrus	—	—	—	—
Neocortex	1[b]	—	—	—

[a]AD, afterdischarge.
[b]Deep temporal stimulation near limbic structures.

TABLE 3. *Emotions elicited by electrical stimulation: Fear 42, anger 1, emotional distress 2*

Stimulated structure	No AD[a] or AD confined to stimulated structure	AD		
		Limbic spread only	Limbic + neocortical spread	Neocortical spread only
Amygdala	17	3	3	—
Hippocampus	9	5	1	—
Parahippocampal gyrus	1	1	3	—
Neocortex	2[b]	—	—	—

[a]AD, afterdischarge. [b]Probably limbic responses: Stimulation was deep, applied near limbic structures from which identical, but stronger, emotional response (fear) was evoked on stimulation.

shows similar results for mnemonic experiential phenomena. These were split about evenly between déjà vu illusions and memory flashbacks. Only one of these was elicited by temporal neocortical stimulation which was applied to deep neocortex close to limbic structures. All others were elicited by limbic stimulations, with 20 of the 34 mnemonic responses being evoked by amygdaloid stimulation, mostly either without afterdischarge or with only a local afterdischarge confined to the area that had been stimulated. Table 3 shows that the anatomical substrate for emotional responses was surprisingly similar to those of perceptual and mnemonic experiential phenomena. Of the 45 emotional responses, 42 were fear, one anger, and two forms of emotional distress of a different kind. The amygdala again was the structure from which most of the affective responses were elicited, most often without an afterdischarge, or only with one confined to the stimulated area.

To discuss the significance of these findings it is necessary to define more clearly the characteristics of the experiential responses elicited by temporal lobe stimulation. A few of our observations will illustrate these.

The first is that of the already mentioned 20-year-old man in whom amygdaloid stimulation had reactivated a memory of an experience he had at the seaside.

Earlier, amygdaloid stimulation at a lower intensity of 1 mA given without warning had elicited another experiential response: As the stimulation was turned on, the patient's face assumed an astonished look and he reported that he had reexperienced a frightening event from his childhood which happened while he was at a picnic in Brewer Park in Ottawa. He described it as follows: "A kid was coming up to me to push me in the water. It was a certain time, a special day during the summer holidays and the boy was going to push me into the water. I was pushed down by somebody stronger than me. I have experienced that same feeling when I had 'petit mals' before." This response occurred without an afterdischarge. This again was an integrated experiential response encompassing perceptual, mnemonic, and affective components. In this patient many diverse experiential responses were elicited by limbic, but never by neocortical, stimulations. Thus, for instance, upon stimulating his left amygdala at 1 mA, he had a feeling "as if I were not belonging here, which he likened to being at a party and not being welcome. There was no afterdischarge. Right hippocampal stimulation at 3 mA induced anxiety and guilt," "...like you are demanding to hand in a report that was due 2 weeks ago...as if I were guilty of some form of tardiness." There was afterdischarge in the region of the right hippocampus and deep temporal neocortex.

Another 32-year-old male patient upon stimulation in the left amygdala at 1.5 mA reported that it felt "like someone talking to a child." It was a female voice and he thought it could have been that of his wife, but he could not understand what was being said. He believed this was an evocation of an old memory. Again there was no afterdischarge.

A third patient, a 32-year-old man, experienced at the beginning of his seizures most vivid déjà vu illusions amounting to an illusion of prescience. At the same time he became very depressed and anguished. Once, during the early part of a seizure recorded by telemetry, a nurse came in with a flashlight. When asked by her whether he had a seizure, he replied: "Yes, and you are coming in right now, it is all part of it, I mean as soon as I pressed it [i.e., the "seizure button"], I almost did not, because I knew you were going to come in. It is as if I were reliving all that is happening now. I just knew that you were going to come in with the flashlight on. In a minute there will be more people, as if it all happened before, just reliving all this." He became very anguished. The seizure discharge involved the limbic structures of the right temporal lobe with spread to temporal neocortex after a considerable delay. The same "déjà vu" experience and anguish were later elicited by right amygdaloid stimulation.

Finally, I would like to relate a yet unpublished sexual experiential response recently observed by my colleage Dr. L. F. Quesney. It was produced by right amygdaloid stimulation in a 40-year-old woman. Upon stimulation of the right amygdala, the patient looked perplexed and was reluctant to talk about what she felt. She had an abdominal feeling like nausea, but in addition she experienced a pleasant feeling in her vulva and on the inner surface of her thighs, as if she were having sexual intercourse. She did not see her partner, but knew it was "X," the boyfriend with whom she had had her first sexual intercourse at age 16, and subsequently many times more. She affirmed that the experience was an evocation of an old memory, and although she subsequently had had intercourse with other men, she was positive that the feeling evoked by amygdaloid stimulation was the feeling of having sexual relations with her old boyfriend "X." The stimulation was followed by afterdischarge involving the amygdala and other limbic structures of the right temporal lobe with spread to temporal neocortex 13 sec later. She volunteered that she had the same sexual experience at the onset of her spontaneous seizures.

It is characteristic of these experiential phenomena that the patients consider them to be similar to real life events, and yet they somehow remain fragmentary. They lack the continuous forward motion in time of true life events, and, although the patient is subjectively intimately involved in them, he is nevertheless a somewhat passive bystander, never having the illusion that he actively participates in these events. Another characteristic of these phenomena is that they most often are set in what might be called a "social context" in the broadest sense of the term, or better perhaps in an "ethological" context. These experiential hallucinations are not events totally disconnected from the patient's life experience; he does not look on them with total detachment, they relate to things or events to which he is not indifferent; they often involve his feelings and his personal memory. They frequently bear some relationship with familiar situations or situations with an affective meaning. They frequently touch on some aspect of his relationship with other people, either known specifically to him, or not.

How should we explain these phenomena? We should first deal with the problem of whether they are the result of some ictal "paralysis" of temporal lobe mechanisms. Most likely this is not the case for reasons detailed in an earlier publication (6). If we accept the fact that they represent some kind of positive expression of the function of the structures activated by epileptic discharge, or electrical stimulation, the question of their anatomical substrate becomes of paramount importance. How can we account for the fact that involvement of the limbic structures of the temporal lobe appears to be essential for the evocation of all aspects of these experiential phenomena, be they perceptual, mnemonic, or affective? In view of the well-known anatomical compartmentalization of the brain mechanisms responsible for these functions, with perception and also some aspects of memory represented in the temporal neocortex, and with affect integrated at the limbic level, one would not expect this. Although this organization undoubtedly reflects a true pattern of topographic representation of brain function, it remains nevertheless true that the distinction between what constitutes perception, memory, and affect is, at least at the introspective level, highly artificial. We experience these phenomena as unified events. It is therefore not too unlikely that somewhere in the brain the contributions of the various areas involved in the elaboration of the components of these experiential mechanisms coalesce. I would like to propose that the site where this occurs is the limbic system, and in particular the amygdala. Visual and auditory perceptual data are first analyzed in the appropriate areas of the temporal neocortex. The objective features of what constitutes a percept are put together there. Subsequently, perhaps also at the neocortical level, this percept is matched with past experience.

Finally, the information is conveyed to the amygdala where affective tone is attached to it. I would like to suggest that this involvement of affect is necessary to make a perception or memory emerge into consciousness, thus enabling it to be experienced as an event "one is living or has lived through." The affective tone attached to perception and memory need not be overwhelmingly intense. All of our everyday experiences of which we become aware are probably endowed with some, if ever so slight, affective coloring. Considering that at any time of our waking existence our brain is being bombarded by a bewildering number of often disconnected sensory data, of which many must at least have the potential to reactivate information stored in memory, the conclusion becomes inescapable that some selection process must be at work which extracts from this ongoing sensory bombardment, as well as from the memory stores, those data that respond to some behavioral need, either actual or potential. What is being selected must be meaningful in some kind of behavioral context; i.e., it must be capable of activating motivational mechanisms, and therefore it will involve affect. Thus affect (not necessarily in the form of an intense emotion) and its anatomical substrate, the limbic structures of the temporal lobe, in particular the amygdala, are important links in the mechanism of selection of what enters into our stream of consciousness. Limbic structures thus are likely to play an important role in determining which sensory data and which memories at any given time emerge into consciousness. The experiential phenomena elicited by temporal lobe discharge or stimulation represent an inadvertent and inappropriate activation of this mechanism, which under these abnormal circumstances operates out of its normal context and in a rather crude manner.

Another interesting feature of experiential phenomena elicited by temporal lobe discharge is the curious absence of certain aspects of perception and memory evoked by such discharge or temporal lobe stimulation. First there is the striking absence of somatosensory hallucinations having an experiential quality. Also absent is the experience of propositional speech, either receptive or expressive. Some patients hear someone talk, but they never relate the content of a conversation. Temporal lobe epileptic discharge or stimulation never elicits the experience of the reenactment of a behavioral sequence moving forward in time, which may have been part of a past experience. However, it often elicits the perceptual and mnemonic context within which such a behavior did or could take place, but the behavioral sequence itself never becomes part of the hallucinated experience. And, as Penfield and Perot (26) so perceptively pointed out, epileptic discharge never evokes a memory of a self-directed effort or action. How can we explain the absence of these aspects of perceptual and mnemonic data in experiences evoked by temporal lobe discharge or stimulation? The answer to this question can, at the present, only be speculative and based on the following considerations.

Behavior depends on two different facets of perception and memory. The one we have been discussing so far is concerned with determining the motivational significance of a situation and is thus involved in the identification of a specific behavioral context. I propose to call this aspect of perception and memory "ethotropic," because it is directed toward the identification of such a behavioral context. This is the aspect of subjective experience which can be activated by temporal lobe epileptic discharge or stimulation. The other facet of perception and memory fulfills an entirely different, though equally important, role in behavior, namely, that of becoming an instrument of the execution of behavior. We may therefore call this aspect of perception and memory "instrumental." Carrying out a certain behavior requires, for instance, the accurate location of objects in space; objects have to be manipulated and locomotion must be induced and directed toward the pursuit of a goal, which in itself may not be fixed in space, thus requiring the continuous updating of spatial information. This requires continuous feedback from somatosensory, visual, and auditory cues. It also requires inner processing to devise behavioral strategy. In man a potent tool in this regard is propositional speech. These "instrumental" aspects of perception and memory and of higher cortical function are never evoked by temporal lobe epileptic discharge or stimulation. This most likely explains why somatosensory hallucinations having experiential qualities similar to those evoked in the visual and auditory modalities never are part of the experiential phenomena evoked by temporal lobe epileptic discharge or stimulation, for somatosensory perception is almost totally "instrumental" rather than "ethotropic." This may also explain why the experience of propositional speech in any form and the memory or the experience of being in the process of carrying out or planning a certain type of activity are not part of temporal lobe-evoked experiential phenomena. It may also be the reason why the experiences evoked by temporal lobe discharge remain fragmentary despite their vividness. They put the patient who experiences them in a certain behavioral context with the immediacy of experience that occurs when one finds oneself in such a context in everyday living, but they leave him there and do not carry him, not even in a fragmentary way, through a sequence of actions associated with the attendant ongoing perceptual feedback that continuously updates the behavioral context in which in real life action takes place. This absence of what we may call the "instrumental" aspects of perception and memory suggests that their cerebral substrate is not temporal and not limbic, but that other brain areas are primarily involved in their elaboration. Some evidence that a dichotomy along these lines is at least present for the visual modality has been provided by the work of Mishkin and his associates (11,19,20). They have shown that visual information handed on from the striate cortex to other areas of the neocortex through anteriorly directed connections at some point follows two divergent pathways, with one taking a ventral course channeling visual information toward the inferior temporal neocortex. This system is involved in the identification of objects and in the retention of these objects in memory. It subserves what I have here called "ethotropic" perception and memory. Another dorsal pathway carries visual information toward the parietal cortex. This system subserves the function of locating objects in extracorporeal space, a function that is vital for the "instrumental" aspects of perception and memory. The concept of a distinction between "ethotropic" and "instrumental" memory is to some extent, although not fully, parallel to that of "declarative" and "procedural" memory discussed by Winograd (31) and Squire (28).

REFERENCES

1. Chow, K. L. (1961): Anatomical and electrophysiological analysis of temporal neocortex in relation to visual discrimination learning in monkeys. In: *Brain Mechanisms and Learning*, edited by J. F. Delafresnaye, pp. 449–468. Blackwell, Oxford.
2. Dewson, J. H., III, and Cowey, A. (1969): Discrimination of auditory sequences by monkeys. *Nature*, 222:695–697.
3. Gloor, P. (1978): Inputs and outputs of the amygdala: what the amygdala is trying to tell the rest of the brain. In: *Limbic Mechanisms. The Continuing Evolution of the Limbic System Concept*: edited by K. E. Livingston and O. Hornykiewicz, pp. 189–209. Plenum Press, New York/London.
4. Gloor, P. (1972): Temporal lobe epilepsy: Its possible contribution to the understanding of the functional significance of the amygdala and of its interaction with neocortical-temporal mechanisms. In: *The Neurobiology of the Amygdala*, edited by B. E. Eleftheriou, pp. 423–457. Plenum Press, New York/London.
5. Gloor, P., Olivier, A., and Quesney, L. F. (1981): The role of the amygdala in the expression of psychic phenomena in temporal lobe seizures. In: *The Amygdaloid Complex*, edited by Y. Ben-Azi, pp. 489–498. Elsevier/North Holland Biomedical Press, Amsterdam, New York, Oxford.
6. Gloor, P., Olivier, A., Quesney, L. F., Andermann, F., and Horowitz, S. (1982): The role of the limbic system in experiential phenomena of temporal lobe epilepsy. *Ann. Neurol.*, 12:129–144.
7. Jackson, J. H. (1879): Lectures on the diagnosis of epilepsy. Lecture III. *Medical Times and Gazette*, 1879, 1:141–143. (Reprinted In: *Selected Writings of John Hughlings Jackson, Vol. 1 On Epilepsy and Epileptiform Convulsions*, edited by J. Taylor, pp. 295–307. Hodder and Stoughton, London, 1931.)
8. Jackson, J. H. (1880/81): On right and left-sided spasm at the onset of epileptic paroxysms, and on crude sensation warnings and elaborate mental states. *Brain*, 3:192–206.
9. Jones, E. G., and Powell, T. P. S. (1970): An anatomical study of converging sensory pathways within the cerebral cortex of the monkey. *Brain*, 93:793–820.
10. Kimura, D. (1963): Right temporal-lobe damage. Perception of unfamiliar stimuli after damage. *Arch. Neurol.*, 8:264–271.
11. Macko, K. A., Jarvis, C. D., Kennedy, C., Miyaoka, M., Shinohara, M., Sokoloff, L., and Mishkin, M. (1982): Mapping the primate visual system with 2-^{14}C deoxyglucose. *Science*, 218:394–397.
12. Massopoust, L. C., Jr., Barnes, H. W., and Verdura, J. (1965): Auditory frequency discrimination in cortically ablated monkeys. *J. Audit. Res.*, 5:89–93.
13. Milner, B. (1966): Amnesia following operation on the temporal lobes. In: *Amnesia*, edited by C. W. M. Whitty and O. O. Zangwill, pp. 109–133. Butterworths, London.
14. Milner, B. (1961): Les troubles de la mémoire accompagnant des lésions hippocampiques bilatérales. In: *Physiologie de l'Hippocampe*, pp. 257–272. Editions du Centre National de la Recherche Scientifique, Paris.
15. Milner, B. (1958): Psychological defects produced by temporal lobe excisions. *Res. Publ. Assoc. Res. Nerv. Ment. Dis.*, 36:244–257.
16. Milner, B. (1968): Visual recognition and recall after right temporal lobe excision in man. *Neuropsychologia*, 6:191–210.
17. Mishkin, M. (1972): Cortical visual areas and their interactions. In: *Symposium on the Brain and Human Behavior*, edited by A. G. Karczmar and J. C. Eccles, pp. 187–208. Springer Verlag, New York/Heidelberg/Berlin.
18. Mishkin, M. (1966): Visual mechanisms beyond the striate cortex. In: *Frontiers in Physiological Psychology*, edited by R. Russell, pp. 93–119. Academic Press, New York.
19. Mishkin, M., Lewis, M. E., and Ungerleider, L. G. (1982): Equivalence of parietopreoccipital subareas for visuospatial ability in monkeys. *Behav. Brain Res.*, 6:41–55.
20. Mishkin, M., and Ungerleider, L. G. (1982): Contribution of striate inputs to the visuospatial functions of the parieto-preoccipital cortex in monkeys. *Behav. Brain Res.*, 6:57–77.
21. Mullan, S., and Penfield, W. (1959): Illusions of comparative interpretation and emotion. *Arch. Neurol. Psychiat.*, 81:269–284.
22. Nauta, J. H. (1972): The central visceromotor system: A general survey. In: *Limbic System Mechanisms and Autonomic Function*, edited by H. Hockman, pp. 21–38. Charles C. Thomas, Springfield, Ill.
23. Penfield, W. (1951): Memory mechanisms. *Arch. Neurol. Psychiat.*, 67:178–191.

24. Penfield, W. (1955): The permanent record of the stream of consciousness. Proc. 14th Internat. Congr. Psychol. Montréal, 1954, Acta Psychol. (Amst). 11:47–69.
25. Penfield, W., and Milner, B. (1958): Memory deficit produced by bilateral lesions in the hippocampal zone. *Arch. Neurol. Psychiatry*, 79:475–497.
26. Penfield, W., and Perot, P. (1963): The brain's record of auditory and visual experience—a final summary and discussion. *Brain*, 86:595–696.
27. Rémillard, G., Andermann, F., Testa, G. F., Gloor, P., Aubé, M., Martin, J. B., Feindel, W., Guberman, A., and Simpson, C. (1983): Sexual ictal manifestations predominate in women with temporal lobe epilepsy: A finding suggesting sexual dimorphism in the human brain. *Neurology*, 33:323–330.
28. Squire, L. R. (1982): The neuropsychology of memory. *Ann. Rev. Neurosci.*, 5:241–273.
29. Turner, B. H., Mishkin, M., and Knapp, M. (1980): Organization of the amygdalopetal projections from modality-specific cortical association areas in the monkey. *J. Comp. Neurol.*, 191:515–543.
30. Ungerleider, L. G., and Mishkin, M. (1982): Two cortical visual systems. In: *The Analysis of Visual Behavior*, edited by D. J. Ingle, M. A. Goodale, and R. J. W. Mansfield, pp. 549–586. MIT Press, Cambridge, Mass.
31. Winograd, T. (1975): Frame representations and the declarative/procedural controversy. In: *Representation and Understanding. Studies in Cognitive Science.* Edited by D. G. Bobrow and E. A. Collins, pp. 185–210. Academic Press, New York/San Francisco/London.

*The Limbic System: Functional Organization and
Clinical Disorders*, edited by B.K. Doane and
K.E. Livingston. Raven Press, New York © 1986.

Contributions of Cerebral Depth Recording and Electrical Stimulation to the Clarification of Seizure Patterns and Behavior Disturbances in Patients with Temporal Lobe Epilepsy

Mark Rayport, Shirley M. Ferguson, and W. Stephen Corrie

*Departments of Neurosciences and Psychiatry, Medical College of Ohio,
Toledo, Ohio 43699*

A unique and remarkable characteristic of this volume, in addition to the excellence of the chapters presented herein, is the intellectual lineage of the participating authors. Each of us in the progression of science stands on the shoulders of predecessors. In the *Second Limbic System Symposium*, Paul MacLean (11) elegantly acknowledged our collective intellectual debt to Papez. I wish, in turn, to acknowledge my own intellectual indebtedness to him, Paul Yakovlev, and Kenneth Livingston in the elucidation of the functional anatomy of subcortical brain systems.

Livingston and Escobar (10) emphasized the cortical projections of the limbic system. It was apparent at once that these limbic frontal and temporal cortices corresponded to the white areas of the myelogenetic brain map of Flechsig (6,7). These white areas bear the higher sequential numbers (38–45), indicating later myelinization. Other high numbers (37–40) appear in the uniquely human cortical areas of Broca and Wernicke (1). Is it possible to draw any inference from the existence of late-myelinizing phylogenetically recent neocortical projection areas of the ancient limbic system? Are these limbic neocortices regulatory or modulatory to the subcortical limbic system? If so, would such projection areas have a role as a cortical substrate of the modulation or control of biologically driven, survival-of-self-or-species behavior in increasingly socially interdependent, culture-producing *Homo sapiens*?

I turn without further delay to the role of stereoelectroencephalography and electrical brain stimulation in the understanding of seizure patterns and behavioral alteration in patients with drug-refractory epilepsy. This chapter and the subsequent one by Ferguson et al. may be regarded as a two-part study of which the first will have a neurological emphasis and the second, a neuropsychiatric emphasis. Each will make reference to certain patients from our respective neurosurgical and neuropsychiatric viewpoints.

It is known that depending on the type(s) of seizures, 20% to 70% of epilepsy patients on antiepileptic drugs remain subject to recurrent seizures despite skillful, serum-level-monitored therapy (5,12,19). A significant number of such persons with drug-refractory seizures can be helped by neurosurgical intervention for seizure control.

Currently, the two major types of neurosurgical intervention for seizure control are excision of the primary epileptogenic cortex (13,14), of which anterior temporal lobectomy is the widely known example (9,15,16), and interventions designed to limit the spread of epileptic discharge through the brain, corpus callosum section being the operation of this type receiving active attention at present (3,4,25). Beyond their dissimilar theoretical bases, these two types of neurosurgical interventions differ significantly in four other major respects: criteria of patient selection, morbidity, mortality, and availability of outcome statistics (Table 1). To be eligible for cortical resection, a patient must have partial (focal) seizures; the primary epileptogenic cortical focus must be localized; its location must be in a safely operable location. Cortical resection has low morbidity and negligible mortality (9,15). Corpus callosum section (CCS), in our hands, has been utilized only in patients with generalized or multifocal seizures. The rather forbidding morbidity and mortality of CCS in the three original series (4,24,26) have markedly declined in recent years with the two-stage approach (18,25). The outcome statistics of cortical resection are well known, thanks, in particular, to a series of classic publications from the Montreal Neurological Institute (MNI) by Penfield and by Rasmussen (13–15). The MNI reports showed that nearly 40% of expertly selected cases of temporal lobectomy became seizure-free postoperatively. In contrast, the outcome probabilities of the operations aimed at limiting the spread of epileptic discharge are not yet established. After CCS, the postoperative absence of seizures pooled from published reports was only 20% (4,24,25). In our own series of 10 callosotomies in multifocal or generalized seizure cases, none are seizure-free (18).

Electroencephalographic (EEG) studies hold a central role in demonstrating and localizing an epileptic focus and therefore in defining operability. Throughout the 1950s, the diagnostic EEG techniques utilized were surface recording at extracranial and cortical levels. Beginning in the 1950s, the French group led by Jean Talairach

TABLE 1. *Comparison of neurosurgical interventions for seizure control (1941–1977)*

Criterion of comparison	Resection of primary epileptogenic cortex	Reduction of spread of seizure discharge
Indication	Unifocal seizures	Poorly defined
Basis of case selection	Demonstration of site of origin	Poorly defined
Operative technique	Well understood	Evolving
Outcome statistics	Well known	Unknown
Morbidity	Near zero	Significant
Mortality	Low	Significant ($\geq$10%)

developed an exceptionally precise human stereotaxic technique for depth electrode placement and introduced and developed the concept and practice of "stereoelectroencephalography" (SEEG) (2,20,21,23). In the 1960s, working at the Albert Einstein College of Medicine, I evolved the hypothesis that the outcome statistics of cortical excision for seizure control were a function of the electrophysiological methodology employed in case selection. Specifically, that the relatively low results of temporal lobectomy (37% seizure-free) published in the literature were consequent to reliance on extracranial EEG and interictal recording techniques for selection of surgical candidates. In other words, the existing statistics were not so much a goal to be emulated as, in fact, a statement of the limitations of outcome benefits resulting from reliance on interictal extracranial EEG for surgical case selection and electrocorticography under acute operating room conditions for localization of the epileptogenic focus on the basis of *inter*ictal discharges. Acting on this belief, I worked with Talairach during my sabbatical year from the Albert Einstein College of Medicine, acquiring command of his acute stereotaxic technique and showing that it was also suitable for microelectrode recording of human single neurons (17).

When I resumed epilepsy surgery at the Medical College of Ohio in the early 1970s, I continued the implementation of the following surgical philosophy:

1. The availability of multitechnical diagnostic capabilities for electrophysiological detection and localization of the epileptogenic cortex, including extracranial EEG, chronic subdural recording, and SEEG with chronically implanted multicontact depth electrodes and electrical brain stimulation would avoid the biasing influence of strong unitechnical preferences that would confine the data base to interictal recording and one particular level of electrode placement, e.g., extracranial, epidural, subdural, or intracerebral.

2. Insofar as the objective of neurosurgical treatment was the elimination of seizures and not of interictal spikes, preoperative EEG localization for surgical case selection must rely primarily on recording during spontaneous occurrence of the patient's habitual seizures.

3. Each patient would be an individual case study in brain pathophysiology, pathomorphology, and behavioral pathology, receiving those modalities of comprehensive investigation applicable to the preoperative understanding of his/her intractable epilepsy problem inclusive of the localization of the seizure mechanism.

4. Since epilepsy pervades both the brain and the life of the afflicted person, a multidisciplinary team inclusive of behavioral specialists would be more effective in helping such persons and in learning about epilepsy.

The practical application of this philosophy is demonstrated in the flow diagram (Fig. 1) of the clinical material for the present neurological/neurosurgical report, which consists of 55 patients with drug-refractory epilepsy who completed the comprehensive preoperative assessment between 1975 and 1982. In 24 (42.9%), the data base showed electroclinical concordance with localizing extracranial EEG; of these, 21 (38.2%) were operated on by cortical resection. Five of the 55 (9.1%)

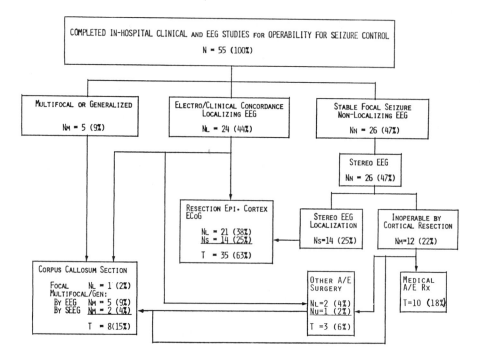

FIG. 1. Flow diagram of the clinical material in this report outlining the epileptological findings in 55 consecutive patients with drug-refractory seizures (1975–1982): (NM) number of multifocal or generalized epilepsy cases; (NL) number of cases with electroclinical concordance and localizing extracranial EEG; (NN) number of cases of partial seizures with stable focal seizure pattern and nonlocalizing extracranial EEG studies inclusive of intensive seizure monitoring with closed-circuit video recording (ISM); (Ns) number of cases with a single epileptogenic focus demonstrated by peri-ictal recording during SEEG/ISM; (A/E) antiepilepsy.

were found to have multifocal or generalized epilepsy and underwent corpus callosum section. The remaining 26 (47.3%) had a stable clinical partial seizure pattern and nonlocalizing extracranial EEG studies. These patients were further studied with SEEG.

Three representative cases are succinctly outlined.

CASE 1

WIC, a 23-year-old single left-handed teacher of handicapped children, sought another medical opinion in regard to her intractable seizures, which first appeared at the age of 9 years. Etiological possibilities included mother's exposure to German measles while pregnant with the patient and an episode of flu in childhood characterized by delirium, marked pyrexia, coma of a few hours' duration, then inability to recognize familiar people for several hours. Neurological examination uncovered an awkward tandem gait and right homonymous hemianopia of which the patient had been unaware and for which there was no history. A computer tomography (CT) scan of the head elsewhere 1 year earlier had demonstrated a hypodense area near the upper left calcarine cortex and a small rounded hyperdensity in the midline postero-superior to the pineal region.

Her seizure pattern consisted of illusion of unfamiliarity, deviation of eyes to the right, receptive dysphasia, amnesia, and behavioral automatism.

Interictal extracranial EEG recording demonstrated bilateral anterior temporal, nasopharyngeal and sphenoidal spikes, with greater voltage on the left. Intravenous pentetrazol activation resulted in increased spiking in the sphenoidal leads bilaterally with somewhat greater voltage on the left. At this point in the workup, her case was presented to a visting senior academic neurologist who encouraged us to proceed with a left anterior temporal lobectomy. However, we were concerned about the electroclinical discordance between a clinical seizure pattern consistent with a posterior temporoparietal localization, and EEG tracings indicative of a mesial anterior temporal localization with uncertain lateralization.

Interictal SEEG recording revealed active bilateral anterior hippocampal spikes, more numerous on the right than on the left, and moderately active left mesial parietal spikes. Intravenous pentetrazol activation produced a seizure originating in the left hippocampus. However, during spontaneous seizures, ictal electrical discharge with suppression onset was recorded from the left mesial parietal cortex at electrode P7 (Figs. 2 and 3). Intracarotid amobarbital injections showed that the right hemisphere was dominant for language. The preoperative seizure classification was partial complex seizures, left mesial parietal.

In 1977 a left parieto-occipital craniotomy was performed, and epileptogenic cortex including an atrophic gyrus was excised from the left superior parietal lobule (Fig. 4). A

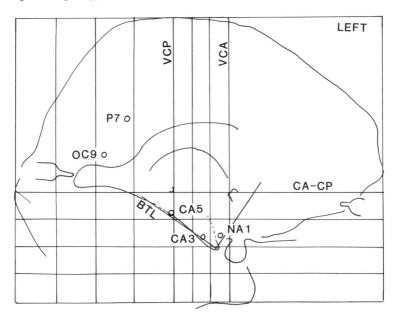

FIG. 2. Case WIC (25 February 1977). Left stereotaxic map showing location of chronically implanted depth electrodes: NA1, left amydgala; CA3, left anterior hippocampus; CA5 left posterior hippocampus; P7, left parietal neocortex; OC9, left parieto-occipital neocortex. BTL, basal temporal line (21); CA-CP, line joining the anterior and posterior commissures (22); VCA and VCP, verticals erected on CA-CP at the anterior and posterior commissures.

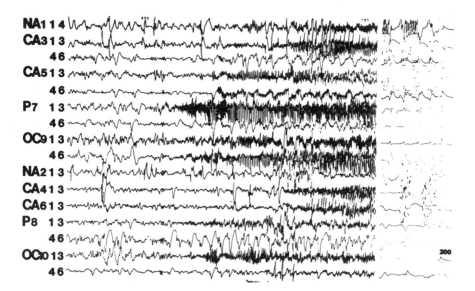

FIG. 3. Case WIC.SEEG recording during a spontaneous clinical seizure. The even-numbered electrodes (NA2, CA4, CA6, P8, and OC10) are the right homologues of the left-sided electrodes (NA1, CA3, CA5, P7, and OC9) identified in the caption of Fig. 1. The numerals 1-3 and 4-6 refer, respectively, to the inner and outer clusters of three contacts each on 5-mm centers. Thus, P7 (1-3) subtends cortex of the medial surface of the left parietal lobe whereas P7(4-6) spans the cortex of the lateral surface of the same lobe. The electrical discharge at the onset of a spontaneous seizure begins in P7(1-3) and spreads to OC-9(1-3) and (4-6), then to CA5(1-3) and CA3(1-3), and to NA1(1-4).

small (2×2 cm) incidental calcified falx meningioma was wholly removed. The excised cortex showed astrocytosis of unknown cause.

The patient has remained seizure-free in the 7 years since surgery, is married and raising a family.

CASE 2

COD, a right-handed 16-year-old white male, was referred for neurosurgical reassessment of his intractable seizures. The first seizure manifestations were behavioral in type and were interpreted in retrospect as having appeared at approximately 8 years of age. Possible etiologic events included an episode of choking at 3 years and a minor fall at 4 years. At the age of 15 years, a cerebellar stimulator was implanted elsewhere for seizure control, without benefit.

His seizure pattern consisted of a behavioral prodrome of irritability and aggressive behavior lasting hours to days. The ictus was ushered in by an epigastric aura with fear, visual illusions (persons he might be looking at would look to him like monsters), and inability to understand; he would stare, scream, attack, or run. Interictal extracranial EEG tracings and ictal conditions showed bilateral independent spike-wave discharges maximal in the nasopharyngeal and anterior temporal derivations bilaterally. His seizures were classified as partial complex, temporolimbic in origin, not lateralized. We believed that he had a single seizure pattern.

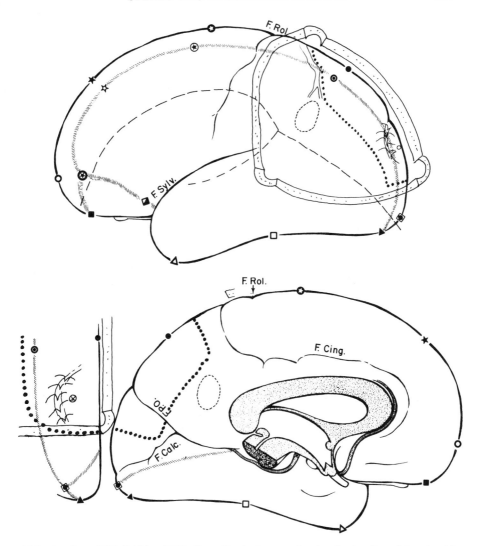

FIG. 4. Case WIC (24 May 1977). Operative brain map showing the location of the atrophic gyrus in parieto-occipital cortex corresponding to the hypodense CT scan lesion, the extent of the cortical excision *(heavy dotted line)* and of the incidental falx meningioma *(short dash line)*. The free margins of the falx cerebri and incisura tentorii and the sinus rectus are outlined *(long dash lines)*.

SEEG (Fig. 5) demonstrated a very active interictal spike focus in each hippocampal formation. SEEG tracings during spontaneous seizures immediately revealed two bilaterally independent seizure onsets originating in the hippocampal formations, characterized electrographically by a suppression onset and correlated respectively with two distinct clinical seizure patterns not detected in the preimplantation workup. With seizures originating in the right medial temporal structures, he would cry out, "Help, it hurts" and roll or turn to the right (Fig. 6). During left mesial temporal discharge, he thumped his left leg, did not

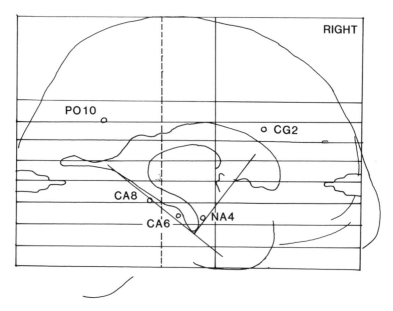

FIG. 5.   Case COD (16 July 1976). Map of right stereotaxic electrode implantation. The electrode and contact identifications are described in the captions of Figs. 2 and 3.

speak, but might groan (Fig. 7). Intracarotid amobarbital injections showed the left cerebral hemisphere to be dominant for language.

He was discharged as inoperable. A few months later he was found dead in his room approximately 1 hr after he had returned to his bed after a known seizure. The cerebellar autopsy findings have been reported elsewhere (8).

CASE 3

PAB, a separated white woman and mother, was referred from another state psychiatric facility at the age of 27 for evaluation of intractable seizures with behavioral symptomatology. She had suffered a head injury at 16 months of age. Chronic seizures began in early childhood.

Her seizure pattern was characterized by an epigastric aura with fear and the feeling that she "was going to be attacked," followed by a "buzzing" sensation (as in a beehive), inability to understand or to speak, and visual illusions and hallucinations. During the ictus, the patient would run, often into dangerous situations. In the postictal period, she might attack other individuals.

Interictal extracranial EEG recordings demonstrated bitemporal independent spikes. Her seizures were classified as partial complex seizures of temporolimbic origin, not lateralized. SEEG revealed bilateral interictal hippocampal spikes and spike bursts of greater voltage and frequency on the right. SEEG discharge during spontaneous seizures originated in the right hippocampus and amygdala.

In 1975 the patient underwent right anterior temporal lobectomy including the amygdala and pes hippocampi. For the past 9 years she has been seizure-free on medication and behaviorally improved.

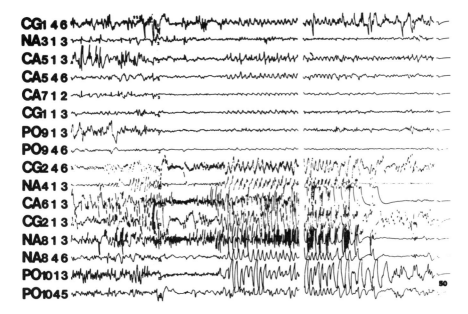

FIG. 6. Case COD SEEG recording during a spontaneous clinical seizure. The ictal discharge arises in the right hippocampus CA4(1-3) and amygdala NA2(1-3). The electrode code further is explained in the captions of Figs. 2 and 3. The gap in the tracing represents a 34-sec interval.

The overall results of SEEG were (Table 2): SEEG generated a localization of the discharging lesion in four cases, one left parietal, in whom this localization would otherwise have been missed, and three cases with bitemporal extracranial EEG discharges who would not have to come to surgery without depth electrode recording. Three of these have been seizure-free for 8, 7, and 2 years, respectively.

SEEG confirmed aspects of the pre-SEEG workup in eight cases and made a definitive localization possible. All eight cases have been operated on. One of the two frontal cases continued to have seizures. The other six had temporal excisions and have been seizure-free from 1 to 7 years. In eight other cases, SEEG yielded clear evidence that they were multifocal and inoperable by cortical excision. Two cases with bifrontal seizures had a preponderance of their seizures emanating from one side. They were both operated on, without significant benefit. Of the multifocal cases, two underwent corpus callosum section, two died after one of their recurring seizures emanating from one side. They were both operated on, without significant benefit. Two multifocals cases underwent corpus callosum section, two died after one of their recurring seizures, and two remain on ineffective medications.

Electrical brain stimulation (EBS) was carried out in 21 (84.0%) of the 25 (84.0%) SEEG cases. In two, EBS generated the information which led to temporal lobe surgery. In 12 others, the results of EBS confirmed the remainder of the data base: half of these were unifocal, the others bilateral. In two cases, EBS reproduced the spontaneous seizure but the remainder of the electrographic data base was not

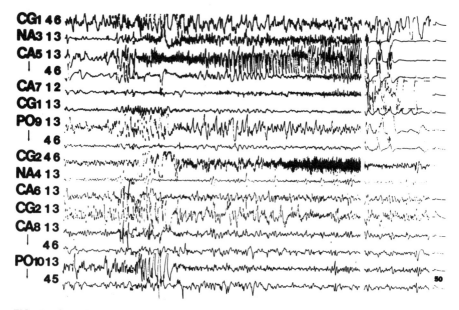

FIG. 7. Case COD SEEG recording during a spontaneous clinical seizure. The ictal discharge is seen arising in the left hippocampus CA3(1-3) and amygdala NA(1-4). The electrode code is further explained in the captions of Figs. 2 and 3. The gap in the tracing represents a 25-sec interval.

TABLE 2. *Depth electrode studies*

SEEG	25
Subdural EEG	1
	N = 26
Definitive surgery	
Focal resection	14
Corpus callosum section	2
RF Amygdalotomy	1
Cerebellar stimulator	1
	N = 18 (69.2%)

adequate to formulate a confident localization. In two cases, EBS did not yield any subjective reports. The contribution of SEEG is summarized in Table 2.

Our results with control of intractable partial complex seizures of temporal lobe origin in 21 consecutive cases, of whom 8 (38.1%) were studied preoperatively with SEEG, show 18 (85.7%) cases are seizure-free, but two have not yet completed a 2-year follow-up. If the seizures were to resume in these 2 patients, the percentage of seizure-free cases would be 76.2%.

CONCLUSIONS

1. SEEG recording of spontaneous seizures is an appropriate method for the localization of the seizure mechanism in patients with a stable clinical seizure

pattern resistant to anti-epileptic medication who have nonlocalizing ictal and interictal extracranial EEGs.

2. Electrical brain stimulation assists in localizing the seizure mechanism and also clarifies the role of a discharging lesion in previously ill-understood peri-ictal and ictal behavior.

3. The resulting seizure control in 85.7% of 21 consecutive cases of partial complex seizures of temporal or parietal lobe origin closely studied before neurosurgical intervention with the individually appropriate EEG modalities during spontaneous seizures and with EBS appears to confirm the hypothesis that the probability of obtaining seizure control by cortical excision is a function of the adequacy of the preoperative workup.

REFERENCES

1. Bailey, P., and von Bonin, G. (1951): *The Isocortex of Man*. pp. 6–7. University of Illinois Press, Urbana.
2. Bancaud, J., Talairach, J., Bonis, A., Schaub, C., Szikla, G., Morel, P., and Bordas-Ferer, M. (1965): *La stéréo-électroencéphalographie dans l'épilepsie. Informations neuropathophysiologiques apportees par l'investigation fonctionelle stéréotaxique*. Masson, Paris.
3. Bogen, J. E. and Vogel, P. J. (1962): Cerebral commissurotomy in man. Preliminary case report. *Bull. LA Neurol. Soc.*, 27:169–172.
4. Bogen, J. E., and Vogel, P. J. (1975): Neurologic status in the long term following complete cerebral commissurotomy. In: *Les syndrômes de disconnexion calleuse chez l'homme*. pp. 227–251. Hop. Neurol., Lyon.
5. Corrie, W. S., Rayport, M., and Ferguson, S. M. (1981): The initial response to an antiepileptic drug predicts its ability to produce long-term freedom from seizures. Presented at the Epilepsy International Symposium, Kyoto, Japan, September 18, 1981.
6. Flechsig, P. (1898): Neue Untersuchungen über die Markbildung in den menschlichen Grosshirnlappen. *Neurol. Centrlbl.*, 17:977–996.
7. Flechsig, P. (1920): *Anatomie des menschlichen Gehirns und Rückenmarks auf myelogenetischer Grundlage*. G. Thieme, Leipzig.
8. Gilman, S., Bloedel, J. R., Lechtenberg, R. (1981): *Disorders of the Cerebellum*, pp. 388–389. F. A. Davis Co., Philadelphia.
9. Jensen, I. (1975): Temporal lobe surgery around the world. Results, complications, and mortality. *Acta Neurol. Scand.*, 52:354–373.
10. Livingston, K. E., and Escobar, A. (1971): Anatomical bias of the limbic system concept. A proposed reorientation. *Arch. Neurol.*, 24:17–21.
11. MacLean, P. D. (1978): Challenges of the Papez heritage. In: *Limbic Mechanisms: The Continuing Evolution of the Limbic System Concept*, edited by K. E. Livingston and O. Hornykiewicz, pp. 1–15. Plenum Press, New York.
12. Meinardi, H., van Heycop ten Ham, M. W., Meijer, J. W. A., and Bongers, E. (1977): Long-term control of seizures. In: *Epilepsy, The Eighth International Symposium*, edited by J. K. Penry. Raven Press, New York.
13. Penfield, W., and Erickson, T. C. (1941): *Epilepsy and cerebral localization*. Charles C Thomas, Springfield, Ill.
14. Penfield, W., and Jasper, H. (1954): *Epilepsy and the Functional Anatomy of the Human Brain*. Little, Brown & Co., Boston.
15. Rasmussen, T. (1975): Cortical resection in the treatment of focal epilepsy. In: *Neurosurgical Management of the Epilepsies*, edited by D. P. Purpura, J. K. Penry, and R. D. Walter. *Adv. Neurol.*, 8:139–154. Raven Press, New York.
16. Rasmussen, T. B. (1983): Surgical treatment of complex partial seizures: results, lessons and problems. *Epilepsia, 24 [Suppl. 1]*: S65–S76.
17. Rayport, M. (1972): Single neurone studies in human epilepsy. In: *Neurophysiology Studied in Man*. pp. 100–109. Excerpta Medica, Amsterdam.

18. Rayport, M., Ferguson, S. M., and Corrie, W. S. (1983): Outcomes and indications of corpus callosum section for intractable seizure control. *Appl. Neurophysiol.*, 46:47–51.
19. Rodin, E. A. (1968): *The Prognosis of Patients with Epilepsy.* Charles C Thomas, Springfield, Ill.
20. Talairach, J., Bancaud, J., Szikla, G., Bonis, A., Geier, S., and Vedrenne, C. (1974): *Approche nouvelle de la neurochirurgie de l'épilepsie. Méthodologie stéréotaxique et résultats thérapeutiques.* Neurochirurgie 20 *(Suppl. 1).*
21. Talairach, J., David, M., and Tournoux, P. (1958): *L'exploration chirurgicale stéréotaxique du lobe temporal dans l'épilepsie temporale.* Masson, Paris.
22. Talairach, J., David, M., Tournoux, P., Corredor, H., And Kvasina, T. (1957): *Atlas d'anatomie stéréotaxique.* Masson, Paris.
23. Talairach, J., Szikla, G., Tournoux, P., Prossalentis, A., Covello, L., Iacob, M., Mempel, E., Buser, P., and Bancaud, J. (1967): *Atlas d'anatomie stéréotaxique du télencephale. Etudes anatomo-radiologiques.* Masson, Paris.
24. Van Wagenen, W. P., and Herren, R. Y. (1940): Surgical division of commissural pathways in the corpus callosum. Relation to spread of an epileptic attack. *Arch. Neurol. Psychiatry*, 44:740–759.
25. Wilson, D. H., Reeves, A. G., and Gazzaniga, M. S. (1982): "Central" commissurotomy for intractable generalized epilepsy: series two. *Neurology*, 32:687–697.
26. Wilson, D. H., Reeves, A. G., Gazzaniga, M., and Culver, C. (1977): Cerebral commissurotomy for the control of intractable seizures. *Neurology*, 27:708–715.

The Limbic System: Functional Organization and Clinical Disorders, edited by B. K. Doane and K. E. Livingston. Raven Press, New York © 1986.

Brain Correlates of Aggressive Behavior in Temporal Lobe Epilepsy

Shirley M. Ferguson, Mark Rayport, and W. Stephen Corrie

Departments of Neurosciences and Psychiatry, Medical College of Ohio, Toledo, Ohio 43699

The focus of this chapter is on the nature and probable mechanisms of aggressive behavior in the person with temporolimbic epilepsy. The use of clearly stated definitions is essential in a study of aggressive behavior.

The term "aggression," according to the *Oxford American Dictionary* (2), denotes the act of making an unprovoked attack. "Aggressiveness" will be used to indicate behavior characterized by a continuous disposition to verbal or nonverbal attack on others, self, or things.

The term "aggressivity" has come into increasing usage recently. Not listed in the major dictionaries, it appears to us as a reasonable professional neologism in need of a nonredundant definition. It is proposed that aggressivity be defined as a behavior disturbance characterized by an intermittent propensity to verbal or nonverbal aggression against others, self, or things.

Current brain assessment technology brings the investigator closer to the mind–brain interface. Still, there is a need for equally rigorous behavioral description in order to define the intervening variables between brain function and behavior. The experimental literature demonstrates variability of response to limbic stimulation, depending on past experience and present context of the animal (1). The uniqueness and complexity of certain partial complex seizures and of nonictal behavior in the seizure patient support this observation.

The behavioral literature of epilepsy during the 1960s and 1970s was dominated by attempts at parsimonious explanations for the aggressive behavior of the temporolimbic patient. Suggested mechanisms ranged from deprived sociocultural background combined with early onset of seizures (7), histopathologic involvement of limbic structures (mesial sclerosis) (3), a basic defect in learning (9), to a "pathophysiologic mechanism separate from that of the seizure disorder" (6). The importance of context in determining the nature of the spontaneous or evoked response has been emphasized (4). More recently, St. Hilaire et al. (8) demonstrated two definite cases of epileptic aggressive behavior in patients with depth electrodes. Ramani and Gumnit (5) concluded that ictal aggression is rare and that episodic aggressive behavior in epileptic patients is essentially an interictal phenomenon.

Response of the environment to aggressive behavior provides an operational measure of the significance and seriousness of the alteration. Thus, our patients have been admitted to such institutions as state psychiatric hospitals from weeks to years, children's psychiatric hospitals, developmental centers, schools for the emotionally disturbed, and group homes. Some have been expelled from schools, jailed, or placed on probation. In other cases there has been considerable disruption of family life with injuries to family members, the patient having to live away from the family, a spouse threatening divorce, and fruitless psychotherapy.

Our own data from patients with intractable seizures have led us to a multifactoral hypothesis that recognizes a significant incidence of aggressive behavior in epileptic patients and emphasizes the interaction of extrinsic and intrinsic factors in its production. Relevant extrinsic factors include interactions with other persons, with the setting, or with ongoing events. Relevant intrinsic factors are (a) pathophysiologic activity of epileptic neuronal populations; (b) higher nervous function impairment due to fixed anatomical brain lesions and/or to intermittent functional lesions related to epileptic neuronal discharge; (c) significant psychodynamic themes of the individual.

It would follow from the above that the mechanisms of aggressive behavior vary from one patient to another and, therefore, must be clarified in the individual case, especially if definitive therapeutic intervention is contemplated.

METHODOLOGY

1. Definition of the clinical seizure pattern(s) and behavioral symptomatology and their interrelationship in the life setting was obtained by interviews with patient and eyewitnesses and by observation of spontaneous seizures during outpatient visits, hospitalization, and intensive seizure monitoring.
2. Comparison of the above with responses to electrical brain stimulation.
3. Continuation of longitudinal behavioral and neurological observations after cortical resection for control of drug-refractory seizures.

CLINICAL MATERIAL

Among 183 patients with partial epileptic seizures formally classified according to the International Classification of Seizures on the basis of neurological, neuropsychiatric, extracranial EEG, neuroradiological, and neuropsychological data, 109 had temporolimbic seizures. Aggressive behavior as previously defined was present in 91 (83%) of these. Temporal lobe operations for seizure control were carried out on 43 (47%) who had aggressive behavior.

FINDINGS

Extrinsic Factors

Repreated aggressive responses of a punitive or taunting nature by the environment may result from the misidentification of seizure manifestations as "bad" or strange behavior. Aggressive manifestations in the patient may develop in response. For illustration, one case will suffice.

BRW was referred for study at 11 years of age with a 6-year history of seizures unresponsive to treatment. His aura consisted of a sensation in his throat followed by brief loss of contact and postictal dysphasia. Scalp electroencephalogram (EEG) confirmed a left temporal epileptic focus.

The patient was the first child of a rigid, narcissistic clergyman who had been proud of his young son previously when he appeared to be precocious, and attentive to his father's every word. Several seizures had occurred for over 1 year before the child was brought to medical attention. When the child did not respond to him as usual, the father took it as a personal affront, as a sign of inattentiveness and disrespect, and repeatedly punished the child verbally and physically. Even after recognition of a seizure disorder, the father communicated his disappointment and displeasure at the imperfections of his child. Similar experiences occurred at school at the hands of teachers and students. If found outside the classroom at an inappropriate time, he would be scolded and punished. In actuality, he might be trying desperately to find his belongings, abandoned at the time of the seizure, and was unable to communicate satisfactorily because of his postictal dysphasia. He was defenseless. His peers also reacted negatively to him because of his behavior—avoiding him or taunting him. He became dysphoric and paranoid—thinking that his classmates were listening to the clicks of his locks to learn the combination so that they could steal his belongings. In response, he had outbursts of anger with attack behavior, which further distanced him from his environment.

Although extrinsic factors in this case appeared to account for the aggressive behavior, intrinsic brain factors were also operational.

Intrinsic Factors

Ictus-Related Aggressive Symptomatology

Aggressive symptomatology was observed in relation to the various phases of the obvious clinical temporolimbic seizure.

During the prodrome

The prodromal period could be brief, occurring just before the aura. In other patients, it lasted for hours, being in fact much longer than the seizure.

Example 1. BAD, a 35-year-old electrician, had held a responsible factory job for 2 years. If his apprentice made an error or attacked a problem incorrectly, BAD would patiently point out the mistake and assume the teacher role in explaining the task. In contrast, he had days during which his behavior was foreign to his usual manner of relating and indicated to him that he might later have a seizure: "When I get up, I know that I am going to have trouble. I have what I call 'the blahs'." He might increase his medication on that day. His altered personality was manifested by his being unusually sharp and nasty, swearing at his apprentice, so that punishment instead of education occurred. In the evening, a seizure often developed with conscious olfactory onset proceeding to a generalized convulsion. The next day, the patient was ready to meet the work and personal demands of his job without the acid behavior that had preceded his seizure.

Example 2. FER, a 24-year-old single man, underwent a left temporal lobectomy after localization by scalp EEG studies.

His first seizure at the age of 6 years was a major motor attack. A chronic temporolimbic seizure disorder began at the age of 11 years. At the age of 12, aggressive behavior became prominent, and by the age of 15, because of attacks on family members with dangerous objects such as knives, psychiatric hospitalization was necessary. Between the ages of 15 and 21, he attended a school for the emotionally disturbed, a college for the emotionally handicapped, and was studied on the research ward of a state hospital. He was seen by a total of six psychiatrists outside of the institutions. Study in a national neurological center led to the conclusion that his seizure disorder was inoperable.

From the age of 21 to 24, he lived in a state institution for epileptics, until referred to us with the persisting chief complaints of drug-refractory seizures and aggressivity.

The seizure onset consisted of receptive aphasia and speech arrest; then he stared and became rigid. The family had noted, and inhospital observations confirmed, that aggressive behavior would precede a seizure by hours to days. Following periods of demanding, impulsive, aggressive behavior, the patient would have one or more seizures and show higher function impairments. For instance, one day while in the hospital, he wanted coffee. Instead of waiting for the nurse to bring it to him, he went into the hall and grabbed the coffee pot. He tussled with the nurse, with the result that coffee was spilled on her. When we saw him after this episode, his speech was not as clear as usual, and, later, he had several seizures. The following morning, he was confused, restless, and irritable; disoriented for time; did not recognize certain personnel; and showed retrograde amnesia. On return to his former state, he related that he remembered the examiner's visit the day after the accident: "You were familiar, but I didn't know your name. I was in a fog."

At operation, an astrocytoma was discovered in the left fusiform gyrus. The left temporal lobectomy included also the amygdala and anterior hippocampus. At last follow-up, 12 years later, he was 36. He had no behavioral problems, although he had an occasional moment of aphasic arrest. He had been holding a civil service job in the capital of his state and served on the board of directors of the local epilepsy association. He wrote in a letter: "Helping those individuals who are mentally disturbed is like a dream come true. Assisting others who are less fortunate means more to me than money."

In this case, aggressive behavior, clearly coinciding with the prodromal period of his seizures, had serious behavioral consequences and was eradicated by removal of the epileptic focus.

During the aura and ictus

During the behavioral automatism for which the patient is amnesic, there may be a motor response consistent with the experience of the aura, or an externalization of repressed or suppressed feelings. Aggressive content may be consistent with a patient's psychodynamic patterns and reflect long-standing central conflicts over the expression of aggressive impulses. The time parameters for the aggressive behavior may vary—sometimes referring to past events and, in other cases, to the present, with ictal acting out of ongoing feelings of anger and depression.

Example 3. JAB, a 36-year-old married unemployed man, had suffered from focal seizures since adolescence, following surgery for a brain abscess in the right temporal lobe.

His seizures began with an aura of fear, which he described as "awesome terror." A similar fearful experience had occurred many times in reality when, following the death of his mother and soon after his brain operation, he would wait up for his father's return from an evening out. Watching at the window, afraid that something had happened to his father, the boy would experience a feeling of terror. When the father appeared over the hill, the boy felt great relief and was able to sink into sleep. Following his aura, which appeared to replicate his terrifying adolescent experiences, the pateint would become subject to his ictus for which he would be amnesic. His ictal behavior consisted of screaming, frightful grimacing, overbreathing, stalking around the room, and threatening. This seizure pattern was totally disruptive to all plans for wage earning and normal social interaction. Despite 9 years of psychoanalysis, these episodes continued. Following operation (J. Ransohoff, MD), he remained seizure-free.

Example 4. One patient, LUE, was surprised at his amnesia-associated aggressive behavior, such as striking his spouse or attempting suicide. The patient later realized that he had been annoyed at his wife or had been depressed over some ongoing difficulties. However, when he was fully aware, he was in control and was not aggressive toward himself or others.

During the postictal period

This period may be brief or extend over days. The most prominent aggressive manifestation is what we have termed "selective aggressivity." The aggressive behavior is not a result of general confusion and not random, but directed toward certain individuals or things and therefore relating to preexisting feelings and experiences. The patient may later characterize the target person as an individual with whom negative interaction had previously occurred. The patient would readily also say that at other times when not under the influence of seizure discharge, he would not have become aggressive.

Examples 5–7. "After a seizure, I never see things the way they are."
"I never hurt a woman or anybody who has been good to me."
Another patient, ELR, would become automatic and walk from one location to another. On one occasion, he remembered being on his hospital ward and was not clear, shortly thereafter, as to how he had reached the place where he found himself, a ward downstairs from his. While trying to figure this out and still mildly confused, he was approached by a person who had been nasty to him at some previous time but now made a gesture to help him. The patient turned on him and attacked him viciously.

One may postulate that affective or limbic evaluation without adequate cortical input and modulation accounts for this type of selective aggression.

Interictal Period

Aggressive symptomatology may occur during what has been called the "interictal" period. This may more correctly be called the peri-ictal period, postictal, or preictal. For instance, subtle seizure activity may be shown to occur in conjunction with previously unexplained behavioral outbursts. If those close to the patient are pressed by inquiry or instructed so as to better observe, or if the examiner himself can make his observations at first hand, it may be found that the objectionable behavior is associated with a single or with multiple minimal seizures. The sequence of events may show that seizure activity has indeed been occurring.

Example 8. GEP, a 25-year-old office worker, had focal seizures localized to the right temporal lobe. She was reported to have attacked her mother on one occasion and had been difficult to subdue for several hours. The antecedent circumstances were not out of the ordinary. The patient and her parents had all returned from work as usual at the end of the day. The patient stated that she was hungry, but, instead of exercising her usual patience until the evening meal could be prepared, she demanded food and proceeded to fight with and strike her mother. In retrospect, the patient's father stated that he had noticed that the patient had been very briefly out of contact and that it was then that the hyperactive behavior had begun. This same patient was observed by the examiner to have similar, though verbal, aggressive outbursts following minimal seizures. In the course of a responsible conversation conveying her appreciation for having found a congenial job, after long unemployment caused by her seizure disorder, she paused almost imperceptibly and stared slightly. Then, both the tone and content of her conversation switched to one of belligerency with paranoid ideation—insisting that she would have to leave the job because of prejudice and describing various negative attitudes exhibited toward her.

This patient was expressing instinctual demands or suppressed feelings, unmodified by cortical evaluation and regulation.

Undetected Higher Cerebral Function Deficits

Example 9. VAG, an 11-year-old girl, had become a severe behavior problem at home because of contrariness and temper outbursts. When asked, for instance, to cooperate in a household task, she would often seem to do the opposite of what was requested. The tense, perfectionistic mother considered the child willful and stubborn and reacted accordingly with strong reprimand. The child, not understanding and unable to describe her unusual experience, would respond with severe temper outbursts. On close observation she was found to have intermittent receptive dysphasia and auditory hallucinated commands. A glioma was demonstrated in her left posterior temporal lobe. After its removal this behavior disappeared.

In other patients higher function deficits affecting memory and speed and efficiency of thinking may persist for days after a seizure. An aggressive response may occur when the patient is pressured by the environment.

Example 10. ROJ, a 25-year-old man, described alteration of his thought processes which persisted for a prolonged time after a seizure: "It's like shoveling snow uphill with a pitchfork." If someone would at this time hurry him or pressure him, an aggressive response might occur.

Postoperative Observations

Postoperative observations have helped to clarify the relationship between aggressive behavior and seizure discharge.

Example 11. Preoperatively, FEM, a 42-year-old laborer, had been chronically irritable. On several occasions, he had become acutely and dangerously paranoid after a series of small seizures. Immediately after operation and during 3 years of observation, he maintained improvement, which he described as follows: "If I get angry now, I just walk away. I don't get into fights the way I did."

Example 12. After a right temporal lobe resection, XAQ, a 12½-year-old girl who had shown aggressive behavior since the onset of the seizure disorder at the age of 5 years, showed no more temper tantrums. Her family said that her personality had returned to what it had been when she was 5; that she was again "sweet and loveable."

Examples 13–15. Other patients say that "things don't bother me the way they used to," or, "I feel better. I don't argue the way I used to," or, "I don't feel mad inside."

Brain Stimulation Responses

Responses behaviorally significant in regard to aggressivity will be described in two patients in the context of clinical history and personal longitudinal observations.

Example 16. COD, a 16-year-old boy, was referred for neurosurgical evaluation because of aggressive behavior and seizures dating from the age of 8 years. His earliest seizures were interpreted as "nightmares." Awakening in the night, he would be found sitting up, staring, screaming, and would attack anyone who would approach. Later he reported dreams of attack by guns and knives. Such episodes subsequently appeared during the day. He also manifested extended periods (hours to days) of irritable behavior during which he attacked people and things. Within a year the behavior problem grew to major proportions, and the boy was admitted to a children's general hospital where it was necessary to keep him in a caged bed. A second hospitalization elsewhere was abruptly curtailed when his behavior was so disruptive that the family was asked at 11 P.M. to take him home. By the age of 10, he required admission to a children's psychiatric hospital where he remained for 4 years. At the age of 15, a cerebellar stimulator was implanted elsewhere with no benefit. At 16, he was admitted to the Medical College of Ohio Hospital for evaluation for possible neurosurgical control of refractory partial epilepsy and behavior.

Close scrutiny of seizure onset and behavioral difficulty indicated a close association: (a) Prior to a seizure, easy irritability and abusive behavior occurred in response to small stimuli and lasted from hours to as long as 2 days. (b) During his aura, he experienced an epigastric sensation with fear associated with visual illusions—the faces of people in sight would look like those of monsters ready to attack—and receptive aphasia. (c) During the ictal/postictal periods, he would stare, scream, run, attack. (d) After a seizure, he would be tractable and apologetic.

During electrical brain stimulation, rapid shifts from pleasant, reasonable behavior to fearful, paranoid, aggressive behavior were observed during electrically induced afterdischarge.

In a prestimulation period, the patient arrived in the EEG laboratory mentally clear and well oriented, stating that he was, "in the hospital, in the recording place, here for a test." Stimulation of the *right amygdaloid nucleus* produced a subjective response of disorientation, misidentifications, and paranoid aggressive content: He gave the location as "a garage," identified the doctors present as "police who are after robbers who stole a thousand dollars."

He made pawing movements if one approached. On stimulation of the *right hippocampus*, the location was again, "the garage," but the staff was classified as "family members—cleaning up together."

On a different occasion he arrived in the EEG laboratory in a pleasant mood, looked around and commented on the equipment. Stimulation of the left hippocampus produced a clinical seizure that began with a look of great fear. He then sat, drew himself up, retreated toward the head of the bed, and began to thrash against his restraints. He could not speak.

This patient showed two mechanisms of aggressivity: (a) He had a prodrome with a raised level of irritability and attack behavior in response to minor stimuli; and (b) during spontaneous seizures and on brain stimulation, aggressivity occurred. During the aura, in response to paranoid ideation, he was ready to attack, and in response to the experience of fear and threatening visual illusions, he tried to flee.

Example 17. PAB, a 27-year-old woman, was transferred for study from a psychiatric facility elsewhere, where she had been detained for 4 years because of aggressive behavior.

Her first seizure had occurred at 16 months of age following head trauma. At 2 years, she was described as placing a hand on her upper abdomen, presumably indicating an epigastric sensation, at the onset of her spells. At 10 years, irritability and rage outbursts appeared: "Sometimes, no one knew why she was mad." The seizures and behavior resulted in erratic school attendance. At 18 she was assigned to a sheltered workshop where she met a man near 60 whom she married. At 20, after bearing two children, she was admitted to a psychiatric hospital in her home state because of aggressive behavior toward herself and others. She remained there for 4 years. At the age of 25, the patient was moved to our psychiatric facility to be within the orbit of our epilepsy group for possible surgical treatment.

Her seizure pattern was as follows: *Aura:* Epigastric sensation with fear, a paranoid feeling (that she was going to be attacked); visual illusions (walls about to fall); and inability to speak. *Ictus:* She would run, sometimes encountering dangerous situations. *Postictally:* She attacked other patients.

After a short period of time in the hospital, the patient met with significant rejection by patients and staff. She was considered unpredictable in mood, manipulative, not trustworthy, overly complaining and aggressive. Diagnostically, she was regarded by some staff members as a patient suffering from psychosis and/or a character disorder, who also had seizures. Observations on the psychiatric ward helped to identify an organic mechanism for some of these characteristics: (a) One day the patient was found with bruises in an unexpected location on the hospital grounds. The patient stated that while out walking, she had been attacked by a man and had been bruised in the struggle to escape. Fortunately, an objective observer's version was available. A nurse stated that she saw the patient walking on the grounds within sight of a male patient. Suddenly the patient began to run at top speed, tripped, picked herself up, and ran into the nearest building. This sequence was consistent with the description of her seizures. (b) The patient would get into frequent fights with other patients. Close observation showed that the individuals attacked were those with whom the patient had had previous negative interactions and that this aggressive behavior occurred following a recognized seizure. (c) The patient was seen during a prolonged period (days) of detachment when she would complain of feeling afraid, as she pointed to her epigastrium. She would give her location as "a hotel" and identify the nurses as "maids." An EEG obtained during this time showed increased temporal spike activity.

During study with stereotaxically implanted depth electrodes, marked fluctuations in the patient's mood state were observed on the neurosurgical unit. One day she arrived in the EEG laboratory morose, sullen, and irritable, exhibiting no spontaneous conversation. The next day she was spontaneous and pleasant, talking freely. She asked, "How is it you change? Yesterday, you looked sad; today you are happy. On some days, I feel on top of the world. On other days, I feel terrible, as if the world is against me."

On stimulation of the *left hippocampus*, the patient had an epigastric sensation with fear. She stated that "people look different." Looking at one of the medical staff, she said, "He is double his weight and strength," or "He is small. I could hold him in my hand. I hear people fussing. It is so fast, I can't keep up. The voices are tangled as if someone is trying to overtalk you." On stimulation of the *right hippocampus*, she stated that "voices are screaming." This was followed almost immediately by her statement that, "The tone of voice is soft and pleasant." She then described a feeling of fear and said, "I'm afraid; I don't like to talk. I would like to get away. The words are twisted."

On stimulation of the *right amygdala*, she became dysphoric and irritable: "I feel afraid, someone is after me. I'm going to be captured."

The rapid fluctuations in affect and perception during brain stimulation were similar to those appearing in her spontaneous behavior which had resulted in a negative reaction from her environment.

Following right temporal lobe excision, which included the amygdala and hippocampus, her emotional lability and aggressivity were eliminated. It was possible for gradual rehabilitation to occur. She was helped to separate from the institutional setting and progressed to a sheltered workshop and competitive work. She resided first in a group home, later at the YWCA, and, then, in her own apartment. She expressed appreciation for her improvement in letters, poems, and during radio interviews, which are a part of her active work in support of the cause of patients with epilepsy.

DISCUSSION

Mechanisms of aggressivity may be related to the following.

1. *Location of the discharging abnormality:*

   a. The neural structures primarily related to aggressive expression in which the onset may be an awareness of a heightened state of irritability unrelated to any particular event or thought process.

   b. Outside the primary neural structures for the expression of aggressive feeling but in the circuitry or locations whose disruption leads to higher function impairments and diminution in neocortical control mechanisms for emotional expression.

   c. In structures responsible for specific higher functions such as those related to speech, and thus producing intermittent disturbances in auditory reception. Consequent misunderstandings arising in interaction with people in the patient's environment may lead to aggressive outbursts.

2. *Intensity of the seizures:*

   a. Clear-cut clinical seizures: (i) during the *prodrome*, which may occur over hours or days with manifestations of a shift in mood and/or increased irritability and aggressivity. (ii) During the *aura*, which may last for seconds or minutes with fearful or anger-provoking content or with vivid hallucinatory experiences associated with pleasurable experiences but leading to action, to rebuff in the puzzled environment, and then to reactive aggressiveness in response to frustration. (iii) During the *ictus*, which may last for seconds or minutes during which a behavioral automatism may occur. This may be related to the content of the aura so that a feeling of fear may lead to fleeing or attacking and a feeling of terror may lead to an acting out or dramatizing of that feeling; or to psychodynamic conflicts with the direct expression of hostility, which is usually suppressed or repressed. (iv) During the *postictal period*, which may last for hours or days, primary thinking processes may gain ascendancy and result in the direct expression, motor or verbal, or unmodified feelings or in a direct response to instinctual demands.

    b. Minimal seizures may occur during a period previously interpreted as the *interictal period*. Clinically, this is manifested by a sudden unexpected shift in behavior or verbal response, such as a disruptive thrust of aggressivity in a patient reasonable only the moment before.

3. *Frequency of seizures:* Fluctuations of behavior and adjustment in relation to the frequency of seizures, major and/or minor. Increased frequency of seizures may lead to increased irritability and impaired higher functions, with consequent misinterpretations and aggressivity.

    The fate of symptomatology after operation then is clearly related to the mechanisms involved in the individual case. The content of the aggressive behavior may well be appropriate to the patient's mentation as a result of seizure discharge and/ or his psychodynamic pattern.

CONCLUSIONS

1. There is a significant incidence of aggressive behavior in patients with temporolimbic epilepsy.
2. Aggressive behavior in some patients with temporolimbic epilepsy may result from temporary disconnection of medial limbic structures from cortical sites necessary for reality-oriented evaluation and control.
3. Interference with higher nervous functions may also play an important role.
4. Definition of the mechanisms of aggressive behavior in the individual patient is essential for evolving an accurate therapeutic plan which may include medication, psychotherapy, environmental manipulation, and/or surgery.

REFERENCES

1. Delgado, J. M. R. (1967): Aggression and defense under cerebral radio control. In: *Aggression and Defense: Neural Mechanisms and Social Patterns*. edited by D. C. Clemente and D. B. Lindsley, pp. 171–193. University of California Press, Berkeley.
2. Ehrlich, E., Flexner, S. B., Carruth, G., Hawkins, J. M. (eds) (1980): *Oxford American Dictionary*. Oxford University Press, New York, p. 14.
3. Falconer, M. A. (1967): Surgical treatment of temporal lobe epilepsy. *NZ Med. J.*, 66:539–542.

4. Kaada, B. (1967): Brain mechanisms related to aggressive behavior. *UCLA Forum Med. Sci.*, 7:95–133.
5. Ramani, V., Gummit, R. J. (1981): Intensive monitoring of epileptic patients with a history of episodic aggression. *Arch. Neurol.*, 38:570–571.
6. Rodin, E. A. (1973): Psychomotor epilepsy and aggressive behavior. *Arch. Gen. Psychiatry*, 28:210–213.
7. Serafetinides, E. A. (1965): Aggressiveness in temporal lobe epileptics and its relation to cerebral dysfunction and environmental factors. *Epilepsia*, 6:33–42.
8. St. Hilaire, J. M., Gilbert, M., Bouvier, G., Barbeau, A. (1980): Epilepsy and aggression: two cases with depth electrode studies. In: *Epilepsy Updated: Causes and Treatment.* edited by P. Robb pp. 145–176. Yearbook Medical Publishers, Chicago.
9. Taylor, D. C. (1969): Aggression and epilepsy. *J. Psychosom. Res.*, 13:229–236.

The Limbic System: Functional Organization and Clinical Disorders, edited by B. K. Doane and K. E. Livingston. Raven Press, New York © 1986.

Radiological Studies in Epileptic Psychosis

Michael R. Trimble

National Hospital for Nervous Diseases and Institute of Neurology, Queen Square, London, WC1N 3BG United Kingdom

The relationship between epilepsy and psychosis has been recognized for many years, and at least two divisions may be suggested. The first is a peri-ictal psychosis, in which patients present with hallucinations, delusions, and disturbed behavior in association with ongoing electrical activity in the brain. In the second, a chronic psychosis emerges interictally. Reports of interictal psychosis were common in the past century, but in the early part of this century they largely disappeared from the literature, several authors even suggesting an antagonistic relationship between epilepsy and psychosis. Although the latter was probably incorrect and based to some extent on a misinterpretation of the literature by succeeding authors (18), a resurgence of interest in the epileptic psychosis occurred with the reports of Hill (9), Pond (12), and Slater and Beard (13). Because of the close resemblance of schizophreniform psychosis to process schizophrenia, Slater and Beard (13) referred to it as a schizophreniform psychosis of epilepsy. Others have disagreed (2), and some have even argued, reintroducing the antagonism literature, that there is little evidence for such increased association (14).

It has been argued elsewhere (16,17), that one of the problems of the literature has been that most authors have used clinical impressions, and little attempt has been made at a precise quantification of the phenomenology of psychopathology in epilepsy using modern techniques of psychiatric assessment. In a recent study, in which the mental state of a group of patients with epilepsy and psychosis prospectively referred to us was described, the clinical signs and symptoms were rated by using the Present State Examination (PSE) of Wing (11). The PSE is a semistructured interview with high interobserver reliability, and it was designed for more accurate assessment and measurement of psychiatric symptomatology, especially the psychoses. In that study, all the patients presented had been psychotic for at least 1 month and were psychotic at the time of the assessment. The psychosis occurred in a setting of clear consciousness, and in addition to their psychiatric examination, several other tests were carried out, including electroencephalography (EEG) and computed axial tomography (CAT). To compare the presentation of epileptic psychosis with schizophrenia, 11 nonepileptic psychotic patients, all of whom had received a clinical diagnosis of schizophrenia, were used as controls.

Of the 24 patients with epilepsy and psychosis, 17 had complex partial seizures and a clinical history and EEG abnormalities compatible with a diagnosis of temporal lobe epilepsy. In seven, the seizure type was generalized, and a diagnosis of primary or secondary generalized epilepsy was made. The PSE subclass categories indicated that 11 of the temporal lobe group were classified as nuclear schizophrenia (NS), six having other forms of psychosis. None of the generalized group received a diagnosis of NS, the latter being composed of symptoms regarded by Schneider as "first rank," in the sense that they are highly likely to be diagnostic of schizophrenia. They include various specific forms of thought disorder, such as intrusion, broadcasting, commentary and withdrawal, specific hallucinations, namely, auditory hallucinations (discussing the patient in the third person), and delusions of control or alien penetration.

Thirteen of the sample received a diagnosis other than NS, six came from the temporal lobe group. Affective disorders were noted in both samples, although paranoid psychoses were more common in temporal lobe patients.

Twenty patients in this study had CT scans performed using an EMI 5005. Cuts of 13 mm were made at normal resolution and radiological assessments included visual inspection of the scan, as well as linear measurements, the latter being performed with a transparent ruler to the nearest 0.5 mm. Subjective assessments of the subarachnoid spaces were rated on a scale of 0 to 3, interobserver reliability having previously been established. The width of the anterior horns, septum caudate distance, the cellae media distance, and the third ventricle size were estimated as described by Gyldensted and Kosteljanetz (7,8). The Evans ratio was measured according to the original descriptions (4) and the posterior fossa structures according to the method of Koller et al. (10).

Evaluation of the CT scans was made blind to the psychiatric diagnoses, and details of the results are presented elsewhere (17a). Visual inspection revealed gross abnormalities in eight of the scans, four showing mild atrophy. In the NS sample, focal lesions were seen in three scans. One had bilateral low-density temporal lobe lesions with greater changes on the left, one had similar lesions with greater changes on the right, and one had a left-sided lesion compatible with earlier resection of an angioma. In the other psychotic patients, there was one left-sided lesion, one right-sided frontal lesion, and one patient with bilateral abnormalities. In the nonepileptic schizophrenia group, no focal lesions were seen, and two were reported as having mild atrophy.

The quantitative data on the scans revealed no differences on cortical assessments in epileptic patients with the different forms of psychosis. All the measurements were large when compared with the normal values quoted in the literature, with the exception of the combined cellae media size and the Evans ratio. From the normative data provided, the most interesting discrepancy was the bilateral septum caudate distance which, in the epileptic NS group, was 17.7 mm (± 3.7 mm) in comparison with quoted values of 14.9 mm. In a small sample ($N = 5$) of epileptic nonpsychotic patients simultaneously radiologically evaluated in this study, the measurement was 13.6 mm (± 3.8 mm), again smaller than in the psychotic group.

No differences in quantitative measurements were noted between the left and right side of the brain in patients with epilepsy and a Catego diagnosis of NS for the width of the anterior horns, septum caudate distance, and the size of the cerebral sulci or cellae media distance.

COMMENT

These CT scan data should be seen in the light of the reports of Slater and Beard (13) and the more recent paper of Toone et al. (15). Using pneumoencephalography, Slater showed a high frequency of atrophic processes in his epileptic psychosis group, especially affecting the central white matter. Toone et al., in a comparison of patients with epileptic psychosis with a group that were nonpsychotic but had epilepsy, noted 44% of the former to have abnormalities (mainly atrophy), with a tendency for a diagnosis of schizophrenia to be associated with left-sided lesions. In our sample some 50% of the total epileptic patients with psychosis have structural lesions and a third of these, atrophy. In the subgroup categorized as NS, all the focal lesions were on the left side, but in two cases the abnormalities were bilateral. These figures are too small to allow comment on the relationship of the laterality of structural lesions to the clincial presentation of psychosis, but the presence of abnormalities in our study is of a similar frequency to those reported by Toone et al.

Quantitative assessments reveal little further information, although it is of interest that the bilateral septum caudate distance is greater in all the psychotic samples and is greatest in the NS group. This hints at involvement of basal ganglia structures in these psychotic states, especially in the group presenting with symptoms of NS.

From the data it would seem that the psychosis that phenomenologically resembles NS occurs in association with temporal lobe epilepsy, but that gross structural lesions on a CT scan, or evidence of atrophy, particularly cortical atrophy, are not clearly associated with its presentation. If gross disturbance of structure is not necessary, we can then attempt to look at function within the central nervous system in such patients using the new technique of positron emission tomography (PET).

PET IN EPILEPTIC PSYCHOSIS

Several methods have been employed to study cerebral blood flow and metabolism in epilepsy. Engel et al. (3) have introduced the 18-fluoro-2-deoxyglucose technique to assess metabolism and have noted focal decreases of glucose uptake during the interictal period in partial epilepsy. These data have been replicated at the Hammersmith Hospital, London, in studies in which we have obtained data on epileptic patients with partial epilepsy using the oxygen 15 inhalation technique. By this method, measurements of the regional cerebral blood flow (rCBF), regional oxygen metabolism ($rCMRO_2$), and the relationship between blood flow and metabolism, the regional oxygen extraction ratio (rOER) were assessed (1). In our studies we demonstrated that these changes in flow and metabolism seen interictally are not confined to the temporal lobes and affect other structures, including the basal ganglia and frontal cortex. In addition, even in patients with unilateral lesions, the contralateral temporal hemisphere appears affected.

We recently carried out a study examining two groups of psychotic epileptic patients, one of which ($N = 6$) was receiving neuroleptic medication at the time of the investigation. The second ($N = 6$) was free from this class of drug, some of the patients never having received neuroleptics in their lives. The psychosis was rated using the PSE, all of the patients having complex partial seizures, secondary generalization occurring in some of them. Age matched data from nonpsychotic epileptic patients ($N = 5$), and age matched nonepileptic volunteer controls ($N = 5$), were available.

The scan procedure has been fully outlined elsewhere (1,5) and will not be presented here. In the majority of patients planes were scanned at OM + 2, + 4, + 6, and + 8, and all were corrected for attenuation by the corresponding transmission scans. Tracer equations that relate steady-state measurements to tissue blood flow, and oxygen extraction ratios, were used to calculate absolute quantitative values of the rCBF, rOER, and rCMRO$_2$.

Following a computer printout of the data, 5.0 cm^2 regions of interest were chosen corresponding to the frontal and occipital regions on slices OM + 4 and OM + 6, respectively. Three areas were measured from the temporal cortex, each 1.5 cm^2 in a continuous strip of slice OM + 4. Additional areas examined included the basal ganglia and a frontotemporal bridge, representing an island of cortical tissue between the frontal and temporal areas on slice OM + 4.

When the frontal, temporal, and occipital areas were examined in this study, all three epileptic samples showed consistently lowered values compared with nonepileptic volunteers, replicating the findings of the first study. (Full details of results are found in ref. 1.) When the psychotic nonneuroleptic-treated group and the nonpsychotic epileptic groups were compared, the former had lower rCMRO$_2$, lower rOER, and higher rCBF in the majority of areas examined. Significantly lower rOERs were recorded from the following regions: left frontal, temporal and frontotemporal bridge, and right frontal and temporal. When the psychotic nontreated, and the nonpsychotic epileptic patients were examined for laterality differences, lower values for the rCBF and rCMRO$_2$ were seen on the left side across the entire temporal cortex in the former, particularly significant in the more posterior zones. Such differences were not recorded for the nonpsychotic sample, with the exception of the anterior temporal rCMRO$_2$.

The treated psychotic patients generally showed lower rCBF values compared with the nontreated, which were significant in the frontal and anterior temporal areas. This resulted in the rOER being higher in the treated group.

COMMENT

Differences between psychotic and nonpsychotic epileptic patients, in whom the length of time of epilepsy, IQ, and age were not significantly different, have been shown in this study using PET as a method of investigating cerebral function *in vivo.* Although the numbers of patients examined is small, and the differences between the groups not great, the pattern of change is consistent, and the differences highly significant in some regions. Of particular interest is the lower rOER in selected regions in psychotic patients, perhaps reflecting real metabolic differences, and the bias toward left-sided decrements of both flow and metabolism in the psychotic group. In that the majority of these latter patients had a syndrome that would be categorized as NS, the results are in keeping with our other study of phenomenology, where a bias toward left-sided lesions and the presentation of NS symptoms were recorded (11).

Although clearly further studies need to be carried out, in particular examining patients with different forms of psychosis, the use of newer techniques such as the CT scan and PET in investigating limbic system structure and function in patients is clearly proving of interest. Our data from radiological studies suggest that the epileptic psychoses most probably represent disturbance of function rather than of gross structure. Further, epileptic psychoses should be seen in the light of new data, particularly from animal models, in which disturbances of limbic system function are being associated with abnormal behavior and the role that epileptic mechanisms play in these is being studied.

SUMMARY

Two radiological studies of epileptic psychosis are presented. In the first, a group of patients had CT scans evaluated by quantitative techniques, and their results are presented in comparison with normative data from other samples. In the second, PET using the oxygen-15 inhalation technique was used to compare cerebral blood and metabolic data in a group of epileptic psychotic patients with normal nonepileptic and nonpsychotic epileptic controls.

The data suggest that the development of epileptic psychosis is not dependent on gross structural lesions, but is more related to disturbance of function, as revealed by such techniques as PET.

REFERENCES

1. Bernardi, S., Trimble, M. R., Frackowiak, R. J. S., Wise, R. J. S., and Jones, T. (1983): Inter-ictal study of partial epilepsy, using positron emission tomography and the oxygen-15 inhalation technique. *J. Neurol. Neurosurg. Psychiatry*, 46:473–477.
2. Bruens, J. H. (1971): Psychoses in epilepsy. *Psychiat. Neurol. Neurochirurg.*, 74:174–192.
3. Engel, J., Kuhl, D. E., Phelps, M. E., and Mazziotta, J. C. (1982): Inter-ictal cerebral glucose metabolism in partial epilepsy and its relation to EEG changes. *Ann. Neurol.*, 12:510–517.
4. Evans, W. A. (1942): An encephalographic ratio for estimating the size of the cerebral ventricles. *Am. J. Dis. Child.*, 64:820–830.
5. Frackowiak, R. J. S., Lenzi, G. L., Jones, T., and Heather, J. D. (1980): Quantitative measurement of regional cerebral blood flow and oxygen metabolism in man using ^{15}O and positron emission tomography. *J. Comput. Assist. Tomogr.*, 4:727–736.
6. Gallhofer, B., Trimble, M. R., Frackowiak, R. J. S., Gibbs, J., and Jones, T. (1985): A study of cerebral blood flow and metabolism in epileptic psychosis using positron emission tomography and oxygen. *J. Neurol. Neurosurg. Psychiatry*, 48:201–206.
7. Gyldensted, C. (1977): Measurement of normal ventricular system and hemispheric sulci in 100 adults with compared tomography of the brain. *Neuroradiology*, 14:183–192.

8. Gyldensted, C., and Kosteljanetz, M. (1976): Measurements of the normal hemispheric sulci with computer tomography: A preliminary study on 44 patients. *Neuroradiology*, 10:205–213.
9. Hill, D. (1953): Psychiatric disorders on epilepsy. *Med. Press*, 229:473–475.
10. Koller, W. C., Glatt, S. L., Perlik, S., Huckman, M. S., and Fox, J. H. (1981): Cerebellar atrophy demonstrated by computed tomography. *Neurology*, 31:405–412.
11. Perez, M. M., and Trimble, M. R. (1980): Epileptic psychosis: Diagnostic comparison with process schizophrenia. *Br. J. Psychiatry*, 137:245–249.
12. Pond, D. A. (1957): Psychiatric aspects of epilepsy. *J. Ind. Med. Prof.*, 3:1441–1451.
13. Slater and Beard, A. W. (1963): The schizophrenia—like psychoses of epilepsy. *Br. J. Psychiatry*, 109:95–150.
14. Stevens, J. (1975): Interictal clinical manifestations of complex partial seizures. *Adv. Neurol.*, 11:85–107.
15. Toone, B. K., Garralda, M. E., and Ron, M. A. (1982): Psychosis of epilepsy and the functional psychoses: A clinical and phenomenological comparison. *Br. J. Psychiatry*, 141:256–261.
16. Trimble, M. R. (1983): Inter-ictal psychopathology in epilepsy. In: *Recent Advances in Epilepsy*, edited by Pedley and B. S. Meldrum, pp. 211–229. Churchill Livingston, Edinburgh.
17. Trimble, M. R., and Perez, M. M. (1982): The phenomenology of the chronic psychoses of epilepsy. In: *Temporal Lobe Epilepsy, Mania, Schizophrenia and the Limbic System*, edited by W. P. Koella and M. R. Trimble, pp. 98–105.
17a. Trimble, M. R., Perez, M. M., Murray, N. M. F., and Reider, I. (1985): Epileptic Psychosis: An evaluation of PSE profiles. *Br. J. Psychiatry*, 146:155–156.
18. Wolf, P., and Trimble, M. R. (1985): Biological antagonism in epileptic psychosis. *Br. J. Psychiatry*, 146:272–276.

The Limbic System: Functional Organization and Clinical Disorders, edited by B. K. Doane and K. E. Livingston. Raven Press, New York © 1986.

Clinical Pictures and Courses of Four Cases with Limbic Epilepsy: A Special Reference to Their Relationship to EEG Patterns

Sadao Hirose and Shunkichi Endo

Department of Neuropsychiatry, Nippon Medical School, Sendagi, Bunkyo-Ku, Tokyo, Japan

A variety of mental symptoms may appear in epileptic patients. A correlation between epilepsy and psychosis has been recognized since the nineteenth century. According to Parnas and Korsgaard (7), in 1875 and 1876 Samt described different types of psychotic reactions among epileptics, including nine cases with chronic psychotic conditions. Many reports concerning the psychotic states of epileptics have since appeared. In 1963 Slater et al. (8) reviewed the literature on chronic psychotic states, closely resembling schizophrenia clinically, that appear in epileptic patients. They described 69 epileptic patients in whom such psychoses appeared. They found that the age of onset of schizophrenia was related to the age of onset of epilepsy and that, in some instances, there was a tendency for psychosis to appear when the frequency of seizures was diminishing. Psychosis most commonly had an insidious onset, although it could also be episodic, acute, or subacute; and its course tended to be chronic. Delusion formation of a typically schizophrenic kind appeared in all but two patients. Also common were hallucinatory experiences, affective disturbances, disturbances of volition and catatonic phenomena, and thought disorders. In keeping with the characteristics of the symptomatology, they referred to these as schizophrenia-like psychoses of epilepsy. They also suggested that various brain lesions could be taken as the etiological factor in both epilepsy and psychosis.

Since then it has been a common opinion among psychiatrists that epileptic psychosis is fundamentally a nonspecific organic psychosis, where epilepsy plays a part only insofar as it might lead to organic cerebral disease (1). Landolt (5) described forced normalization of the electroencephalogram (EEG) as a reaction to organic damage brought about by epilepsy.

On the other hand, recent progress in the study of limbic system dysfunction has focused on the etiological relationship between temporal lobe epilepsy—or more properly, "limbic epilepsy" (2)—and epileptic psychosis. Flor-Henry (1) stated that epilepsy of the nondominant temporal lobe is associated with manic-depressive symptoms, whereas in the dominant temporal lobe, epilepsy leads to schizophrenic-like disturbances. He also stated that epileptic psychoses are fundamentally related to the epileptic process and are not nonspecific psychoses resulting from structural damage.

In recent years violent assaultive behavior has been found to be related to limbic system dysfunction. In 1970 Mark and Ervin (6) found four characteristic symptoms to be common in patients with limbic brain disease or temporal lobe epilepsy and violent episodes in their histories. They referred to this set of symptoms together as the "dyscontrol syndrome."

In this report we describe the clinical pictures and courses of four cases with limbic epilepsy, two of whom had recurrent psychotic episodes and the others, attacks of impulsive self-injury. We also investigate the relationship between clinical pictures and EEG patterns.

CLINICAL EXAMPLES

Case 1: Y. M.

A 58-year-old female first developed a confusional state with perplexity at the age of 22. She had had a punctilious, hardworking, obliging, and stubborn personality. There was no familial predisposition to mental disorders or epilepsy. Since 1948 she had been hospitalized several times and each time was diagnosed as schizophrenic by several psychiatrists because she periodically showed schizophrenic features such as a hallucinatory paranoid state with psychomotor excitement or stupor. She had received electroconvulsive therapy (ECT) and insulin coma treatment repeatedly with full recoveries but had relapsed each time. One year after her first psychotic episode, grand mal and absence seizures spontaneously occurred in 1949.

In March 1958 she visited Matsuzawa Mental Hospital and was subjected to orbitoventromedial undercutting by Hirose because no sustained recovery was obtained by psychotropic drugs and anticonvulsants. After the operation she was markedly improved both in schizophrenia-like symptoms and in epileptic seizures.

In November 1967 she had an attack of status epilepticus after she stopped taking anticonvulsant agents, but immediately recovered after resuming medication. This was the first convulsive attack after the operation. Since then she has had no attacks of convulsion or absence.

In August 1976 she appeared in a dream-like state with auditory hallucinations, delusions of reference, and perplexity. She believed herself to be hypnotized and that people were making her critical. She was admitted to our clinic and recovered with treatment by haloperidol. In February 1980 she was readmitted to our clinic in a dreamy state, preceded by a state of drowsiness wherein she felt herself to be in a battlefield and heard the sounds of shots. During this admission haloperidol was effective in treating her psychotic symptoms, and she was discharged from our clinic in April 1980. After discharge she sustained a state of remission with a small dose of haloperidol and anticonvulsant medication.

During the long-term follow-up of 25 years, we observed the close relationship between her clinical features and EEG patterns, which are summarized in Table 1. Landolt's "forced normalization" of EEG was seen concurrently with the psychotic state, as shown in Fig. 1, and the EEG showed a low voltage fast record without any paroxysmal discharges or other epileptic abnormalities, while various minor EEG abnormalities of epileptic nature were observed during remission. Figure 2 shows focal spike-wave complex (SWC) in the right temporal and frontal areas. This focal discharge was found in the EEG recorded in the state of drowsiness which was followed by a dreamy state during her last admission. Figure 3 shows her computed tomography (CT) scan 21 years following orbitoventromedial undercutting. There are wedge-shaped low-density areas bilaterally in the orbitomedial

TABLE 1. *Various EEG patterns and related clinical features in the long-term followup of case 1*

Diffuse irregular SWCs were seen after status epilepticus in 1967
Various minor EEG abnormalities of epileptic nature such as 4–5 Hz diffuse phantom
 SWC, irregular sharp waves (left occipital predominant), and 4–5 Hz slow-wave bursts of
 short duration (sometimes with larval spikes) were seen in the state of remission
Landolt's "forced normalizations" of EEG were observed concurrently with the
 psychotic state
In 1980 a focal SWC in the *right* temporal and frontal areas was found in the EEG
 recorded in the state of drowsiness, followed by a dreamy state

---

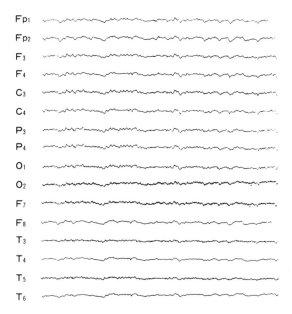

FIG. 1. Forced normalization of EEG of case 1 in the state of psychosis. Low-voltage fast record without any kind of paroxysmal discharges or other epileptic abnormalities. Calibrations, 1 sec and 50 μV.

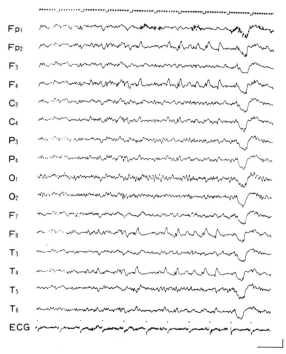

FIG. 2. Focal SWC in the *right* temporal and frontal area of case 1 in the state of drowsiness. Calibration, 1 sec and 50 μV.

frontal regions, which demonstrate the operative lesions. However, no ventricular dilatation or cortical atrophy can be observed.

Case 2: Y. T.

A 32-year-old housewife first visited our clinic in September 1982. She was thought to be suffering from deteriorating schizophrenia because of symptoms such as abulia, blunting of affect, negativistic attitudes, ideas of reference, and so on. However, EEG examination revealed epileptic abnormalities such as sporadic bilateral spikes or sharp waves in the parietal and occipital areas, with background activity which included a large number of diffuse theta waves. Her epileptic fits began at the age of 10. In a fit, she suddenly ceased her activity and became astatic for a short time. Although these fits often occurred more than ten times a day, she spontaneously recovered without medication after several years. They were considered to be atypical petit mal attacks. Since remission she has had no further epileptic attacks. However, at the age of 21 she had a psychotic episode and was sent to a mental hospital with the diagnosis of schizophrenia. She had visual and auditory hallucinations, religious and mystic experiences, delusional mood, thought-broadcasting, and ideas of reference. She was in a state of emotional turmoil with anxiety, phobias, and depression. She recovered within a week with treatment that

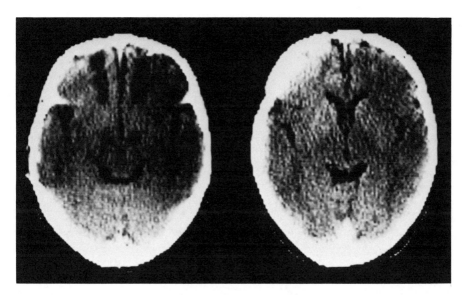

FIG. 3. Case 1: A computed tomography scan 21 years after orbitoventromedial undercutting shows a wedge-shaped low-density area in bilateral orbitomedial frontal regions, which demonstrate operative lesions. However, no ventricular dilatation and cortical atrophy can be observed.

included chlorpromazine, levomepromazine, and ECT. She could recall her abnormal experiences during the psychotic episode. Subsequently, she experienced seven episodes of a similar psychotic state over a period of 5 years. The duration of these episodes ranged from a week to 2 months. After the age of 25, she had no definite psychotic episodes, showing occasional transient mood changes which resembled a mild form of so-called epileptic ill humor. She gradually developed personality deficits similar to a chronic, deteriorating schizophrenic patient. She lost interest in domestic duties and in her hobbies. She often spent time lying on her bed and neglected her husband and daughter. Moreover, she often quarreled with her husband. She became "lazy," and her visits to the hospital became irregular. She had not gone to the hospital for 1½ years before her visit to our clinic.

During the 2-month admission in our clinic, she did not show any positive schizophrenic symptoms such as hallucinations, delusions, and so on, but she showed abulia, blunting of affect, passive and indifferent attitude, and, occasionally, ideas of reference with respect to the nursing staff. However, she gradually improved with treatment by carbamazepine and diazepam and was discharged. In this patient, haloperidol was ineffective.

The sleep EEG recorded 2 weeks after admission still showed high-voltage SWC, but no focal abnormality was observed, as shown in Fig. 4. The last EEG, recorded 8 days before her discharge when she was relatively improved, showed low-voltage fast activity with no paroxysmal discharges. Retrospective investigation of her previous EEG revealed no EEG abnormalities consistent with her mental states.

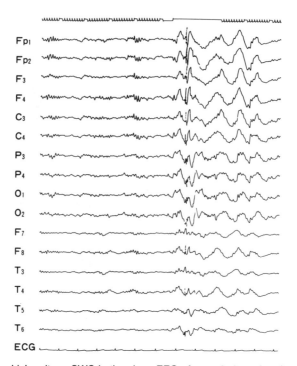

FIG. 4. Diffuse high-voltage SWC in the sleep EEG of case 2, 2 weeks after the admission. Calibration, 1 sec and 50 μV.

Her EEG usually showed bilateral irregular SWC in frontal and frontoparietal areas, regardless whether she was psychotic or not. She showed a focal left anteriotemporal and anterior EEG abnormality of 6 Hz SWC only once when she was in a state of remission. At that time, 6 years after her first psychotic episode, the diagnosis of psychomotor epilepsy was confirmed in another psychiatric clinic.

Case 3: S. B.

A 19-year-old female was admitted to the Department of Cardio-Thoracic Surgery of our hospital and received an emergency thoracotomy to remove a needle from the right ventricle of her heart, which she had stabbed through her left chest wall in a self-injurious act during a state of epileptic ill-humor on June 26, 1982. Since the age of 12, she had had absence seizures or arrests with development of automatisms. She was diagnosed as epileptic in several hospitals, and in one hospital she was found to have a right-sided EEG abnormality. She then received various kinds of anticonvulsants. However, her fits were never adequately controlled, because of irregular medication. She often refused to take drugs because they made her irritable. Whenever she stopped taking medications, she would have attacks. From the age of 14 onward, grand mal seizures occurred and frequently developed into status epilepticus.

During the year before admission for emergency thoracotomy, her irritable state became prominent. She became very aggressive and behaved violently toward her family in the period of ill-humor, which was brought about by the use of anticonvulsants.

On July 8, 1982 she was referred to our psychiatric ward from the Department of Cardio-Thoracic Surgery, after the thoracotomy. Various combinations of anticonvulsants, including carbamazepine 600 mg/day, were tried, but these failed to relieve her state of ill-humor until haloperidol was added, along with the reduction of all anticonvulsants, except carbamazepine. On the ward she was irritable, uncooperative, and aggressive toward nurses and other patients. She sometimes had ideas of reference regarding them and behaved violently against them. On July 27 she injured herself again by stabbing a Japanese red-lacquered chopstick through her right flank abdominal wall and also by stabbing several injection needles into various parts of her body.

Figure 5 shows the sewing needle at the right ventricle of her heart. The chest tube had already been inserted to treat a sucking hemopneumothorax before the thoracotomy. Figure 6 shows the 20-cm inserted chopstick, and also one can see several needles. After removal of the chopstick, it was verified radiographically that the tip of the chopstick had penetrated into the abdominal cavity.

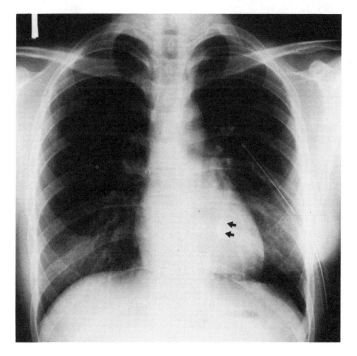

FIG. 5. Case 3: S. B., a 19-year-old female with self-inflicted needle wound. The *arrow* shows the sewing needle at her right ventricle of heart. The chest tube was already inserted for sucking hemopneumothorax before the thoracotomy.

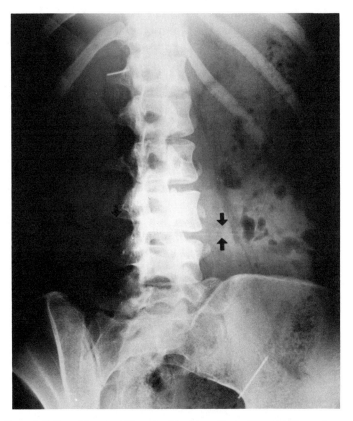

FIG. 6. Case 3: S. B., a 19-year-old female. She injured herself by stabbing a Japanese chopstick through her right flank abdominal wall and also by stabbing several injection needles into various parts of her body. The *arrow* shows the inserted 20-cm chopstick.

Figure 7 shows the focal spikes in the right anteriotemporal and temporal areas with a phase reversal in bipolar leads in the EEG recorded during the state of illhumor. She could not tell us when she stabbed herself, even after her recovery.

A month after admission all anticonvulsants except carbamazepine were discontinued, and haloperidol was increased to the dose of 18 mg/day. She gradually became quiet. She no longer showed any aggressive behavior and, after a trial of staying with her family, she was discharged. Remarkable improvement in the EEG was seen, and 8 to 9 Hz irregular alpha was the dominant activity, with low-voltage fast activity and a few theta waves. No paroxysmal discharges were observed in the state of remission.

Case 4: M. S.

A 24-year-old unmarried woman was referred to our clinic from a mental hospital for orbito-ventromedial undercutting because the operation was expected to im-

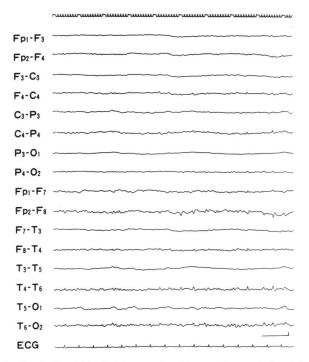

FIG. 7. Focal spikes in the *right* anteriotemporal and temporal areas in the state of ill-humor of case 3: A phase reversal in bipolar leads. Calibration, 1 sec and 50 μV.

prove her uncontrollable impulsive conduct and self-injury. She had an early history of severe otitis media and measles, with frequent attacks of febrile convulsions. At the age of 16 she had autonomic seizures and absence seizures, which sometimes developed into grand mal episodes. She received no treatment for these seizures. She had had a circumstantial, viscous, selfish, explosive, and impulsive personality; and these traits gradually became conspicuous. After her graduation from a senior high school she got a job, but she showed various problem behaviors such as disappearance from her home and a suicidal attempt. At the age of 21, when she was disappointed in love, she went to her lover's home and forced him to meet her. Then she injured herself by cutting her finger with a knife and attempted suicide by taking sedatives. At the age of 22, she suddenly disappeared from her home without apparent reason and repeated her suicidal attempt. She was subsequently confined to a mental hospital, and her EEG revealed that she had a borderline record of 4 Hz bilateral theta bursts in the frontal and central areas during hyperventilation, with a low threshold value to pentalenetetrazol. Despite treatment with a combination of anticonvulsants and antipsychotic drugs such as chlorpromazine, haloperidol, chlorprothixene, and antidepressants, she showed no improvement and repeatedly injured herself by stabbing sewing needles into her body; namely, in the elbow, abdomen, breast, and so on. Moreover, she attempted suicide by swallowing detergent and jumping from the top of a staircase. She had been hospitalized several times, and she was referred to our clinic in June 1972. At the time of admission, she was quiet and showed no impulsive behavior. As shown in Fig. 8, irregular SWCs of short duration were seen in her EEG during hyperventilation. After that she became hypochondriacal and complained of headache and nausea. She often lay in bed. In these hypochondriacal states, the EEG showed improvement. As shown in Fig. 9, sharp waves and dysrhythmias were reduced, and irregular diffuse SWCs during hyperventilation were no longer observed. She also showed a state of mild euphoria for a week, and the same EEG pattern was seen, along with a slightly lowered threshold with megimide provocation. She said that her self-injuries and suicidal attempts were performed during her uncontrollable feelings of irritability, loneliness, and nihilistic mood which suddenly overtook her and which usually continued for a few days. She underwent orbito-ventromedial undercutting and was followed for 2 months after the operation, and she no longer showed mood changes or ill-humor. Her EEG showed a large amount of sharp waves and slow bursts (sometimes with larval spikes) during hyperventilation, which

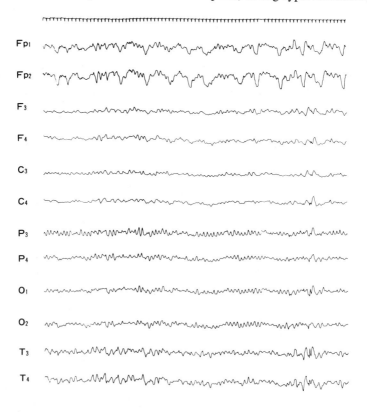

FIG. 8. Irregular SWC of short duration appearing during hyperventilation in the state of remission of case 4. Calibration, 1 sec and 50 μV.

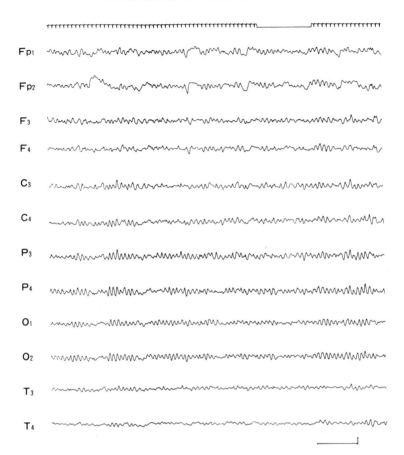

FIG. 9. Improved EEG in the hypochondriacal state of case 4. Sharp waves and dysrhythmias are reduced and SWC is no longer observed. Calibration, 1 sec and 50 μV.

resembled the EEG pattern recorded at the time of admission to our clinic. In 1975, 3 years after the operation, she married, and her explosive behavior was reduced.

SUMMARY AND DISCUSSION

Table 2 shows some details of two cases with psychotic episodes, and two cases with impulsive self-injuries, including ages of onset of epilepsy and psychotic or ill-humored episodes, duration of each episode, clinical pictures, and their EEG correlates.

In three cases the epileptic seizures precede the psychotic or ill-humored episodes. Recently, Parnas and Korsgaard (7) noted that the range of time interval between the age of onset of epilepsy and psychosis was very broad, and in many studies these relationships were not considered of any importance. In our cases the

TABLE 2. *Some details of two cases with psychotic episodes and two cases with impulsive self-injuries*

Case No.	Name	Age	Sex	Age of Onset of Epilepsy	Age of Onset of Episode	Duration of Episode	Symptoms	EEG Correlates
1.	Y.M.	58	F	23 years	22 years	1-4 months	Catatonic features, excitement, stupor, auditory hallucination, delusion of reference, confusion, perplexity	'Forced normalization' in the state of psychosis
							Sleepy tendency followed by a dreamy state	Right-sided SWC in frontal and temporal areas
2.	Y.T.	32	F	10 years	21 years	1 week-2 months	Catatonic features, visual and auditory hallucination, delusional mood, thought-broadcasting, religious and mystic experiences, anxiety, fear, depression	Bilateral epileptic discharges in both psychotic state and remission Left-sided SWC in F and aT in remission
3.	S.B.	19	F	12 years	16 years	2 months*	Irritability, aggressive behavior to others, frequent impulsive self-injuries	Right-sided spikes in aT and T in the state of ill-humor Improved EEG with no paroxysmal discharge in remission
4.	M.S.	24	F	16 years	19 years	A few days	Irritability, depressive feeling of loneliness and sadness, ideas of suicide, frequent impulsive self-injuries, suicidal attempts	'Forced normalization' of incomplete form in the state of ill-humor Irregular SWC in remission

* The episode of ill-humor was usually brought by administration of anticonvulsants, but this time the episode was improved by the medication of haloperidol and discontinuation of anticonvulsants except carbamazepine.

range of this time interval is broad: 11 years in a case with psychotic episode (case 2); 4 years and 3 years in two cases with the episode of ill-humor (cases 3 and 4). Case 1 is an exceptional one, in which the onset of psychosis preceded the epilepsy, and thus misdiagnosis was made by several psychiatrists.

The duration of psychotic episodes in two cases ranged from 1 week to 5 months, and most of them fell between 1 and 2 months. Considering a report of Hirose (3) in 1972 that the operative lesion had caused slight degeneration and gliosis of the dorsomedial nucleus, intralaminar nuclei of the thalamus, and uncinate fasciculus in two brains of well-improved patients who had undergone orbito-ventromedial undercutting, it is interesting that in case 1 the duration of many episodes after the operation became shorter, with remarkable improvement in epileptic seizures. In case 3 the episode of ill-humor lasted nearly 2 months and seemed to be interrupted with treatment by haloperidol and discontinuation of anticonvulsants except for carbamazepine.

The symptomatology of our two cases with psychotic episodes resembled each other, showing acute or subacute onset of catatonic features with confusional coloring, hallucinations, and delusions. However, in case 1, episodes of a dreamy state were usually preceded by a state of drowsiness. In one of the dreamy states, the patient felt as if she were in a battlefield. A right-sided focal EEG abnormality was found only in one of these states of drowsiness. In case 2, not only auditory hallucinations but also visual hallucinations were seen. Religious and mystic experiences with affective coloring such as anxiety, fear, and depression occurred as characteristic symptoms throughout all episodes of this case.

In cases 3 and 4, with frequent impulsive self-injuries, there were some differences in symptomatology. The former showed impulsive, aggressive behavior toward herself and others. In the latter, irritability was accompanied by depressive feelings such as loneliness or sadness, and her aggressiveness was directed toward herself.

In this case study, interest has been focused on the relationship of EEG patterns to the clinical features and their courses in each case to draw out possible causal factors for the episodes of psychosis of ill-humor. In case 1[1], forced normalization of the EEG was seen concurrently with the episodes of psychotic features, as proposed by Landolt (5), who took this phenomenon to be a manifestation of excessive reaction of normal tissues of the brain to the damaged brain function with lesional changes in the brain. Therefore, it is interesting to speculate that the direct manifestation of limbic epilepsy during the psychotic episodes in this case was the state of drowsiness which was followed by a dreamy state, accompanied by a right-sided EEG focus in frontal and anteriotemporal areas. Forced normalization of EEG of incomplete form was also observed in case 4 (Fig. 9), as EEG improvement without SWC during the hypochondriacal state of the patient, in contrast to the appearance of SWC in remission. However, this phenomenon was

---

[1]Case 1 was reported by Hirose (4) at the *First International Symposium on Limbic Epilepsy and the Dyscontrol Syndrome* in Sydney, 1980, and also at the Thirteenth Epilepsy International Congress in Kyoto, 1981.

not seen in case 2 with psychotic episodes or in case 3 with impulsive self-injuries in the state of ill-humor. Besides case 1, focal EEG abnormalities in frontal and anteriotemporal areas were observed in cases 2 and 3. Whereas in case 3, a right-sided focus in the anteriotemporal area was connected with the state of ill-humor, and a remarkably improved EEG without focal discharges was seen in the state of remission. In case 2 the left-sided SWC in anteriotemporal and frontal areas was observed only once in the EEG recorded during remission, and usually bilateral, irregular SWCs in frontal and frontoparietal areas were seen, regardless whether EEGs were recorded in the psychotic episodes or in remission. During hospitalization in our clinic, the patient showed bilateral spikes or sharp waves, and at the time of her discharge she showed low-voltage fast EEG without any paroxysmal patterns.

From those EEG findings it might be concluded that the phenomenon of forced normalization, which was observed in three of four cases, does relate to the nonfocal discharges and does not relate to the focal discharges in the frontotemporal region. These focal discharges seemed to relate to the state of drowsiness in case 1, an episode of ill-humor in case 3, and only in case 2 was it seen concurrently with the state of remission. Therefore, it seems that there are two types of EEG correlates in epileptic episodes: one of them is the manifestation of seizure discharges themselves, and the other is the manifestation of a certain pathogenetic factor related to the epileptic process. In our cases, the former can be applicable to the frontotemporal focal discharges and the latter to the forced normalization of EEG during psychotic episodes, which is still an intriguing phenomenon. As to the correlation between laterality of epileptogenic focus and the type of psychopathology, a dominant hemispheric EEG focus was observed in only one case (case 2) out of two cases with schizophrenia-like psychotic episodes, in accordance with the findings of Flor-Henry (1). Cases 1 and 2 had nondominant hemispheric EEG foci.

In conclusion, no unequivocal relationships between EEG correlates and the clinical states were found in our cases, studied longitudinally and very carefully. EEG forced normalization in the episodes relates only to nonfocal epileptic discharges. Focal discharges in frontotemporal regions showed interindividual differences in relation to the clinical states. Accordingly, accumulation of many more cases studied longitudinally and carefully will be needed. In such a way, we might find a key to resolve the inconsistencies in statistical and transversal studies.

ACKNOWLEDGMENT

Our thanks are due to Dr. Iwao Kubota in the Department of Neuropsychiatry, and to Dr. Yasuhiro Yamamoto, in the Department of the Critical Care Medicine at Nippon Medical School, for their enthusiastic assistance.

REFERENCES

1. Flor-Henry, P. (1969): Psychosis and temporal lobe epilepsy: A controlled investigation. *Epilepsia*, 10:363–395.

2. Girgis, M. (1981): *Neural Substrates of Limbic Epilepsy*. Warren H. Green, St. Louis.
3. Hirose, S. (1972): The case selection of mental disorder for orbitoventromedial undercutting. In: *Psychosurgery*, edited by Hitchcock et al., pp. 291–303. Charles C Thomas, Springfield, Ill.
4. Hirose, S. (1981): Long-term followup of psychosurgical operations in epilepsy with explosive behavior and episodic confusional states in atypical psychoses. In: *Limbic Epilepsy and the Dyscontrol Syndrome*, edited by Girgis and Kiloh, pp. 267–280. Elsevier, Amsterdam.
5. Landolt, H. (1958): Serial EEG investigations during psychotic episodes in epileptic patients and during schizophrenic attacks. In: *Lectures on Epilepsy*, edited by de Haas, pp. 91–133. Elsevier, Amsterdam.
6. Mark, V. H., and Ervin, F. R. (1979): *Violence and the Brain*. Harper & Row, New York.
7. Parnas, J., and Korsgaard, S. (1982): Epilepsy and psychosis. *Acta Psychiat. Scand.*, 66:89–99.
8. Slater, E., Beard, A. W., and Glithero, E. (1963): The schizophrenia-like psychoses of epilepsy. *Br. J. Psychiatry*, 109:95–150.

The Limbic System: Functional Organization and
Clinical Disorders, edited by B. K. Doane and
K. E. Livingston. Raven Press, New York © 1986.

Psychological Methodology Versus Clinical Impressions: Different Perspectives on Psychopathology and Seizures

*C. Stark-Adamec and **R. E. Adamec

*Psychology Department, University of Regina, Regina, Saskatchewan, Canada S4S OA2
and **Psychology Department, Memorial University of Newfoundland,
St. John's, Newfoundland, Canada A1B 3X9

THE CONTROVERSY

Background

A controversy of considerable durability, in both the psychiatric and neurological literatures, revolves around the issue of whether psychosocial problems are an inevitable concomitant of seizure disorders. One approach to the issue, exemplified in the work by Dodrill et al. (12) and by Tan (29), has been to document adjustment difficulties in patients with epilepsy: emotional adjustment, interpersonal adjustment, vocational adjustment, financial status, adjustment to seizures per se, and overall psychosocial functioning. According to their data, emotional adjustment (sexual problems, tension and anxiety, guilt, depression) was one of the two main areas of difficulty for seizure patients. Our research explores this particular area in more depth and may provide clues to the brain mechanisms involved in the etiology of the emotional difficulties—without, of course, negating social contributors to the difficulties.

Another approach, exemplified in the work by Bear (e.g., ref. 7), has been to argue that temporal lobe epileptics suffer from a unique syndrome of psychopathology. As the limbic system is involved in the integration of subjective emotional states with memory and cognition (15), and as temporal lobe epilepsy (TLE), or complex partial seizures (CPS) as it is now called, is defined as episodic sequences of altered perception and behavior which are thought to be initiated by abnormal, recurrent discharging of cells deep in the temporal lobe (i.e., in the limbic system) (13,16), on a neurophysiological level one would predict that patients with CPS would be likely to experience psychological problems, particularly in the emotional sphere. Research using animal models of epileptogenesis (reviewed in ref. 2) lends support to this prediction: it has been demonstrated that repetitive limbic system discharges can produce lasting alterations in emotional response to a variety of environments (e.g., 1–4). However, in the clinical literature, the evidence for a syndrome of behavioral change and psychopathology in CPS is equivocal.

The "18-Trait" Syndrome

After a careful search of the literature to determine the characteristics that have been associated with CPS, Bear and Fedio (8) came up with a list of 18 "traits." They then constructed five items per "trait" label and added a 19th "trait" of 10 items from the *MMPI Lie Scale* to yield a 100-item self-report questionnaire. A purportedly parallel questionnaire was developed to be filled out by a rater (someone who knows the patient well). On the basis of the responses of 48 people (15 right-focus CPS patients; 12 left-focus CPS patients; 12 secretaries and research assistants at the National Institutes of Health, NIH; 9 patients at NIH under treatment for neuromuscular disorders), they reported being able to detect, with a high degree of accuracy, not only whether a patient had CPS, but also whether the focus was on the left or the right side of the brain—with left-focus patients "tarnishing" their image and showing more paranoia and anger, and right-focus patients "polishing" their image.

Problems with the "18-Trait" Approach

Unfortunately, there are more than a few serious methodological and interpretive flaws in the research published by Bear and his colleagues. Since these have been discussed in detail elsewhere (26), they are only highlighted here.

1. The dichotomous true/false response alternative used by Bear is notorious for being the most unreliable response format (23). This may be one of the reasons that other investigators (e.g., Hermann and Riel, ref. 18; Mungas, ref. 21; Rodin, Schmaltz, and Twitty, ref. 24) have been unable to replicate the NIH results.

2. The 18 traits are conceptually derived units rather than *also* being statistically derived units—putting in question the validity of summing items within a trait. For instance, their *altered sexuality* trait consists of two items reflecting increased sexual interest, two reflecting decreased sexual activity, and one reflecting same-sex sexuality—all of which, in the Bear and Fedio scoring system, get added together.

3. The results of their principal components analysis, performed on the "traits", were misinterpreted, with the result that considerable theoretical significance was attributed to what is, in fact, an artifact of the statistical procedure used (see ref. 19 for a discussion of the properties of principal component analysis).

4. Their conclusion that left-focus patients "tarnish" their image while right-focus patients "polish" their image was based, in large part, on the discrepancies between rater reports and self-reports when, in addition to the fact that the formats of the assessment instruments differed in two important respects, 46 of their 100 items were not, in fact, parallel in meaning. If one asks different groups of people different questions, it is not surprising that the resulting patterns of answers would differ.

5. The discriminant function analysis that yielded such high degrees of accuracy of prediction was applied inappropriately, with far too small a subject-to-variable

ratio. The accuracy of prediction was further artificially inflated by the failure to utilize any of the conservative classification procedures, and the results of the analysis—particularly in the Bear (7) publication—were misinterpreted (see ref. 14 for a discussion of the abuses of discriminant function analysis).

6. The sample sizes were far too small for the scope of the generalizations that were made.

SCOTT LABORATORY APPROACH TO THE ISSUE

Our approach has been to ask whether patients with a variety of seizure disorders experience psychiatrically relevant problems. Although Bear's research leaves much to be desired, our decision was that the items constructed for his questionnaire could prove useful in examining the issue of psychosocial concomitants of seizure disorders. Having first determined that the items were scalable—i.e., that they covered attitudes, beliefs, and behaviors that people would want to qualify their responses to—we changed the response format from true/false to a 7-point, "not at all applicable" through to "extremely characteristic" scale, added an item, and, in general, improved the scale construction methodology.

Using our modification of the Bear and Fedio questionnaire, we found that our 101 items were reducible to 26 dimensions (cluster analysis—average distance linkage method; ref. 27). Interestingly, only six of Bear and Fedio's 18 traits are closely reproduced (i.e., hold together as independent and cohesive clusters) when large samples are used. Psychiatric patients obtain higher scores than nonpatients on 24 of these 26 dimensions (MANOVA), indicating that our questionnaire may be tapping psychiatrically relevant issues. Our preliminary results indicated that both sides of the controversy are right and that both sides are equally wrong, i.e., that approximately 20% of seizure patients are virtually indistinguishable from psychiatric patients, but that 30% of seizure patients are "misclassified" as non-patients (jackknifed discriminant function analysis; ref. 27).

CHRONIC ILLNESS CONFOUNDS

One possible explanation of the similarities between psychiatry patients and seizure patients lies in the fact that they are both "patients," i.e., we may have been tapping into a "sick person syndrome." To begin to explore this possibility, we compared the responses of 70 seizure patients, 92 psychiatric patients, 28 dialysis patients, and 447 nonpatients (MANOVA with age covaried) on our questionnaire (28). Dialysis patients were chosen as our first chronic medical condition contrast group as chronic hemodialysis is known to be associated with a variety of psychological problems (10,11,20).

Dialysis patients resembled nonpatients on 16 of our 26 composite indices (clusters) and scored significantly *lower* than nonpatients on three indices: *increased interest in sex, elation, and emotional* (Fig. 1). It makes sense, given their situation, that they would not be experiencing an increased interest in sex and that they would not be as elated as people who do not have a life-threatening medical condition.

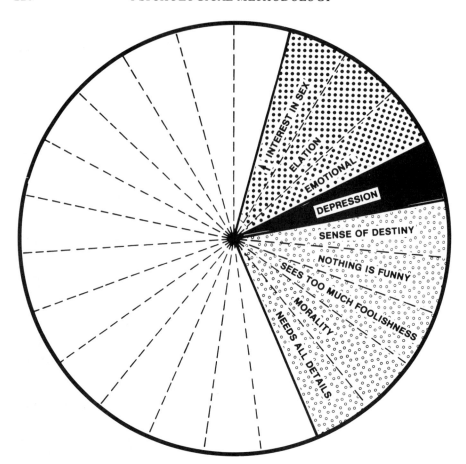

FIG. 1. Pattern of dialysis patient scores on 26 indices: (□) dialysis equal to nonpatients; (●) dialysis less than nonpatients and patients; (■) dialysis greater than nonpatients and less than patients; (○) dialysis greater than nonpatients and equal to patients.

Their lowered emotionality may be reflecting the adaptive denial mechanisms described for these patients.

Dialysis patients scored significantly higher than nonpatients and resembled psychiatric and seizure patients on five indices: *a sense of destiny, finding that nothing is funny, seeing too much foolishness in the world, being annoyed or disturbed by law-breakers or rule-breakers (justice/morality)*, and *needing all details* (Fig. 1). It should be noted, however, that all groups differed on the *depression* dimension, with psychiatric patients reporting the most depression, followed by seizure patients, then dialysis patients, and then nonpatients. This pattern of results is of interest as, intuitively, it is not all that unexpected that the patient groups would resemble each other on these dimensions. Yet, an "inflated" sense of personal destiny, humorlessness, "hypermorality," a "compulsive" need for details, and sadness have been attributed to complex partial seizure patients as a function of their specific neuropathophysiology (7,8). This pattern of elevated scores across dialysis, seizure, and psychiatric patients would suggest that these dimensions are more strongly related to general aspects of chronic medical illness than to the neuropathophysiology associated with complex partial seizures.

Deleting the five indices on which dialysis patients did not differ from psychiatric and seizure patients but did differ from nonpatients—i.e., not deleting *depression*— seizure patients differed significantly (MANOVA) from nonpatients on 16 dimensions: *religiosity, depression, depression +, emotional, moody, unforgiving of self, hatred, temper, own life story important*, philosophical*, powerlessness*, confusion*, repetitiousness*, dependence*, hot-headedness*,* and *writing compulsion* (Fig. 2). On eight of these indices* (*) they also scored as high as psychiatric patients.

It must be remembered, however, that these comparisons are based on group means and that the mean does not accurately reflect individuals at the extremes of the distributions. Using the discriminant functions derived from 14 of the indices (Table 1), the conservative jackknifing procedure "correctly" classified 35.7% of the seizure patients, 66.3% of the psychiatry patients, and 86% of the nonpatients. Within the seizure patient group, 32.9% scored so low on the indices that they were "misclassified" as nonpatients. On the other hand, 31.4% of the seizure patients scored so high on the indices that they were "misclassified" as psychiatry patients. Clearly, seizure patients do not constitute a homogeneous group. It is clear from this analysis that of these three groups, they are the *least* homogeneous.

To summarize up to this point, our results indicate that although seizure patients, as a group, experience psychosocial problems, *part* of the pattern of elevated scores may be a function of the stresses associated with chronic medical conditions—i.e., the five dimensions on which dialysis patients differed from nonpatients and resembled the other patient groups. (We will, of course, be adding other samples of patients with chronic medical conditions to determine more precisely those dimensions affected by long-term medical illnesses.) The attribution of Bear and Fedio's *particular* 18-trait personality syndrome to patients with complex partial seizures would, thus, not seem entirely justified.

SYNDROME SPECIFICITY

Bear (5) has stated that "... the critical observation in defining a syndrome is the regular, simultaneous occurrence of multiple symptoms, medical or behavioral, in the same patient" (p. 48). He further contends that while psychiatric patients may exhibit elements of his syndrome, only patients with seizure disorders involving the temporal lobe would show *all* the elements of the syndrome (5,6,9). Mungas (21,22), on the other hand, maintains that what Bear's instrument measures is a very *nonspecific* psychopathology.

It was possible for us to address this issue directly (25). First, we considered that a "syndrome" with 26 elements in it would make it virtually impossible to find

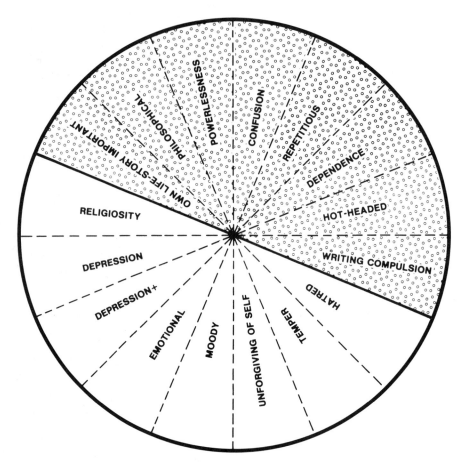

FIG. 2. Sixteen indices on which seizure patients score higher than nonpatients (omitting five indexes on which dialysis patients score higher than nonpatients: (○) seizure patients equal to psychiatric patients; (□) seizure patients less than psychiatric patients.

TABLE 1. *Discriminant analysis: 26 indices; jackknifed classification (14 indices)*

Actual group	Classification (%)		
	Seizures	Psychiatry	Nonpatients
Seizures	35.7	31.4	32.9
Psychiatry	18.5	66.3	15.2
Nonpatients	9.0	5.0	86.0

Total Percent "Correct," 65.6.

anyone who would be suffering from the syndrome, i.e., who would score high on all 26 indices. So, to be generous, we utilized the second-order clusters, of which there were 11 (Table 2). If Bear is correct, a large percentage of seizure patients should score high (mean second-order cluster score greater than 4) on all 11 components of the "syndrome," whereas virtually no psychiatric patients should score high on all 11 elements. As Bear might have predicted, only 1% of the psychiatric patients scored high on 10 or 11 of the elements (female; substance-use disorder, mixed). However, only 1.4% of the seizure patients scored high on 10 or 11 of the elements (male; CPS with secondary generalization but no clear EEG evidence of epilepsy).

Considering that perhaps our criterion for a syndrome might still be too stiff, we loosened it so that it would only be necessary for a person to score high on more than 50% of the elements to be considered to have manifested the "syndrome". Of the seizure patients, 31.4% scored high on more than half the elements. (It should be noted that these high-scoring seizure patients were CPS patients, CPS patients with secondary generalization, *and* primary generalized seizure disorder patients.) However, an even greater percentage of psychiatric patients—44.5%— scored high on more than half the elements of the syndrome. Furthermore, with 11 dimensions and the possibility of scoring high, medium, or low on each of them, there are 78 possible combinations, e.g., high on six, low on two, moderate on three versus high on seven, low on one, moderate on three, and so on. The 70

TABLE 2. *Eleven second-order clusters*

1. Own life story important
2. Interprets deeply
   Philosophical
   Powerlessness
   Sense of destiny
   Religiosity
3. Increased interest in sex
   Elation
4. Depression
   Depression +
   Emotional
   Moody
   Unforgiving of self
5. Confusion
   Repetitious (to & off the point)
6. Dependence
7. Temper
   Hotheadedness
   Hatred
8. Nothing is funny
   Sees too much foolishness
9. Decreased sexual activity
10. Morality
    Needs all details
11. Diary important
    Writing compulsion

seizure patients exhibited 34 different combinations of high/medium/low scores on the 11 second-order clusters. Taken together, these data do not provide a very impressive argument for specificity. This, incidentally, is without taking into account the pattern of scores across clusters. It is not just the combination, it is the permutation of scores that is important when considering the possible existence of a syndrome. There are 8.7×10^{36} permutations of the 11 components: *None* of the patients with the same combination had the same permutation. Even allowing for the fact that a medical definition of a syndrome may be considerably looser than a statistical definition of a syndrome, the data do not support Bear's operational definition of a particular 18-trait syndrome of psychopathology specific to complex partial seizure patients.

Another way to look at the specificity issue is to test for differences within the predefined groups according to diagnosis. The psychiatry patients were grouped according to the *DSM-III* classification system into major categories of schizophrenic disorders (*DMS-III* 295; 7.2%); affective disorders (*DSM-III* 296; 24%); anxiety disorders (*DSM-III* 300; 20%); personality disorders (*DSM-III* 301; 31%); substance use disorders (*DMS-III* 303/305; 7.2%); and adjustment disorders (*DSM-III* 309; 9.6%). The MANOVA results were clear and unequivocal; *DSM-III* diagnostic groups do not differ on any of the 11 second-order clusters. The seizure disorder patients were grouped according to three diagnoses: complex partial seizures (CPS) (22%), CPS with secondary generalization (38%), and primary generalized (40%). Once again the MANOVA results were clear and unequivocal: patients with these three seizure diagnoses do not differ on any of the 11 second-order clusters.

Nevertheless, there are MANOVA differences between psychiatric patients and nonpatients, between seizure patients and nonpatients, between these patients and dialysis patients, and both differences and nondifferences between seizure patients and psychiatric patients on these second-order clusters. Once again, using a jackknifed discriminant function analysis, almost equal proportions of seizure patients get "misclassified" as psychiatric patients (38.6%) as get "misclassified" as nonpatients (35.7%).

If there is a syndrome, it is not as specific as claimed, but it is also not as nonspecific as claimed. The really interesting question is not whether seizure patients suffer from or are free of psychopathology, but, more importantly, how might one predict *which* seizure patients would likely be at risk for psychopathology, and what factors might be responsible for this increased risk.

PREDICTION

A clue to one of the factors that may differentiate these subgroups has recently been provided by Hermann et al. (17). They were conducting retrospective research on 14 patients with generalized epilepsy, 14 CPS patients with olfactory and gustatory auras, and 11 CPS patients with fear auras. They found that the *paranoia, psychasthenia, schizophrenia,* and *social introversion* scales of the MMPI were significantly higher for the CPS-fear-aura patients than for either of the other two groups. Furthermore, all CPS patients with psychopathology had fear auras, although not all fear-aura-CPS patients had psychopathology. In other words, CPS patients who have fear auras may be more at risk for psychopathology than are CPS patients with gustatory or olfactory auras or than patients with primary generalized epilepsy. The fear aura is of particular interest since it is believed that this preictal or paraictal event indicates a spread of discharge into anterior temporal lobe structures, including limbic areas such as the amygdala (2). The aura may thus serve as a marker of degree of limbic involvement in the seizure discharge.

Hermann et al. (17), however, were unable to account for the "some but not all" nature of the fear-aura-CPS link with psychopathology. To help sort out our data, as well as those of Hermann et al., we initiated a study investigating aura experiences in relation to the psychological concomitants of CPS in more detail. Both the frequency and intensity of 33 preictal and paraictal events are being studied. Among other factors that are being taken into account are the locus of the lesion or focus (or foci) (when known), age at onset of seizures, chronicity, seizure frequency, and medication.

The potential impact of research in this area is, in part, dependent on the precision with which the seizure diagnosis can be specified. Definitive diagnoses of seizure disorders are difficult to achieve: (a) the clinical and EEG findings may not concur; (b) neurologists may differ in the emphasis placed on the history and clinical symptomatology; or, as frequently happens with CPS patients, (c) the patient may not have an EEG-detectable seizure at the time the EEG is taken. To circumvent the diagnostic problems and to access an uncontestably definitive criterion group of CPS patients, we have initiated collaborative research with the Neurology Service at Hôpital Notre-Dame in Montréal (Dr. J.-M. Saint-Hilaire and I. Rouleau). By studying patients scheduled for temporal lobectomy with simultaneous scalp, cortical, and limbic electrode recordings, we will be validating our questionnaires and putting our theories to the test. These new, collaborative research endeavors will also undoubtedly stimulate additional, testable hypotheses regarding patterns of limbic system dysfunction.

ACKNOWLEDGMENTS

This research is supported by a grant from the National Health Research and Development Programme (NHRDP: 6606-1843-42), Health and Welfare Canada, to Drs. Stark-Adamec, Adamec, and Hicks. The research is being conducted during the tenure of a National Health Research Scholar Award (Stark-Adamec) and an Ontario Mental Health Foundation Scholar Award (Adamec). The aura and criterion group studies are partially assisted by a contribution from the Savoy Foundation for Epilepsy (Stark-Adamec).

We are grateful to Drs. R. Hicks and S. Bruun-Meyer (Psychiatry Service, Wellesley Hospital), Drs. J. Bruni and J. Schneiderman (Neurology Service, Wellesley Hospital), and Dr. Clare Williams and his staff on the Renal Unit at the

Wellesley for providing access to their patients. We are indebted to Mr. J. Martin Graham (Scott Laboratory, Wellesley Hospital) for his statistical expertise, for his dedication to our research effort, and for his many thoughtful contributions to the projects. We would also like to express our appreciation to Ms. Heather Williams (Manager, Sherbourne Health Club) for her assistance in accessing nonpatients through her facility.

REFERENCES

1. Adamec, R. E. (1978): Normal and abnormal limbic system mechanisms of emotive biasing. In: edited by K. E. Livingston and O. Hornykiewicz (Eds.) *Limbic mechanisms: The continuing evolution of the limbic system concept*, pp. 405–455. Plenum Press, New York.
2. Adamec, R. E., and Stark-Adamec, C. (1983): Limbic kindling and animal behavior—Implications for human psychopathology associated with complex partial seizures. *Biol. Psychiatry*, 18(2):269–293.
3. Adamec, R. E., and Stark-Adamec, C. (1983): Partial kindling and emotional bias in the cat, lasting after-effects of partial kindling of ventral hippocampus. I: Behavioral changes. *Behav. Neural Biol.*, 38:205–222.
4. Adamec, R. E., and Stark-Adamec, C. (1983): Partial kindling and emotional bias in the cat, lasting after-effects of partial kindling of ventral hippocampus. II: Physiological changes. *Behav. Neural Biol.*, 38:223–239.
5. Bear, D. M. (1983): Behavioral symptoms in temporal lobe epilepsy. *Arch. Gen. Psychiatry*, 40:467–468.
6. Bear, D. M. (1979): Temporal lobe epilepsy—A syndrome of sensory-limbic hyperconnection. *Cortex*, 15:357–384.
7. Bear, D. M. (1977): The significance of behavioral change in temporal lobe epilepsy. *McLean Hosp. J.*, Special Issue, 9–21.
8. Bear, D. M., and Fedio, P. (1977): Quantitative analysis of interictal behavior in temporal lobe epilepsy. *Arch. Neurol.*, 34:454–467.
9. Bear, D. M., Levin, K., Blumer, D., Chetham, D., and Ryder, J. (1982): Interictal behavior in hospitalised temporal lobe epileptics: Relationship to idiopathic psychiatric syndromes. *J. Neurol. Neurosurg. Psychiatry*, 45:481–488.
10. Beard, B. H., and Sampson, T. F. (1981): Denial and objectivity in hemodialysis patients: Adjustment by opposite mechanisms. In: *Psychonephrology 1: Psychological factors in hemodialysis and transplantation*, edited by N. B. Levy. pp. 169–175. Plenum Medical Book Co., New York.
11. Czaczkes, J. W., and De-Nour, A. K. (1978): *Chronic hemodialysis as a way of life. Brunner/Mazel, New York.*
12. Dodrill, C. G., Batzel, L. W., Queisser, H. E., and Temkin, N. R. (1980): An objective method for the assessment of psychological and social problems among epileptics. *Epilepsia*, 21:123–135.
13. Dreifuss, F. E. (1975): The differential diagnosis of partial seizures with complex symptomatology. In: *Advances in neurology, vol. 11: Complex partial seizures and their treatment*, edited by J. K. Penry and D. D. Daly. pp. 187–199. Raven Press, New York.
14. Fletcher, J. M., Rice, W. J., and Ray, R. M. (1978): Linear discriminant function analysis in neuropsychological research: Some uses and abuses. *Cortex*, 14:564–577.
15. Gloor, P., Olivier, A., Quesney, L. F., Andermann, F., and Horowitz, S. (1983): The role of the limbic system in experimental phenomena of temporal lobe epilepsy. *Ann. Neurol., (in press)*.
16. Goldensohn, E. S. Initiation and propagation of epileptogenic foci. In: *Advances in neurology, vol. 11: Complex partial seizures and their treatment*, edited by J. K. Penry and D. D. Daly, pp. 141–162. Raven Press, New York.
17. Hermann, B. P., Dikmen, S., Schwartz, M. S., and Karnes, W. E. (1982): Interictal psychopathology in patients with ictal fear: A quantitative investigation. *Neurology* (NY), 32:7–11.
18. Hermann, B. P., and Riel, P. (1981): Interictal personality and behavioral traits in temporal lobe and generalized epilepsy. *Cortex*, 17:125–128.
19. Kim, J.-O. (1975): Factor analysis. In: *Statistical Package for the Social Sciences (SPSS)*, edited by N. H. Nie, C. H. Hull, J. G. Jenkins, K. Steinbrenner, and D. H. Bent. pp. 468–514. Second Edition, McGraw-Hill, New York.

20. Levy, N. B. (1981): Psychological reactions to machine dependency: Hemodialysis. In: The psychiatric clinics of North America—The medically ill patient, edited by J. J. Strain. pp. 351–363. W. B. Saunders Company, Philadelphia.
21. Mungas, D. (1982): Interictal behavior abnormality in temporal lobe epilepsy: A specific syndrome or nonspecific psychopathology? *Arch. Gen. Psychiatry*, 39:108–111.
22. Mungas, D. (1983): In reply to Bear (1983). *Arch. Gen. Psychiatry*, 40:468–469.
23. Osgoode, C. E., Suci, G. J., and Tannenbaum, P. H. (1958): *The measurement of meaning*. Urbana, University of Illinois Press.
24. Rodin, E., Schmaltz, S., and Twitty, G. (1983): What does the Bear-Fedio temporal lobe personality inventory measure? *Neurology*, 33(4):[*Suppl.* 2] PP15.
25. Stark-Adamec, C., Adamec, R. E., Graham, J. M., Bruun-Meyer, S. E., and Hicks, R. C. (1983): *Specificity versus nonspecificity of psychosocial problems with complex partial seizures.* Presented at the University of Toronto Department of Psychiatry Research Day, Toronto, September 23, 1983.
26. Stark-Adamec, C., Adamec, R. E., Graham, J. M., Hicks, R. C., and Bruun-Meyer, S. E. (1982): Failures to replicate Bear and Fedio's 18-trait complex partial seizures syndrome: Possible explanations. Rept. to Health and Welfare, Canada.
27. Stark-Adamec, C., Adamec, R. E., Graham, J. M., Hicks, R. C., and Livingston, K. E. (1982): *The psychosocial complexities of complex partial seizures.* Presented at the Canadian Psychological Association Convention, Montreal, June 1982.
28. Stark-Adamec, C., Graham, J. M., Adamec, R. E., Bruun-Meyer, S. E., and Hicks, R. C. (1983): *Sorting out the psychosocial complexities of complex partial seizures.* Presented at the Canadian Psychological Association Convention, Winnipeg, June 1983.
29. Tan, S.-Y. (1982): *Psychosocial functioning of epileptic patients: Findings from a Canadian study.* Presented at the 14th Epilepsy International Symposium, London, England, August 1982.

The Limbic System: Functional Organization and Clinical Disorders, edited by B. K. Doane and K. E. Livingston. Raven Press, New York © 1986.

Does Limbic System Dysfunction Play a Role in Affective Illness?

Robert M. Post

Biological Psychiatry Branch, National Institute of Mental Health, Bethesda, Maryland 20205

In considering whether limbic system function plays a critical role in the affective dysregulation of manic-depressive illness, a series of caveats should be raised. It is likely that as global a function as affective regulation, and one of such evolutionary significance for the animal, will have multiple neurochemical systems encoded on multiple levels of the neuroaxis (48) regulating and modulating its function.

HIERARCHICAL REGULATION OF CNS FUNCTION

Satinoff (96), for example, noted that temperature regulation was hierarchically represented and re-represented at multiple levels of the CNS. Lower centers controlling temperature regulation located in pons, medulla, and spinal cord dealt with primitive responses utilizing wide set-points, with strong stimuli being required for alteration. At higher levels of midbrain and upper pons, tonic inhibition of lower centers was noted. At higher levels of the hypothalamus, temperature responses were more integrated, with a narrower set-point achieved. Higher limbic system areas, such as amygdala, also appeared to be involved with an increasingly finer level of integration and regulation. Finally, at the highest level of neocortical function, the social context of temperature regulation in man is most obviously defined in his homebuilding, manipulation of garments, and utilization of heating and air-conditioning to ensure fine levels of thermoregulation and comfort.

Are we faced with a similar hierarchical level of multiple centers regulating affect? As this is quite likely to be the case, the question raised in this chapter should be shifted from "whether limbic system dysfunction plays a role in affective illness," to "what elements of affective regulation does the limbic system subserve?" Brainstem lesions can alter affect; the pseudobulbar syndrome associated with crocodile tears is a well-known clinical vignette. Sham rage is noted at a hypothalamic level. Multiple studies in animals have documented alterations in affective function with appropriate either stimulation or lesion of a variety of limbic system structures (11,25,47,71). Finally, in a parallel fashion, the impact of our social and communal relationships on our affective tone (presumably mediated, at least in part, through language and other functions represented in our cerebral cortex) is generally accepted.

Although a variety of techniques are currently available for examining the question of whether limbic system dysfunction mediates the affective disorders, relatively few approaches have been robustly studied.

LIMBIC BIOCHEMISTRY AND PHYSIOLOGY

Direct approaches to regional localization of brain function in affective illness need to be pursued in greater depth. One obvious approach, that of biochemical studies of autopsy specimens of patients with affective illness, or, perhaps, of patients who committed suicide (not always related to affective illness), requires further study. There is preliminary evidence that serotonin and/or its metabolites may be low in the brainstem of patients who commit suicide (13,61,74,100), although these data need to be replicated more precisely in controlled studies, and a more systematic exploration of the impact on limbic system structures needs to be pursued. Studies of brain peptides in addition to classical neurotransmitter function may give new and added leverage to this endeavor. Measures of limbic system-specific proteins (58) may become clinically useful. Animal models of depression, such as "learned helplessness" (3,64) may also provide new directions for direct clinical testing in man. A vast literature exists on the effects of stimulation or lesion studies in animals that is highly suggestive that limbic system function and dysfunction is a critical modulator of affect. Because of limitations of space in this chapter, this topic is not further discussed here but the interested reader is referred to volumes such as those of Isaacson (47), Ben-Ari (11), Eleftheriou (25), Myers (71), and Livingston and Hornykiewicz (60).

POSITRON EMISSION TOMOGRAPHY

A technique of considerable promise is that of regional studies of glucose utilization employing positron emission tomography (PET) techniques. Preliminary data in affective illness are promising, but, in contrast to the epilepsies where "hot" spots are evident during seizure discharges and relative hypometabolism evident in the same area during interictal periods, convincing focal areas of abnormality in affective illness have not been demonstrated. Buchsbaum and et al. (15) have suggested that affectively ill patients have a reduced frontal to occipital ratio of glucose utilization (based on higher occipital metabolism) compared with normal controls, similar to that observed in schizophrenia. However, a number of other neuropathological states, such as epilepsy itself and the psychosis of epilepsy (114), are also associated with this relative frontal hypometabolism. These data thus are suggestive that a nonspecific relative hypofrontality may be occurring across a variety of psychopathological entities and that this cannot be construed as specific to either affective illness or schizophrenia.

Preliminary data (15) suggest that more severely depressed patients may have relative hypofunction of both left and right temporal lobes compared with manics, schizophrenics, or normals. More detailed analysis of discrete areas of brain using higher resolution techniques in the future may better reflect limbic structures. In addition, employing unique behavioral or cognitive strategies during the time of deoxyglucose administration may be likely to enhance the appearance of changes in affectively ill patients. Modern PET methodologies have been shown to be sensitive enough to detect alterations in glucose utilization depending on the strategies used for the processing of information (stories or music) in the appropriate auditory areas of cortex in normal volunteers (66). With similarly focused strategies directed at uncovering differences in the processing of affective material, regional alterations may be uncovered.

TEMPORAL LOBE EPILEPSY AS A MODEL OF LIMBIC DYSFUNCTION: POTENTIALS AND HAZARDS

The syndrome of temporal lobe epilepsy (complex partial seizures) provides an important leverage point in discussing limbic system dysfunction in affective syndromes. We discuss this approach and topic with some trepidation. The relationship of psychosis and temporal lobe epilepsy has been one of heated debate over many decades. Both direct and inverse relationships between seizures and psychosis have been postulated; possibly both are correct (114). The critical variables associated with the eruption of psychosis in temporal lobe epilepsy have similarly been hotly debated (45,110). Nonetheless, we think that some of the lessons associated with the study of the relationship of seizures to psychosis may be useful in considering their relationship to affective syndromes.

Table 1 summarizes some of the relevant literature on the incidence of affective illness in patients with complex partial seizures or temporal lobe epilepsy. In seizure patients presenting with psychiatric complaints, we have reviewed a number of

TABLE 1. *Incidence of affective illness in psychiatrically ill patients with temporal lobe epilepsy*

Investigators	N	Affective illness	Schizophrenia-like	Confusional syndromes	Anxiety disorders	Other
Dalby (20)	54	20 (37%)	4 (7%)			30 (55%)
Dongier (23)	236	70 (30%)	49 (21%)	117 (50%)		
Mulder and Daly	62	16 (26%)			36 (58%)	4 (6%)
(70)	(14 dupl.)		20 (32%)			
Flor-Henry (32)	50	9 (18%)	21 (42%)	9 (18%)		11 (22%)
Perez and	16	2 or 5	11 (69%)			
Trimble (78)		(12%) (31%)				
Currie et al. (19)	40	4 (10%)	12 (30%)		7 (18%)	17 (43%)
Pritchard et al.	20	2 or 7	3 (15%)			16 (80%)
(89)	(6 dupl.)	(10%) (35%)				
Shukla et al.	49	5 (10%)	11 (22%)	1 (27%)	6 (12%)	26 (53%)
(103)						
Small et al.	44	2 (5%)	6 (14%)	14 (32%)	6 (14%)	16 (36%)
(107)						
Parnas et al.	25	1 (4%)	3 (12%)			21 (84%)
(75)						
Total	596	139 (23%)	140 (23%)	141 (24%)	55 (9%)	141 (24%)

studies that suggest an approximately equal (23%) incidence of affective syndromes and schizophrenia-like psychosis in patients with psychiatric disorders. The overall incidence of major affective disorders in patients with temporal lobe epilepsy would presumably be much lower, as these figures include only those already presenting with psychiatric illness. Nonetheless, it is of interest that there is a relatively high proportion of patients presenting with affective illness in addition to the more well-accepted schizophrenia-like psychosis. Also noteworthy is the incidence of confusional syndromes and anxiety disorders. Thus, in addition to refocusing attention on major affective syndromes occurring in patients with temporal lobe epilepsy (21,29,93), these data also highlight the relative nonspecificity of clinical psychiatric presentations of patients with temporal lobe epilepsy.

Another approach to this apparent nonspecificity is summarized in Table 2. Here we have, in a rather selective review of the literature, reports of a wide variety of syndromes and symptoms purportedly occurring in association with temporal lobe epilepsy. Although the precise relationship of each of these syndromes or symptoms to seizure disorders or stimulation of temporal lobe-limbic structures is controversial and remains to be elucidated, the "take home" message in this table is that widely diverse syndromes can apparently emerge in association with temporal lobe seizures or their interictal physiological dysfunction. Thus, if only some of these purported relationships withstand the tests of time and rigorous scientific study, they are highly suggestive of the nonspecificity of syndromes associated with temporal lobe epilepsy.

TABLE 2. *Diverse psychiatric manifestations associated with temporal lobe epilepsy*

Syndrome or symptom	Selected references
Affective psychosis	Dongier (23), Dalby (20), Flor-Henry (32)
Schizophreniform psychosis	Slater et al. (104), Kristensen and Sindrup (55), Stevens (109), Sherwin (102), Taylor (112)
Panic-anxiety	Gloor (41), McLachlan and Blume (62), Currie et al. (19), Harper and Roth (43)
Personality changes	Bear and Fedio (8), Bear et al. (9)
Aggression	Serafetinides (98), Ashford et al. (4), Ramani and Gumnit (90), Rodin (94), Delgado-Escueta et al. (22)
Ecstatic seizures (Dostoevsky epilepsy)	Cirignotta et al. (18)
Demonic possession	Mesulam (67)
Religiosity	Waxman and Geschwind (118)
Suicidality	Pritchard et al. (89)
Sexual (orgasmic)	Flor-Henry (33), Mandell (65), Heath (44)
Gelastic	Sackeim et al. (95)
Multiple personality syndrome	Mesulam (67), Schenk and Bear (97)
Transient global amnesia	Tharp (113)
Cognitive perceptual alteration (Psychosensory symptoms)	Dalby (21), Penfield (76), Gloor et al. (41)
Depersonalization (mental diplopia)	Jackson and Stewart (49)

These data immediately raise the question of what are the underlying determinants in the patient and his environment and genetic predisposition that may give some specificity to the behavioral manifestations that might accompany temporal lobe epilepsy. In this regard we are struck by the findings of Belenkov and Shalkovskaya (10) and Kopa et al. (54) who stimulated identical areas of the hypothalamus or thalamus in different behavioral contexts and observed different behavioral responses. When the brain was stimulated while the animal was in a safe area associated with food reward or nonshock, a positive affective response was observed. When the same electrode site was stimulated with identical current in a situation previously associated with fear or stress, a totally different behavioral reaction occurred. Thus, the psychosocial history and environmental context of the organism appeared to interact with the electrophysiological stimulation of the brain.

Perhaps in a similar fashion, behavioral alterations associated with stimulation of identical areas of brain in epileptic patients may differ considerably, based on their developmental histories and psychosocial contexts. Moreover, behavioral consequences of repeated stimulation may be very different from those observed following single stimulation. We have postulated not only that seizures themselves, in some instances, show kindling, but that behavioral manifestations of repeated seizures may also develop in a kindling-like, progressive fashion (81,82). If repeated instances of ictal electrical discharges were altering circuits critical to normal modulation of behavior and affect, one might expect a lag in the appearance of behavioral disturbance following the onset of temporal lobe seizures. While the data summarized in Table 3 are superficially consistent with such a formulation (i.e., there is an average lag of approximately a decade between the onset of seizures and the onset of psychoses), it is possible that this relationship may be an artifact of the usual differences in age of onset of these respective syndromes in the general population (89,105). More systematic investigation of the relationship between seizure onset and the development of affective symptomatology appears indicated.

As in the kindling paradigm, the interval between stimulations may also be important. Therefore, variable effects may occur even when similar areas of the brain are altered during complex partial seizures and their interictal electrophysiology and biochemistry changes. In addition, one should also note that the ictal patterns of local cerebral metabolism studied with positron computed tomography (CT) with 18F-labeled 2-fluoro-2-deoxyglucose "were associated with activation of anatomic structures unique to each patient studied" (30). Thus, there may be great individual variability in anatomical areas and neuronal pathways involved in each individual patient's seizure focus, even when they display relatively classical presentations of psychomotor epilepsy. Moreover, there may be variability of seizure pathway and seizure focus within an individual patient. In addition, when one considers the possible association of behavioral pathology to either the ictal process itself with its increased glucose utilization or the interictal process (hypometabolism and its associated cerebral dysfunction), perhaps there is little wonder of the wide

TABLE 3. *Interval between onset of seizures and psychosis*

Reference	N	Age onset Seizure	Age onset Psychosis	Interval
Yde et al. (119)	(20)	(45)	(29)	(− 16)
	7	13	25	12
Gastaut (38)	83	20.6	31.7	11
Serafetinides and Falconer (99)	12	14.5	27	12.5
Slater et al. (104)	69	15.7	29.8	14.1
Slater and Moran (105)	M	19.3	34	14.8
	F	12	25.2	13.2
Glaser (39)	37	—	—	6
Jus (50)	15	—	—	13
Flor-Henry (32)	50	13	24	11
Bruens (14)	19	13	25	12
Standage (108)	5	15.6	34.7	19.1
Trixler and Nador (115)	7	—	—	14
Kristensen and Sindrup (55)	96	21	34	13
Peters (79)	8	13.4	26.9	13.5
Sugano and Miyasaka (111)	21	14.8	28	13.2
Ramani and Gumnit (91)	10	10.8	16.4	5.6
Total	N = 439	$\overline{X}$ = 15	27.5	11.8[a]
				12.1[b]

[a]Weighted $\overline{X}$ interval.
[b]Unweighted $\overline{X}$ interval.

TABLE 4. *Interictal psychoses and type of epilepsy*

	Centren cephalic	Temporal	Frontal	Others	Total
Confusional	138 (64%)	117 (50%)	11 (52%)	33 (52%)	299 (56%)
Affective	50 (23%)	70 (30%)	8 (38%)	15 (23%)	143 (27%)
Schizophreniform	27 (13%)	49 (21%)	2 (10%)	16 (25%)	94 (18%)
Total	215 (40%)	236 (44%)	21 (4%)	64 (12%)	536

From Dongier (23).

variety of psychiatric syndromes associated with this nonunitary phenomenon of temporal lobe epilepsy.

A further caveat regarding regional localization of function is raised by the study of Dongier (23) as summarized in Table 4. It is obvious that affective syndromes were observed in many types of epileptic seizures, presumably originating at different areas of the brain. Affective syndromes accounted for 30% of the psychiatric manifestations of temporal lobe epilepsy, whereas they constituted 23% of the centren cephalic type, and 38% of the frontal type. Thus, these early findings of the 1960s suggest the possibility that psychiatric manifestations may not be specifically associated with a given seizure type. This point has also been raised by Stevens (110) in her critique of the relationship of personality variables to patients with temporal lobe epilepsy. Many systematic studies comparing temporal lobe epileptics with other seizure types, major differences in personality traits as measured by Minnesota Multiphasic Personality Inventory (MMPI) and other systematic techniques, have not emerged. The same may turn out to be the case for more severe psychopathological syndromes such as major affective disorders. Using modern psychodiagnostic tools and techniques, this issue would appear to deserve reexploration and study, however. This would appear to be an important issue in light of the extremely high incidence of depression reported by Engel and associates (30) in his clinical patients with complex partial seizures. Similarly, Robertson (92) reported a relatively high incidence of depression in their unselected population of temporal lobe epileptics (unselected for psychiatric versus nonpsychiatric problems).

The issue of relative proportion of affective syndromes to seizure type would obviously be of considerable theoretical import. Several issues deserve consideration. In many types of generalized seizures, limbic system structures would appear to be involved, either directly or as an indirect consequence of the generalized seizure disorder. Thus, it is possible that some of the nonselectivity of behavioral manifestations could relate to the fact that limbic structures are impaired in a variety of seizure types. Perhaps some of the more modern techniques of regional glucose utilization may be helpful in further elucidating this issue. Utilizing control groups with focal seizures that clearly do not generalize to limbic structures may also be of particular help. The answer to this question of the relative frequency of affective disorders with seizure type may help substantiate or refute the theory of Hermann (45) that seizures, as an unpredictable event, may be an ideal paradigm for generating "learned helplessness." If this theory were correct, one would, in fact, expect an incidence of affective disturbance quite independent of type of seizure.[1]

Others in this volume have discussed the possible relationship of temporal lobe epilepsy to interictal behavioral disturbance (1,7). Although not further engaging in this controversy, we would like to point out a peculiar aspect of many of the features included in this suggested syndrome (8,12,46) and the affective disorders. Should some elements of this interictal behavioral syndrome be verified, either in the subgroup of patients with temporal lobe epilepsy or in epileptics in a more general fashion, their relationship to affective disorders may deserve further study. Specifically, many features of this syndrome appear to overlap with those described in the affective syndromes of mania and depression. For example, as illustrated in Table 5, hypergraphic religiosity, anger, irritability, aggression, paranoia, circumstantiality, obsessional concern with details of justice and ethics, sense of profundity and importance, and denial, all purportedly part of the interictal behavioral syn-

---

[1]However, severity of seizure and the intensity of the disturbing psychosocial consequences of having a seizure may bear an important impact on the degree of distress and "learned helplessness" that might be associated with the anticipation of possibly having a seizure. In addition, a variety of other variables would also apparently be pertinent, including degree of seizure control.

TABLE 5. *Comparison of symptom picture of the interictal behavioral disorder of temporal lobe epilepsy (TLE) and primary affective illness*

Shared symptoms	
TLE and MANIA	TLE and DEPRESSION
Hypergraphia	Helplessness
Religiosity	Sadness
Anger/irritability	Decreased libido
Aggression	Obsessionalism
Paranoia	Self-criticism
Circumstantiality	Suicidal ideation
Obsessional concern with details of justice and ethics	Apathy
Sense of profundity and importance	
Denial	

Nonshared symptoms	
Hyperactivity	Insomnia and anorexia
Racing thoughts	Psychomotor retardation or agitation
Rapid speech	Decreased memory or concentration
Euphoria	
Decreased sleep	

drome of temporal lobe epilepsy, are familiar signs and symptoms of the manic syndrome. Perhaps it is equally interesting to note the nonshared symptoms. Hyperactivity, racing thoughts, rapid speech, euphoria, and decreased sleep are cardinal signs and symptoms of the manic syndrome and yet are relatively infrequently cited as consistent with the interictal syndrome of patients with temporal lobe epilepsy.

Similarly, many of the descriptors of the interictal personality disturbances of patients with temporal lobe epilepsy are similar to those observed in depression and might include helplessness, sadness, decreased libido, obsessionalism, self-criticism, suicidal ideation, and apathy. Again, an interesting area of nonshared symptoms is apparent in terms of insomnia, psychomotor retardation or agitation, decreased memory or concentration. These nonshared or nonoverlapping symptoms seem to be in the area of psychomotor activation or retardation. Whereas more major affective disorders that include these alterations of psychomotor function are also noted in patients with seizure disorders, they do not appear to be prominent among the descriptions of the interictal personality disturbances. Different neuronal substrates may be involved in the psychomotor alterations of more classical presentations of severe endogenous affective illness that are not typically highlighted in the description of the interictal personality disturbances in patients with temporal lobe epilepsy. Exploring the subtypes of the affective disturbances and their comparison and contrast to classical manic-depressive disorder may prove fruitful.

EPILEPTOID-PSYCHOSENSORY SYMPTOMS IN
PSYCHIATRIC PATIENTS

Although systematic study of the similarities and differences in behavioral disturbances of patients with epilepsy in affective illness may ultimately prove rewarding, we have also begun an investigation utilizing the opposite approach. We asked our nonepileptic psychiatric patients which symptoms they had that were often associated with patients with temporal lobe epilepsy. Dr. Silberman and I devised a psychosensory rating scale comprised of common alterations reported to occur in patients with temporal lobe epilepsy (Silberman et al., 1984). We decided to assess these alterations after hearing many of our patients spontaneously report that they had major psychosensory alterations during the course of their affective episodes. We asked patients about formed and unformed hallucinations in all sensory modalities, sensory perceptual illusions, cognitive illusions (i.e., déjà vu or attributions of special profound meaning), "ictal" type of affective states, time distortions, altered flow of thought, and motor automatisms. If a symptom was reported as positive, the interviewer inquired about the exact nature of the phenomenon and circumstance of occurrence. Those associated with sleep or drowsiness, the use of drugs, or other situations that may have "ordinary" physiological explanations were excluded. The main criteria for judging a symptom as present were its abrupt, paroxysmal nature and its occurrence in the absence of any apparent physiologic or psychological causation.

Forty-four patients with a diagnosis of primary affective disturbance were studied in comparison with 33 epileptic patients with foci in the temporal lobe and 30 control subjects who were recruited from a medical outpatient clinic at the National Institute of Mental Health, where they were being treated for hypertension. Compared with these medical control patients who showed less than two of these para-epileptic symptoms, patients with temporal lobe epilepsy, as expected, reported more than eight. Patients with primary affective illness, however, also showed a high incidence of these symptoms, showing more than seven. These were almost exclusively reported during episodes of affective illness and very few (less than three) were reported during well intervals. Some of the overlapping signs and symptoms are noted in Fig. 1. The para-epileptic symptoms that were significantly present in both affectively ill and epileptic subjects more frequently than controls are illustrated in the converging area of the diagram. Thus, illusions of significance were reported significantly more often in both patient populations compared with the medical controls (66% of the affectively ill patients reported illusions of significance while 27% of the epileptics reported this symptom). Signs and symptoms that were reported significantly more often than controls only in the affective population, such as speeded thoughts in 68%, are so listed (on the left). Epileptic patients showed significantly more symptoms compared with medical controls (on the right) on such items as motor automatisms, speech arrest, vestibular hallucinations, etc.

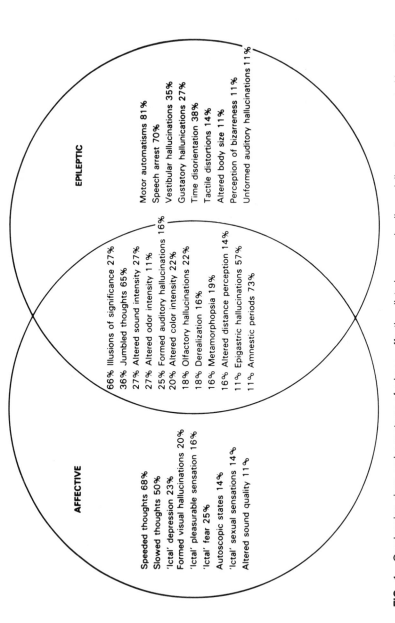

FIG. 1. Overlapping signs and symptoms of primary affective disturbance and epilepsy (all symptoms reported by <10% of controls).

AFFECTIVE

Speeded thoughts 68%
Slowed thoughts 50%
'Ictal' depression 23%
Formed visual hallucinations 20%
'Ictal' pleasurable sensation 16%
'Ictal' fear 25%
Autoscopic states 14%
'Ictal' sexual sensations 14%
Altered sound quality 11%

66% Illusions of significance 27%
36% Jumbled thoughts 65%
27% Altered sound intensity 27%
27% Altered odor intensity 11%
25% Formed auditory hallucinations 16%
20% Altered color intensity 22%
18% Olfactory hallucinations 22%
18% Derealization 16%
16% Metamorphopsia 19%
16% Altered distance perception 14%
11% Epigastric hallucinations 57%
11% Amnestic periods 73%

EPILEPTIC

Motor automatisms 81%
Speech arrest 70%
Vestibular hallucinations 35%
Gustatory hallucinations 27%
Time disorientation 38%
Tactile distortions 14%
Altered body size 11%
Perception of bizarreness 11%
Unformed auditory hallucinations 11%

Thus, there would appear to be a considerable degree of overlap in symptoms commonly reported by epileptic patients and also described by affectively ill patients. These indirect data raise the possibility that similar substrates that mediate these syndromes are being activated in both epileptic and affectively ill patients. However, many reservations need to be raised before this suggestion might be accepted. One is certainly the issue of specificity again. We have now extended this testing to patients with panic-anxiety disorders, and we have found a similarly high incidence of psychosensory/epileptoid symptoms in this group compared with the affectively ill and epileptic patients (116). Moreover, Chapman (16) reported that many of these symptoms occurred in the prodromal phases of acute schizophrenic psychosis. Thus, we would not claim that many of these symptoms are in any way specific to patients with affective illness, but these symptoms that appear to be closely associated with the epileptic aura, the ictal process itself, or its downstream consequences in patients with temporal lobe epilepsy are often reported by psychiatrically ill patients with primary affective illness or panic anxiety states.

It is of interest that Penfield and Jasper (77) reported many of these phenomena associated with electrical stimulation, in a relatively selective fashion, of the temporal cortex but not of other areas of brain. More recently, Gloor and associates (41) reported that many of these phenomena appeared to be elicited by stimulation of amygdala and hippocampus rather than the overlying temporal cortex. Such experiential phenomena were observed during seizure activity that was elicited but also occurred with limbic stimulation (amygdala and hippocampus) which produced no afterdischarge, suggesting that actual ictal activity is not necessary for their occurrence. In light of these data, and in anticipation of our subsequent discussion of the use of anticonvulsants in affective syndromes described below, we would again emphasize that we are not suggesting that our psychiatric patients have an underlying seizure disorder, but that in some instances disregulated neural activity may be occurring in pathways similar to those involved in patients with complex partial seizures.

We present these preliminary data on the occurrence of paroxysmal psychosensory symptoms or para-epileptic symptoms in our affectively ill patients in the hope that they might stimulate further research. It is possible that the neural pathways involved in more discrete symptoms, such as those described in our psychosensory rating scale, will be more amenable to anatomical and physiological dissection (41,42) than more global affective syndromes such as depression or anxiety.

It is of some interest that our affectively ill patients who report a greater number of these symptoms responded best to the classical treatment agent for manic-depressive illness, i.e., lithium carbonate. We are currently exploring whether patients with more of these symptoms also respond to the anticonvulsant carbamazepine, although preliminary review of the data suggest that this may not be the case.

ANTICONVULSANTS IN AFFECTIVE ILLNESS

Another possible approach to the issue of whether limbic system dysfunction is associated with affective illness is the relative efficacy of different anticonvulsants in the treatment of affective illness. If limbic system substrates are critically involved in affective dysregulation, one would predict that anticonvulsants more useful in the treatment of temporal lobe epilepsy in limbic seizure disorders would be the most effective treatment agents in major affective illness. Similarly, drugs that are not particularly effective in the treatment of temporal lobe epilepsy would be predicted to be not useful in affective illness. In assessing the relative efficacy of anticonvulsants in inhibiting amygdala-kindled afterdischarges compared with cortical-kindled afterdischarges, Albright and Burnham (2) found that carbamazepine was the most effective. Moreover, it was the only drug to suppress amygdala afterdischarges better than cortical afterdischarges, the ratio being 55%. Other anticonvulsants in order of efficacy on amygdala versus cortical afterdischarges were, sequentially, sodium valproate (37%), phenobarbital (33%), phenytoin (30%), methsuximide (25%), clonazepam (22%), ethosuximide (14%), and diazepam (0%). It is of interest that there is some convergence in the ability of these agents to suppress amygdala-kindled compared with cortical-kindled afterdischarges and the ability of these agents to be useful in the clinical treatment of temporal lobe epilepsy (80). However, it should again be highlighted that carbamazepine and related drugs used in temporal lobe epilepsy are also highly effective in grand mal seizures (80). Although sodium valproate is not widely accepted as a major treatment agent of temporal lobe epilepsy, the first four agents on the list of Albright and Burnham, and perhaps clonazepam (68), have some recognized value in the treatment of this syndrome. Methsuximide, ethosuximide, and diazepam are not widely considered useful in the clinical treatment of complex partial seizures or temporal lobe epilepsy.

Considerable evidence is now emerging that carbamazepine may be clinically effective in the acute and prophylactic treatment of both manic and depressive phases of primary affective illness (5,6,53,72,85–87). There are some data to suggest that the second anticonvulsant on the rank-order list of Albright and Burnham is also effective in manic-depressive patients. Lambert and associates (57) reported, in open clinical trials, that an analog of valproic acid was useful in the treatment of manic-depressive illness. More recently, Emrich and associates (28) reported that valproic acid alone was a useful antimanic agent in a small number of patients studied in a double-blind fashion. In addition, he reported that valproic acid, when added to previously ineffective doses of lithium carbonate, was useful in the prophylactic treatment of rapid cycling manic-depressive patients (26,27). Other anticonvulsants have not been systematically studied, with the exception of clonazepam, which Chouinard and associates (17) reported was as effective as lithium in the treatment of acute mania. The data with phenytoin are highly controversial; double-blind, placebo-controlled studies are sorely needed to assess the preliminary observations from uncontrolled studies that this agent might be of some use in the treatment of affective syndromes (36,52,56).

As illustrated in Fig. 2, we have recently completed a double-blind, placebo-controlled crossover in a single patient to three different anticonvulsant agents. This patient, described in detail elsewhere (88), responded well to carbamazepine instituted on a blind basis during two separate clinical trials compared with similar periods during placebo medication. In contrast, the patient showed no apparent clinical response to the two other anticonvulsants, phenytoin and valproic acid. These data are of interest from several perspectives. If they are to be substantiated in a larger series of patients, they would suggest that generalized anticonvulsant properties of a given series of drugs are not sufficient to produce clinical improvement during psychotic manic states, as illustrated in this single individual. It is apparent that this patient responded rather selectively to the anticonvulsant carbamazepine but not to the anticonvulsant phenytoin or valproic acid when administered in clinically acceptable dosages achieving plasma levels within the accepted anticonvulsant spectrum. These data suggest that (a) a given individual may respond differentially to anticonvulsants, and (b) some particular aspect of the mechanism of action of carbamazepine and its biochemistry and physiology may be responsible for the clinical improvement achieved in this individual compared with lack of improvement achieved with the two other anticonvulsants.

Further clinical trials of a variety of anticonvulsants in affectively ill patients are clearly required; the preliminary data are not inconsistent with the observations that those agents that are useful in the treatment of major motor and complex partial seizures appear to be among those that are of greater utility in the treatment of primary affective illness. Systematic study of the mechanism of action of carbamazepine and related anticonvulsants useful in the treatment of affective illness, in comparison to classical psychotropic agents useful in the treatment of the syndrome, such as lithium carbonate, should also be a theoretically rewarding avenue of investigation. The common physiological and biochemical properties of the anticonvulsants that are effective in affective illness, in contrast to the other agents, may provide important hints to the mechanism of action of these agents in this psychiatric illness.

ELECTROCONVULSIVE THERAPY AS A LIMBIC ANTICONVULSANT

We and others in this volume have discussed psychopathology occurring in association with seizure disorders and the effectiveness of some anticonvulsants in affective illness. How might one juxtapose these observations with those documenting the unequivocal benefits of electroconvulsive therapy in acute depression and mania (31)? One possible explanation derives from recent work indicating that electroconvulsive seizures (ECS) in rats may paradoxically be potent anticonvulsants, at least for seizures kindled from the amygdala. ECS administered 6 hr before each once-daily stimulation of the amygdala (compared with sham ECS or real ECS given immediately after kindling) markedly suppressed the development

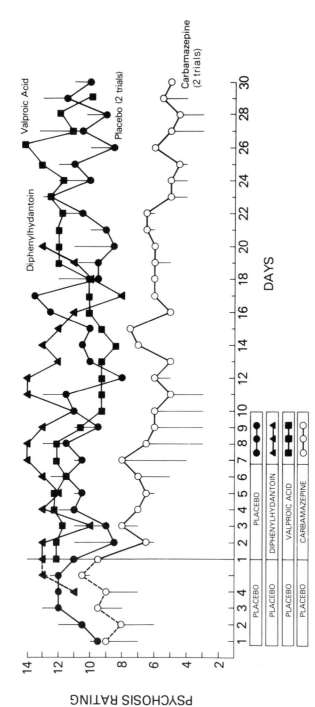

FIG. 2. Carbamazepine but not diphenylhydantoin or valproic acid decreases manic psychosis in a patient with manic-depressive illness.

of kindling (84). Moreover, in a second study, repeated daily ECS for 7 days suppressed the occurrence of completed kindled seizures in a long-lasting fashion. As such, the induction of major motor seizures of electroconvulsive therapy and anticonvulsants such as carbamazepine may have common properties. These data suggest the possibility that the biochemical and physiological effects of electroconvulsive therapy that are associated with its anticonvulsant properties may also be of importance to the therapeutic effects in affectively ill patients.

CONCLUSIONS

The distorted sensory and motor homunculus that illustrates the relative density of sensory and motor fibers innervating different areas of the body has been well mapped out for the sensory and motor areas of the neocortex. Is there an equivalent distribution of anatomical localization of affect, an affective homunculus in brain? We appear to be a long way from such a description. In most instances the techniques outlined in this chapter are relatively indirect in attempts to establish whether or not limbic system dysfunction plays a critical role in affective illness. We are struck, however, that there are several areas of important progress, including new findings that several of the anticonvulsant agents are useful in the treatment of primary affective illness. Moreover, recent technological advances such as the use of computerized axial tomography and PET scan techniques, as well as nuclear magnetic resonance (NMR) may allow more discrete localization of areas of brain pathology and dysfunction.

Perhaps we should end on another note of both caution and promise. Throughout this chapter we have referred to the limbic system as a general region, without referring to any of its discrete parts. Papez (73), MacLean (63) and others have done much to present an integrated if not unified concept of limbic system circuitry and function. All have acknowledged that within this rubric exists a diversity of structures with, at times, opposing functions. Stimulation of the hippocampus may, in fact, produce opposite effects in some instances to stimulation of the amygdala. Moreover, stimulation of one area of the amygdala may produce opposite effects to stimulation of another area, as illustrated in Table 6. This very lack of homo-

TABLE 6. *Reciprocal functions of amygdala subdivisions*

	Dorsomedial	Basolateral	Ref.
Hypothalamic elicited attack	↓	↑	24
Rage, hissing	↑	↓	101, 117, 120
Blood pressure	↑	↓	37, 69
Corticosteroids	↑	↓	106
Feeding	↑	↓	35, 59
Sex	↑	↓	51
Self-stimulation	↑	↓	51
Social reinforcement	↑	↓	34
Playfulness and motor activity	↑	↓	34

TABLE 7. *Opposing aspects of mania and depression*

	Depression	Mania
Mood	Depressed	Elated
Anger, aggression	Self-directed	Other directed
Affect quality	Flat	Labile
Motor activity	Retarded (agitated)	Increased
Speech	Retarded; mute	Excessive
Ideation	Slow, blank	Speeded up
Associations	Restricted	Flight of ideas
Self-concept	Suicidal, worthlessness	Maniacal, grandiosity
Religious preoccupation	Guilty, sinfulness	Ordained, righteousness
Response to social cues, limit setting	Increased	Decreased
Sexual interest, performance	Decreased	Increased
Appetite	Decreased	Increased
Energy, interests	Decreased	Increased
Sleep	Decreased (or increased)	Increased

geneity in limbic system function, however, could provide a comprehensible mechanism for understanding the opposing aspects of manic-depressive illness. As outlined in Table 7, many of the cardinal signs and symptoms of affective illness occur in relatively opposite fashions in manic compared with depressed phases of the illness. Most theories of affective dysfunction and its treatment with single agents such as lithium and carbamazepine have failed to explain in a unitary framework how these agents might be effective in both phases of the syndrome. It is possible that hyperfunction or hypofunction could occur in a given area of the limbic system such as a subdivision of the amygdala, or that a unitary excitatory or inhibitory process could shift slightly to other areas of brain mediating opposing effects on behavior, physiology, and biochemistry. Thus, in this fashion, a unitary pathological process could account for opposite behavioral effects and response to single therapeutic agents such as lithium carbonate or carbamazepine.

REFERENCES

1. Adamec, R., and Stark-Adamec, C. (1983): Limbic hyperfunction, limbic epilepsy, and interictal behaviour: models and methods of detection. *This volume.*
2. Albright, P. S., and Burnham, W. M. (1980): Development of a new pharmacological seizure model: effects of anticonvulsants on cortical- and amygdala-kindled seizures in the rat. *Epilepsia,* 21:681–689.
3. Anisman, H. (1984): Vulnerability to depression: contribution of stress. In: *Neurobiology of Mood Disorders,* edited by R. M. Post and J. C. Ballenger, pp. 407–431. Williams & Wilkins, Baltimore.
4. Ashford, J., Wesson, S., Schulz, C., and Walsh, G. O. (1980): Violent automatism in a partial complex seizure. *Arch. Neurol.,* 37:120–122.
5. Ballenger, J. C., and Post, R. M. (1978): Therapeutic effects of carbamazepine in affective illness: a preliminary report. *Commun. Psychopharmacol.,* 2:159–178.
6. Ballenger, J. C., and Post, R. M. (1980): Carbamazepine (Tegretol) in manic-depressive illness: a new treatment. *Am. J. Psychiatry,* 137:782–790.
7. Bear, D. (1983): Hemispheric specialization and emotional functions: what epilepsy tells us about sensory-limbic connections. *This volume.*

8. Bear, D. M., and Fedio, P. (1977): Quantitative analysis of interictal behavior in temporal lobe epilepsy. *Arch. Neurol.*, 34:454–467.
9. Bear, D., Levin, K., Blumer, D., Chetham, D., and Ryder, J. (1982): Interictal behaviour in hospitalized temporal lobe epileptics: relationship to idiopathic psychiatric syndromes. *J. Neurol. Neurosurg. Psychiatry*, 45:481–488.
10. Belenkov, N. Y., and Shalkovskaya, L. N. (1980): Role of dominant motivation in manifestation of the effects of electrical stimulation of the hypothalamus and limbic region. *Neurosci. Behav. Physiol.*, 10:112–117.
11. Ben-Ari, Y. (1981): *The Amygdaloid Complex, INSERM Symposium #20*. Elsevier/No. Holland Biomedical Press, Amsterdam.
12. Blumer, D. (1975): Temporal lobe epilepsy and its psychiatric significance. In: *Psychiatric Aspects of Neurological Disease*, edited by D. F. Benson and D. Blumer, pp. 171–198. Grune & Stratton, New York.
13. Bourne, H. R., Bunney, W. E., Jr., Colburn, R. W., Davis, J. M., Davis, J. N., Shaw, D. M., and Coppen, A. J. (1968): Noradrenaline, 5-hydroxytryptamine, and 5-hydroxyindoleacetic acid in hindbrains of suicidal patients. *Lancet*, 2:805–808.
14. Bruens, J. H. (1971): Psychoses in epilepsy. *Psychiatry, Neurol. Neurochir.*, 74:175–192.
15. Buchsbaum, M. S., De Lisi, L. E., Holcomb, H. H., Cappelletti, J., King, A. C., Johnson, J., Hazlett, E., Dowling-Zimmerman, S., Post, R. M., Morihisa, J., Carpenter, W., Cohen, R., Pickar, D., Weinberger, D. R., Margolin, R., and Kessler, K. M. (1984): Anteroposterior gradients in cerebral glucose use in schizophrenia and affective disorders. *Arch. Gen. Psychiatry*, 41:1159–1166.
16. Chapman, J. (1966): The early symptoms of schizophrenia. *Br. J. Psychiatry*, 112:225–251.
17. Chouinard, G., Young, S. N., and Annable, L. (1983): Antimanic effect of clonazepam. *Biol. Psychiatry*, 18:451–466.
18. Cirignotta, F., Todesco, C. V., and Lugaresi, E. (1980): Temporal lobe epilepsy with ecstatic seizures (so-called Dostoevsky epilepsy). *Epilepsia*, 21:705–710.
19. Currie, S., Heathfield, K. W. G., Henson, R. A., and Scott, D. F. (1971): Clinical course and prognosis of temporal lobe epilepsy. *Brain*, 94:173–190.
20. Dalby, M. A. (1971): Antiepileptic and psychotropic effect of carbamazepine (Tegretol) in the treatment of psychomotor epilepsy. *Epilepsia*, 12:325–334.
21. Dalby, M. S. (1975): Behavioral effects of carbamazepine. In: *Complex Partial Seizures and Their Treatment, Advances in Neurology, Vol. 11*, edited by J. K. Penry and D. D. Daly, pp. 331–343. Raven Press, New York.
22. Delgado-Escueta, A., Mattson, R. H., King, L., Goldensohn, E. S., Spiegel, H., Madsen, J., Crandall, P., Dreifuss, F., and Porter, R. J. (1981): The nature of aggression during epileptic seizures. *N. Engl. J. Med.*, 305:711–716.
23. Dongier, S. (1959/60): Statistical study of clinical and electroencephalographic manifestations of 536 psychotic episodes occurring in 516 epileptics between clinical seizures. *Epilepsia*, 1:117–142.
24. Egger, M. D., and Flynn, J. P. (1967): Further studies on the effects of amygdaloid stimulation and ablation in hypothalamically elicited attack behavior in cats. In: *Structure and Function of the Limbic System (Progress in Brain Research, Vol. 27)*, edited by W. R. Adey and T. Tokinzane, pp. 165–182. Elsevier/No. Holland Biomedical Press, Amsterdam.
25. Eleftheriou, B. E. (1972): *Advances in Behavioral Biology, The Neurobiology of the Amygdala, Vol. 2*. Plenum Press, New York.
26. Emrich, H. M., Altmann, H., Dose, M., and von Zerssen, D. (1983): Therapeutic effects of GABA-ergic drugs in affective disorders. A preliminary report. *Pharmacol. Biochem. Behav.*, 19:369–372.
27. Emrich, H. M., von Zerssen, D., Kissling, W., and Möller, H. J. (1982): Antimanic action of propranolol and of sodium valproate. Presented at 13th CINP Congress, Tel Aviv, 1982.
28. Emrich, H. M., von Zerssen, D., Kissling, W., Möller, H. J., and Windorfer, A. (1980): Effect of sodium valproate in mania. The GABA-hypothesis of affective disorders. *Arch. Psychiatr. Nervenkr.*, 229:1–16.
29. Engel, J., Jr. (1983): Local cerebral glucose metabolism in epilepsy: clinical and animal investigations. 15th Epilepsy International Symposium, Washington, D.C., p. 101. *(Abstract)*.
30. Engel, J., Jr., Kuhl, D. E., and Phelps, M. E. (1982): Patterns of human local cerebral glucose metabolism during epileptic seizures. *Science*, 218:64–66.

31. Fink, M. (1979): *Convulsive Therapy: Theory and Practice*. Raven Press, New York.
32. Flor-Henry, P. (1969): Psychosis and temporal lobe epilepsy: a controlled investigation. *Epilepsia*, 10:363–395.
33. Flor-Henry, P. (1976): Lateralized temporal-limbic dysfunction and psychopathology. *Ann. NY Acad Sci.*, 280:777–797.
34. Fonberg, E. (1981): Specific versus unspecific functions of the amygdala. In: *The Amygdaloid Complex, INSERM Symposium No. 20*, edited by Y. Ben-Ari, pp. 281–291. Elsevier/No. Holland Biomedical Press, Amsterdam.
35. Fonberg, E., and Delgado, J. M. R. (1961): Avoidance and alimentary reactions during amygdala stimulation. *J. Neurophysiol.*, 24:651–654.
36. Freyhan, F. A. (1945): Effectiveness of diphenylhydantoin in management of nonepileptic psychomotor excitement states. *Arch. Neurol. Psychiatry*, 53:370–374.
37. Gastaut, H. (1952): Correlations entre le systeme nerveux vegetatif et le systeme de le vie de relation dans le rhinencephale. *J. Physiol. (Paris)*, 44:431–470.
38. Gastaut, H. (1956): Etude electroclinique des episodes psychotiques survenant en dehors des crises cliniques chez les epileptiques. *Rev. Neurol.*, 95:588–594.
39. Glaser, G. H. (1964): The problem of psychosis in psychomotor epileptics. *Epilepsia*, 5:271–278.
40. Gloor, P., Olivier, A., and Quesney, L. F. (1981): The role of the amygdala in the expression of psychic phenomena in temporal lobe seizures. In: *The Amygdaloid Complex, INSERM Symposium, No. 20*, edited by Y. Ben-Ari, pp. 489–498. Elsevier/No. Holland Biomedical Press, Amsterdam.
41. Gloor, P., Olivier, A., Quesney, L. F., Andermann, F., and Horowitz, S. (1982): The role of the limbic system in experiential phenomena of temporal lobe epilepsy. *Ann. Neurol.*, 12:129–144.
42. Halgren, E. (1981): The amygdala contribution to emotion and memory: current studies in humans. In: *The Amygdaloid Complex, INSERM Symposium, No. 20*, edited by Y. Ben-Ari, pp. 395–408. Elsevier/No. Holland Biomedical Press, Amsterdam.
43. Harper, M., and Roth, M. (1962): Temporal lobe epilepsy and the phobic anxiety-depersonalization syndrome. *Compr. Psychiatry*, 3:129–151.
44. Heath, R. G. (1964): Pleasure response of human subjects to direct stimulation of the brain: physiologic and psychodynamic considerations. In: *The Role of Pleasure in Behavior*, edited by R. G. Heath, pp. 219–243. Hoeber, New York.
45. Hermann, B. P. (1979): Psychopathology in epilepsy and learned helplessness. *Med. Hypotheses*, 5:723–729.
46. Hermann, B. P., and Reil, P. (1981): Interictal personality correlates of temporal lobe and primary generalized epilepsy. *Cortex*, 17:125–128.
47. Isaacson, R. L. (1974): *The Limbic System*. Plenum Press, New York.
48. Jackson, J. H. (1932): Remarks on evolution and dissolution of the nervous system. In: *Selected Writings, Vol. II*. Hodder & Stoughton, London.
49. Jackson, J. H., and Stewart, P. (1899): Epileptic attacks with a warning of a crude sensation of smell and with the intellectual aura (dreamy state) in a patient who had symptoms pointing to gross organic disease of the right temporal-sphenoidal lobe. *Brain*, 22:534–549.
50. Jus, A. (1966): Troubles mentaux a symptomatologie schizophrenique chez les epileptiques. *Evolut. Psychiatry*, 31:313–319.
51. Kaada, B. R. (1972): Stimulation and regional ablation of the amygdaloid complex with reference to functional representations. In: *Advances in Behavioral Biology, The Neurobiology of the Amygdala, Vol. 2*, edited by B. E. Eleftheriou, pp. 205–281. Plenum Press, New York/London.
52. Kalinowsky, L. B., and Putnam, T. J. (1943): Attempts at treatment of schizophrenia and other non-epileptic psychoses with dilantin. *Arch. Neurol. Psychiatry*, 49:414–420.
53. Kishimoto, A., Ogura, C., Hazama, H., and Inoue, K. (1983): Long-term prophylactic effects of carbamazepine in affective disorder. *Br. J. Psychiatry*, 143:327–331.
54. Kopa, J., Szabo, I., and Grastyan, E. (1968): A dual behavioral effect from stimulating the same thalamic point with identical stimulus parameter in different conditional reflex situations. In: *Biological Foundations of Emotion*, edited by E. Gellhorn, pp. 107–127. Scott, Foresman & Co., Glenview, Illinois.
55. Kristensen, O., and Sindrup, E. H. (1978): Psychomotor epilepsy and psychosis. *Acta Neurol. Scand.*, 57:370–379.
56. Kubanek, J. L., and Rowell, R. C. (1946): The use of dilantin in the treatment of psychotic patients unresponsive to other treatment. *Dis. Nerv. Syst.*, 7:47–50.

57. Lambert, P. A., Carraz, G., Borselli, S., and Bouchardy, M. (1975): Le dipropylacetamide dans le traitement de la psychose maniaco-depressive. *Encephale*, 1:25–31.
58. Levitt, P. (1984): A monoclonal antibody to limbic system neurons. *Science*, 223:299–301.
59. Lewinska, M. K. (1967): Changes in eating and drinking produced by partial amygdala lesions in cat. *Bull. Acad. Pol. Sci. (Biol.)*, 15:301–305.
60. Livingston, K. E., and Hornykiewicz, O. (1978): *Limbic Mechanisms*. Plenum Press, New York.
61. Lloyd, K. G., Farley, I. J., Deck, J. H. N., and Hornykiewicz, O. (1974): Serotonin and 5-hydroxyindoleacetic acid in discrete areas of the brainstem of suicide victims and control patients. *Adv. Biochem. Psychopharmacol.*, 11:387–397.
62. McLachlan, R. S., and Blume, W. T. (1980): Isolated fear in complex partial status epilepticus. *Ann. Neurol.*, 8:639–641.
63. MacLean, P. D. (1954): The limbic system and its hippocampal formation; studies in animals and their possible application to man. *J. Neurosurg.*, 11:29–44.
64. Maier, S. F., and Seligman, M. E. P. (1976): Learned helplessness: theory and evidence. *J. Exp. Psychol. (Gen)*, 105:3–46.
65. Mandell, A. J. (1980): Toward a psychobiology of transcendence: God in the brain. In: *The Psychobiology of Consciousness*, edited by R. J. Davidson and J. M. Davidson, pp. 379–464. Plenum Press, New York.
66. Mazziotta, J. C., Phelps, M. E., Carson, R. E., and Kuhl, D. E. (1982): Tomographic mapping of human cerebral metabolism: auditory stimulation. *Neurology*, 32:921–937.
67. Mesulam, M. M. (1981): Dissociative states with abnormal temporal lobe EEG (multiple personality and the illusion of possession). *Arch. Neurol.*, 38:176–181.
68. Mikkelsen, B., Berggreen, P., Joensen, P., Kristensen, O., Kohler, O., and Mikkelsen, B. O. (1981): Clonazepam (Rivotril) and carbamazepine (Tegretol) in psychomotor epilepsy: a randomized multicenter trial. *Epilepsia*, 22:415–420.
69. Morin, G., Naquet, R., and Badur, M. (1952): Variations of arterial pressure by stimulation of the amygdaloid nucleus and its neighboring structures in the cat. *C. R. Soc. Biol. (Paris)*, 146:747–749.
70. Mulder, D. W., and Daly, D. (1952): Psychiatric symptoms associated with lesions of the temporal lobe. *JAMA*, 150:173–176.
71. Myers, R. D. (1974): *Handbook of Drug and Chemical Stimulation of the Brain*. pp. 627–632. Van Nostrand Reinhold Co., New York.
72. Okuma, T. (1984): Therapeutic and prophylactic efficacies of carbamazepine in manic depressive psychosis. In: *Anticonvulsants in Affective Disorders*, H. M. Emrich, T. Okuma, A. A. Muller (Eds), pp. 76–87, Excerpta Medica, Amsterdam.
73. Papez, J. W. (1937): A proposed mechanism of emotion. *Arch. Neurol. Psychiatry*, 38:725–743.
74. Pare, C. M. B., Young, D. P. H., Price, K., and Stacey, R. S. (1969): 5-Hydroxy-tryptamine, noradrenaline, and dopamine in brainstem, hypothalamus and caudate nucleus of controls and of patients committing suicide by coal-gas poisoning. *Lancet*, 2:133–135.
75. Parnas, J., Korsgaard, S., Krautwald, O., and Jensen, P. S. (1982): Chronic psychosis in epilepsy. *Acta Psychiatr. Scand.*, 66:282–293.
76. Penfield, W. (1975): *The Mystery of the Mind. A Critical Study of Consciousness and the Human Brain*. Princeton University Press, Princeton, New Jersey.
77. Penfield, W., and Jasper, H. (1954): *Epilepsy and the Functional Anatomy of the Human Brain*. Little, Brown & Co., Boston.
78. Perez, M. M., and Trimble, M. R. (1980): Epileptic psychosis-diagnostic comparison with process schizophrenia. *Br. J. Psychiatry*, 137:245–249.
79. Peters, J. G. (1979): Dopamine, noradrenaline and serotonin spinal fluid metabolites in temporal lobe epileptic patients with schizophrenic symptomatology. *Eur. Neurol.*, 18:15–18.
80. Porter, R. J., and Penry, J. K. (1978): Efficacy and choice of antiepileptic drugs. In: *Advances in Epileptology, 1977: Psychology, Pharmacotherapy, and New Diagnostic Approaches*, edited by H. Meinardi and A. J. Rowan, pp. 220–230. Swetz & Zeitlinger, Amsterdam.
81. Post, R. M. (1977): Clinical implications of a cocaine-kindling model of psychosis. In: *Clinical Neuropharmacology*, Vol. II, edited by H. L. Klawans, pp. 25–42. Raven Press, New York.
82. Post, R. M. (1983): Behavioral effects of kindling. In: *Advances in Epileptology: XIVth Epilepsy International Symposium*, edited by M. Parsonage, pp. 173–180. Raven Press, New York.
83. Post, R. M., Ballenger, J. C., Uhde, T. W., and Bunney, W. E., Jr. (1984): Efficacy of carbamazepine in manic-depressive illness: implications for underlying mechanisms. In: *Neurobiology of*

Mood Disorders, edited by R. M. Post and J. C. Ballenger, pp. 777–816. Williams & Wilkins, Baltimore.

84. Post, R. M., Putnam, F. W., Contel, N. R., and Goldman, B. (1984): Electroconvulsive seizures inhibit amygdala kindling: implications for mechanisms of action in affective illness. *Epilepsia*, 25:234–239.

85. Post, R. M., and Uhde, T. W. (1985): Carbamazepine as a treatment for refractory depressive illness and rapidly cycling manic-depressive illness. In: *Special Treatments for Resistant Depression*, edited by J. Zohar and R. H. Belmaker, pp. 281–371. Spectrum Press, New York.

86. Post, R. M., Uhde, T. W., Ballenger, J. C., Chatterji, D. C., Green, R. F., and Bunney, W. E., Jr. (1983): Carbamazepine and its -10,11-epoxide metabolite in plasma and CSF: relationship to antidepressant response. *Arch. Gen. Psychiatry*, 40:673–676.

87. Post, R. M., Uhde, T. W., Ballenger, J. C., and Squillace, K. M. (1983): Prophylactic efficacy of carbamazepine in manic-depressive illness. *Am. J. Psychiatry*, 140:1602–1604.

88. Post, R. M., Berrettini, W., Uhde, T. W., Kellner, C. (1984): Selective response to the anticonvulsant carbamazepine in manic-depressive illness: A case study. *J. Clin. Psychopharmacol.*, 4:178–185.

89. Pritchard, P. B., Lombroso, C. T., and McIntyre, M. (1980): Psychological complications of temporal lobe epilepsy. *Neurology*, 30:227–232.

90. Ramani, V., and Gumnit, R. J. (1981): Intensive monitoring of epileptic patients with a history of episodic aggression. *Arch. Neurol.*, 38:570–571.

91. Ramani, V., and Gumnit, R. J. (1982): Intensive monitoring of interictal psychosis in epilepsy. *Ann. Neurol.*, 11:613–622.

92. Robertson, M. (1983): Depression and epilepsy. Proc. 15th Epilepsy International Symposium, Washington, D.C., Sept. 1983.

93. Robertson, M. M., and Trimble, M. R. (1983): Depressive illness in patients with epilepsy: a review. *Epilepsia*, 24:S109–S116.

94. Rodin, E. A. (1973): Psychomotor epilepsy and aggressive behavior. *Arch. Gen. Psychiatry*, 28:210–213.

95. Sackeim, H. A., Greenberg, M. S., Weiman, A. L., Gur, R. C., Hungerbuhler, J. P., and Geschwind, N. (1982): Hemispheric asymmetry in the expression of positive and negative emotions: neurologic evidence. *Arch. Neurol.*, 39:210–218.

96. Satinoff, E. (1978): Neural organization and evolution of thermal regulation in mammals. *Science*, 201:16–22.

97. Schenk, L., and Bear, D. (1981): Multiple personality disorder and related dissociative phenomena in patients with temporal lobe epilepsy. *Am. J. Psychiatry*, 138:1311–1315.

98. Serafetinides, E. A. (1965): Aggressiveness in temporal lobe epileptics and its relation to cerebral dysfunction and environmental factors. *Epilepsia*, 6:33–42.

99. Serafetinides, E. A., and Falconer, M. A. (1962): The effects of temporal lobectomy in epileptic patients with psychosis. *J. Ment. Sci.*, 108:584–593.

100. Shaw, D. M., Camps, F. E., and Eccleston, E. G. (1967): 5-Hydroxytryptamine in the hindbrains of depressive suicides. *Br. J. Psychiatry*, 113:1407–1411.

101. Shealy, C. N., and Peele, T. L. (1957): Studies on amygdaloid nucleus of cat. *J. Neurophysiol.*, 20:125–139.

102. Sherwin, I. (1982): The effect of the location of an epileptogenic lesion on the occurrence of psychosis in epilepsy. In: *Advances in Biological Psychiatry, Vol. 8: Temporal Lobe Epilepsy, Mania, and Schizophrenia and the Limbic System*, edited by W. P. Koella and M. R. Trimble, pp. 81–97. S. Karger, Basel.

102a. Silberman, E. K., Post, R. M., Nurnberger, J., Theodore, W., Boulenger, J-P. (1985): Transient sensory, cognitive, and affective phenomena in affective illness: A comparison with complex partial epilepsy. *Br. J. Psychiatry*, 146:81–89.

103. Shukla, G. D., Srivastava, O. N., Katiyar, B. C., Joshi, V., and Mohan, P. K. (1979): Psychiatric manifestations in temporal lobe epilepsy: a controlled study. *Br. J. Psychiatry*, 135:411–417.

104. Slater, E., Beard, A. W., and Glithero, E. (1963): The schizophrenia-like psychoses of epilepsy. *Br. J. Psychiatry*, 109:95–150.

105. Slater, E. and Moran, P. A. P. (1969): The schizophrenia-like psychoses of epilepsy: relation between ages of onset. *Br. J. Psychiatry*, 115:599–600.

106. Slusher, M. A., and Hyde, J. E. (1961): Effect of limbic stimulation on release of corticosteroids into the adrenal venous affluent of the cat. *Endocrinology*, 69:1080–1084.
107. Small, J. G., Small, I. F., and Hayden, M. P. (1966): Further psychiatric investigations of patients with temporal and nontemporal lobe epilepsy. *Am. J. Psychiatry*, 123:303–310.
108. Standage, K. F. (1973): Schizophreniform psychosis among epileptics in a mental hospital. *Br. J. Psychiatry*, 123:321–323.
109. Stevens, J. R. (1973): Psychomotor epilepsy and schizophrenia: a common anatomy? In: *Epilepsy: Its Phenomena in Man*, edited by M. A. B. Brazier, pp. 190–214. Academic Press, New York.
110. Stevens, J. R. (1982): Risk factors for psychopathology in individuals with epilepsy. In: *Advances in Biological Psychiatry: Temporal Lobe Epilepsy, Mania, and Schizophrenia and the Limbic System*, edited by W. P. Koella and M. R. Trimble, pp. 56–80. S. Karger, Basel.
111. Sugano, K., and Miyasaka, M. (1980): Epileptic psychosis and the occurring conditions. *Folia Psychiatr. Neurol. Jpn.*, 34:340–342.
112. Taylor, D. C. (1975): Factors influencing the occurrence of schizophrenia-like psychosis in patients with temporal lobe epilepsy. *Psychol. Med.*, 5:249–254.
113. Tharp, B. R. (1979): Transient global amnesia: manifestation of medial temporal lobe epilepsy [letter]. *Clin. EEG*, 10:54–56.
114. Trimble, M. R. (1984): Interictal psychoses of epilepsy. *Acta Psychiatr. Scand.*, 69(Suppl. 313):9–20.
115. Trixler, M., and Nador, G. (1976): Schizophrenia-like psychoses in temporal lobe epilepsy. *EEG Clin. Neurophysiol.*, 41:213–214.
116. Uhde, T. W., Boulenger, J.-P., Roy-Byrne, P. P., Geraci, M. F., Vittone, B. J., and Post, R. M. (1985): Longitudinal course of panic disorder: clinical and biological considerations. *Prog. Neuropsychopharmacol. Biol. Psychiatry*, 9:39–51.
117. Ursin, H., and Kaada, B. R. (1960): Subcortical structures mediating the attention response induced by amygdala stimulation. *Exp. Neurol.*, 2:109–122.
118. Waxman, S. G., and Geschwind, N. (1975): The interictal behavior syndrome of temporal lobe epilepsy. *Arch. Gen. Psychiatry*, 32:1580–1586.
119. Yde, A., Lohse, E., and Faurbye, A. (1941): On the relation between schizophrenia, epilepsy, and induced convulsions. *Acta Psychiatr. Neurol. Scand.*, 16:325–388.
120. Yoshida, M. (1963): Effects of amygdaloid stimulation on emotional responses produced by hypothalamic stimulation in cats. *Psychiatr. Neurol. Jpn.*, 65:863–879.

The Limbic System: Functional Organization and Clinical Disorders, edited by B.K. Doane and K.E. Livingston. Raven Press, New York © 1986.

Episodic Behavioral Disorders and Limbic Ictus

Russell R. Monroe

Department of Psychiatry, University of Maryland, Baltimore, Maryland 21201

The most popular strategy for the study of the behavioral consequences of a limbic ictus in humans has been a comparative evaluation of temporal lobe epilepsy (TLE) versus other forms of epilepsy and/or acute organic brain syndromes, and/or the so-called "functional" psychoses (1). The basic assumption behind this strategy is that TLE, as rigorously defined by focal temporal spikes in the electroencephalogram (EEG) and/or complex psychic seizures, is synonymous with limbic seizures and that deviant behavior, not typical of TLE seizures, is an interictal event. However, to make a truly empirical study of the behavioral consequences of a limbic ictus in the human requires direct observation on subjects with chronically implanted subcortical electrodes. These studies reveal that storms of electrical activity can occur in the limbic system without reflection in nearby structures or on the temporal cortex, let alone in scalp recordings, and that behavioral changes associated with this limbic ictal activity are seldom characteristic of grand mal, petit mal, or psychomotor epilepsy. Such observations remind us that the clinical EEG is an extremely "blunt" diagnostic instrument even when it includes sphenoidal leads and EEG activating procedures. The prevalence of false-negative EEG findings is so high as to call into question the validity of intergroup comparisons and also should remind us that it is not easy to prove what behavior is ictal and what is interictal.

A second strategy are studies on the correlations between behavior and brain activity recorded through implanted subcortical electrodes. This too has obvious drawbacks. Such a drastic procedure limits the number of subjects studied, with perhaps 200 to 300 such patients reported in the literature. Not only that, the cohort studied is very select because these studies are limited to those with an illness so severe as to warrant a drastic therapeutic intervention of either subcortical electrical stimulation or specific extirpation of an epileptogenic focus. Furthermore—fortunately for the patients, but unfortunately for science—precise neuroanatomic confirmation of electrode placement is seldom available.

There is a third strategy, one that I have preferred, which was suggested by observations made on subjects who had spontaneous or induced limbic seizural activity as monitored by subcortically implanted electrodes. The behavioral patterns that correlated with the limbic ictus had consistent characteristics that could be utilized in identifying individuals with, at least, presumptive evidence for limbic epilepsy or what I call an epileptoid episode disorder. The behavioral changes in these patients are intermittent or paroxysmal, demonstrating an abrupt onset and an equally precipitous remission. They experience intense dysphoric affects associated with impulsive action. They describe symptoms suggesting a prodrome or aura of epilepsy, or have symptoms that might be considered *formes frustes* of epilepsy. Other symptoms are characteristic of the acute brain syndrome, such as clouding of sensorium, partial amnesia, illusions, and visual hallucinations. By using such criteria for an epileptoid episodic disorder, one can differentiate these intermittent behavioral aberrations from another intermittent group whose behavior is hysterical and/or manipulative. As a further aid in this discrimination I utilize a drug activation (alpha chloralose) that is particularly effective in eliciting nonspecific EEG abnormalities and, although to some degree increases the false-positives, drastically reduces the false-negatives. Admittedly, this strategy, too, has drawbacks, and the evidence for a specifically defined syndrome associated with a limbic ictus will remain inferential until we have developed a non-intrusive measure of excessive neuronal discharges deep in the brain. The heuristic value of this inferential approach is that certain dramatic behavioral disorders are recognized as an ictal phenomenon that should respond to drugs that raise seizure threshold. The validity of such a concept now rests on the response of such individuals to anticonvulsants.

SPONTANEOUS AND INDUCED LIMBIC ICTUS

The subjects reported here have been reported in more detail elsewhere (2) and were subjects in the Tulane cohorts studied after the original publication, edited by Robert Heath, entitled *Studies in Schizophrenia* (3,4).

Patient 021[1] was a mother and housewife in her mid 20s who already had fixed paranoid delusions. Superimposed on this chronic psychosis were acute episodes which her husband referred to as "spells." These spells were preceded by severe headaches and then by a vacant stare, which alerted those around her that she was about to explode. Hallucinations, both visual and auditory, quickly followed. At this point she would jump out of bed, begin attacking people around her, tearing off her clothes, breaking up the furniture, and pulling on her hair "to get the snakes out of it." During such a confused episode she was disoriented, and following cessation of the attack she had only a hazy recollection of the events. The intense fear and rage during the attack were replaced by a chronic depression and remorse. During the attacks the subcortical electrogram revealed paroxysmal bursts of spikes and spike waves in the limbic system which in this patient, unlike most, was also reflected on the temporal cortex. An intravenous (i.v.) injection of sodium amytal would temporarily relieve symptoms and replace the ictal recording with typical barbiturate spindling. As the drug effect wore off, both the symptoms and the ictal electrogram would return. With spontaneous remission of her "spell" the ictal

---

[1]Patients numbers are those used in ref. 2.

recording was replaced by an interictal record of occasional spikes in the limbic recordings.

Patient 019 was also a chronic paranoid schizophrenic without any superimposed episodic symptoms. Aside from fixed delusions, her outstanding symptoms were the negative or deficit symptoms such as abulia, flatness of affect, and thought disorder. As it had been previously observed in other patients that septal stimulation would often lead to a brightening of the affects, temporary clearing in the thought disorder, and initiative and interest in interpersonal activities, this patient was stimulated daily for a period of several weeks. Instead of brightening, this patient became increasingly irritable, and although she interacted more with her mother, this left much to be desired, as it first consisted of a verbal abuse then threats of physical attacks. There was increasing confusion and some problems with recent memory. The patient claimed she could not remember whether she had taken her medication. With the frequent stimulation the afterdischarges became more prolonged until they outlasted the interval between stimulations. The day of the last stimulation a burst of seizural activity spread to the cortex and the patient screamed out that she was going to pass out. At this time the stimulation procedure was discontinued. Viewed retrospectively, in the light of Goddard's subsequent publications on the kindling phenomenon (5), it would seem that this may represent kindling in the human subject.

As already mentioned, stimulating the septal area would often elicit a pleasurable response, increased alertness, a new participation with the outside world, and an openness or friendliness with those in the immediate environment. Stimulating the tegmentum of the mesencephalon elicited a primitive, frightening rage directed at anybody in the environment, usually the closest person at hand, which would terminate as soon as the stimulating current was shut off. Stimulating the amygdala would elicit a dramatic fight or flight response with more discrimination in that the object toward whom this response was directed was usually somebody in the immediate environment who had a symbolic connection with the patient's past; e.g., "I attacked him because he has a Southern accent like my father." It was interesting that stimulating with the same parameters in the same location would, some days, elicit a fight, and other days, a flight pattern. The response often could be predicted on the basis of events that had occurred during the preceding 24 hr. I mention this because it particularly dramatizes the complementarity of neurologic and psychologic data. Stimulating the hypothalamus elicited physiologic responses suggesting fight or flight, namely, elevation of blood pressure, tachycardia, sweating, piloerection, without any particular cognitive or emotional concomitance of the fight/flight response (6).

The "smell" brain as a phylogenetic antecedent of limbic structures suggested an evaluation of patients when stimulated by strong odors. Not surprisingly, this elicited spindling-type activity in the amygdala and hippocampal area. What was surprising was the observation that certain mild odors would elicit greater activity than more caustic ones. In one man stale beer seemed to be the most potent stimulus, and when asked to associate to this smell he reported an adolescent experience of being homosexually accosted in a bar. Following this lead, such spindling activity could be elicited by memories of being the radio officer on an ammunition ship during World War II, wherein only he and the captain knew of prowling German submarines that any moment could blow them into oblivion. On the other hand, one of his most pleasant early childhood memories of Christmas morning and finding an electric train under the Christmas tree also elicited this spindling. Simple arithmetic calculations immediately terminated such spindling, and, surprisingly, intense painful memories of frustrations during the preceding several weeks did not elicit such activity. This pattern was certainly not an ictal one, but it did represent a spindling hypersynchrony, which raises the question of whether intense, old memories could possibly influence the seizural threshold in the limbic system (7).

Finally, Heath reports a patient who, when impulsively explosive (e.g., thrusting a fist through a window) showed a limbic ictal pattern. However, on another occasion, when impulsively threatening suicide if he was not given a pass out of the hospital, the patient did not show such an ictal pattern. This emphasizes the importance of distinguishing between the epileptoid dyscontrol act and the hysteroid (or motivated) dyscontrol act (4). The clinician who is aware of these epileptoid and hysteroid poles in dyscontrol behavior soon recognizes that the dyscontrol acts of most of his patients are seldom at the extreme ends of the continuum, but fall somewhere between these poles (2).

These observations on patients with chronically implanted subcortical electrodes guided me to the third strategy in studying the behavior consequences of a limbic ictus, that is, an investigation of patients with intermittent paroxysmal disorders, or what I call episodic behavioral disorders, whether they had more conventional evidence (EEG or behavioral) of typical epilepsy, or not (2).

THE DYSCONTROL SYNDROME—OPERATIONALLY DEFINED

My definition of episodic behavioral disorders is that this syndrome represents any precipitously appearing maladaptive behavior, intermittent and recurrent, that interrupts the life-style or the life flow of the individual (2). This behavior represents a discontinuity in terms of space-time relations, there being a sudden change in personality or life-style as compared with the "before" and the "after" patterns of behavior. These episodic behavioral disorders can be either episodic disinhibitions of action or episodic inhibitions of action. Figure 1 summarizes this concept. Within the center square are the main characteristic symptoms of the episodic disorders, that is, the precipitous onset, abrupt remission, intense dysphoric affects, and the lack of residual symptoms during the intervals between episodes. Outside the square, but within the circle, are the diverse symptoms that are not specific for the syndrome, but some or all of these may be represented in a given attack. Depending on which symptoms are predominant, a plethora of diagnoses may be applied to this syndrome even though, as I have proposed, there is a single underlying mechanism, namely, a limbic ictus associated with most of these dis-

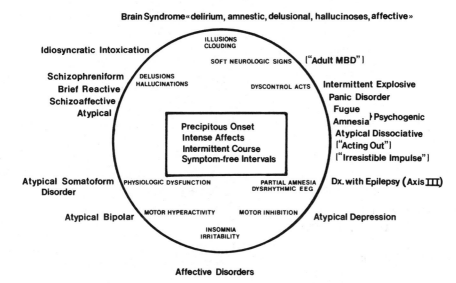

FIG. 1. DSM III assignment of episodic behavioral disorders (axis I); [" "] indicates no provision in DSM III (14).

orders. The possible diagnoses for the episodic syndrome are indicated outside of the circle. The dyscontrol acts is the primary subject of this discussion (2).

Episodic dyscontrol is a subgroup of the episodic behavioral disorders and is defined as an abrupt single act or a short series of acts with a common intent, carried through to completion with at least a partial relief of tension or an immediate gratification of a specific need (2). As a subclass of the episodic behavioral disorders, it shares the characteristic precipitous, maladaptive interruption in the life-style and the life flow of the individual. In the psychiatric literature such labels as "acting on impulse," "impulse neurosis," "irresistible impulse," or "acting out" have been used to classify such behavior (Fig. 2).

The term "dyscontrol" was not an official diagnostic label in *DSM II* nor is it utilized in *DSM III*. However, in the latter the concept of the dyscontrol syndrome was incorporated into the diagnostic criteria for "Disorders of Impulse Control Not Elsewhere Classified," particularly 312.34 Intermittent Explosive Disorder. The diagnosis applies to those individuals who have recurrent paroxysmal episodes of loss of control of aggressive impulses that result in serious assault or destruction of property. The magnitude of the behavior during an episode is grossly out of proportion to any precipitating event. The individuals often describe these episodes as "spells" or "attacks." The symptoms appear abruptly, and regardless of duration, remit almost as quickly. Following each episode there usually is regret or self-reproach at the consequences of the action and the inability to control the impulses. Between episodes there are no signs of generalized impulsivity or aggressiveness. Previously, these individuals might have received the diagnosis of "explosive personality."

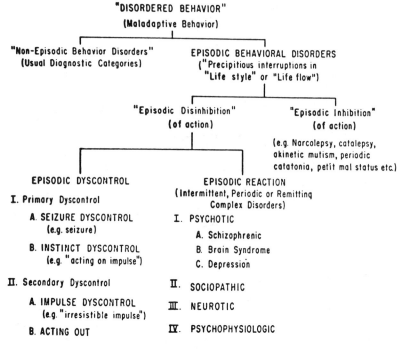

FIG. 2. Disordered behavior (12).

There are usually prodromal affective or autonomic symptoms signaling an impending episode. During the episodes themselves there may be subtle changes in sensorium, and following the episode there is usually a spotty or partial amnesia. The behavior is a surprise to those in the individual's milieu, and even the individual afflicted is often startled by his own behavior, describing the events as resulting from a compelling force beyond his control, even though he is willing to accept responsibility for his actions.

Some individuals claim hypersensitivity to sensory input such as loud noises, rhythmic auditory or visual stimuli, and bright lights. Other features suggesting an organic disturbance may be present, such as EEG abnormalities or minor neurologic signs and symptoms thought to reflect subcortical or limbic system dysfunction. Epilepsy is rarely present, but is nevertheless more common than in individuals without the disorder. Psychiatric history often reveals childhood hyperactivity and accident proneness. The social consequences of the disorder can be disastrous to the individual and to others, leading to incarceration in prison or chronic hospitalization.

Predisposing factors include any toxic agent, such as alcohol, which may lower the threshold for violent outbursts, and conditions conducive to brain dysfunction, such as perinatal trauma, infantile seizures, head trauma, or encephalitis. There is some evidence that the disorder is more common in family members of individuals with the disorder.

The dyscontrol syndrome as I originally defined it, however, covers a whole range of possible impulsive acts, that is, not only aggressive acts but also flight behavior or orgasmic release. As we have already mentioned, electrical stimulation of the limbic area often elicits not only an explosive rage reaction but an equally precipitous panic similar to what is described elsewhere in *DSM III* as a "panic disorder." These panic disorders 300.01 are defined as at least three panic attacks occurring within a 3-week period at times other than during marked physical exertion or a life-threatening situation and in the absence of a physical disorder that could account for this symptom of anxiety. Furthermore, these attacks should not occur only when exposed to a circumscribed phobic stimulus and should include at least four of the following symptoms: dyspnea, palpitations, chest pain, choking sensations, dizziness, feelings of unreality, paresthesias, hot and cold flashes, sweating, faintness, trembling, fear of loss of control. I feel that the bouts of aggressiveness, panic, as well as erotomania, all have a common underlying mechanism, that of a limbic ictus, and, in fact, it is not uncommon to see all three such episodes in one patient. It would be preferable, then, if these were grouped together under a dyscontrol syndrome that would emphasize a possible common therapeutic regimen.

Under *DSM III* the impulse syndromes are considered an Axis I diagnosis because no matter how ego-syntonic the behavior is during the act itself, in retrospect the individual and his asssociates see the act as ego-alien, that is, something quite out of character for the individual actor and out of context for the situation. Thus, the behavior meets the criteria for a symptom. However, in one subgroup of the dyscontrol syndrome, i.e., "acting out," this ego-alien quality is minimized or denied through psychological defense mechanisms, particularly repression in some form. Thus, "acting out" is defined as a dyscontrol act that is so patently inappropriate to the situation and so out of character for the actor and so inadequately explained by the person committing the act that one can only conclude the act is determined by unconscious motives, as an attempt to resolve repressed conflicts (2). As *DSM III* eschews psychodynamic considerations, there is no diagnostic category for "acting out," which must be defined in psychodynamic terms.

There is still another type of dyscontrol behavior not covered in *DSM III*. This syndrome has been labeled in the psychiatric, particularly in the forensic, literature as the "irresistible impulse." In this subgroup of the dyscontrol syndrome, which I have labeled "impulse dyscontrol," the act itself might be quite explosive and often aggressive, but is preceded not only by mounting tension but also by a conscious awareness of the impending action, with the realization of the potential disastrous consequences of such action. This awareness is accompanied by waivering doubt and indecisiveness as to whether to consumate the act or not and is often accompanied by elaborate and bizarre attempts to control the impulse, thus the label "irresistible impulse."

The patient with a dyscontrol syndrome can be mistakenly assigned to the personality disorders under *DSM III*, axis II, but this may lead to serious prognostic and therapeutic errors. It is true that there are individuals with an impulsive lifestyle who see the world as "a series of opportunities, temptations, frustrations, sensuous experiences, and fragmented impressions" (8). There is no distinct category for such individuals in *DSM III*. Most likely, if male they would be assigned to the "antisocial personality" and if female to the "histrionic personality." Or they might be assigned to two other diagnostic categories, i.e., the narcissistic personality or the borderline personality, all four types being described as "dramatic, emotional, or erratic." By definition, the dyscontrol patient does not manifest persistent deviant behavior, rather, such behavior is episodic or intermittent. This differential becomes crucial when one realizes that the dyscontrol syndrome has a good prognosis with psychopharmacologic and/or psychotherapeutic intervention whereas the personality disorders, with their relatively poor prognosis, often suggest a therapeutic nihilism that is decidedly unwarranted for the dyscontrol syndrome.

DYSCONTROL SYNDROME: PHENOMENOLOGICALLY DEFINED

In evaluating dyscontrol acts, one should establish the specificity of the drives or urges behind the act, the coordination and complexity of the motor behavior during the act, and the appropriateness of the motives or goals of the act (Fig. 3). The dyscontrol act is characterized by feeling, "I just did it, I don't know why." It is an experience of having executed a significant action "without a clear and complete sense of motivation, decision, or sustained wish, so that it does not feel completely deliberate or fully intended" (8). Despite this spontaneity and lack of

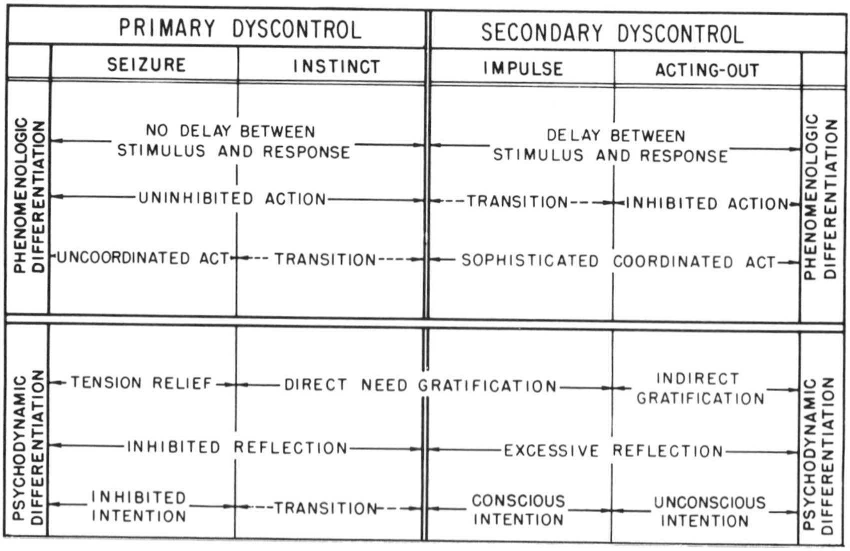

PRIMARY DYSCONTROL		SECONDARY DYSCONTROL		
SEIZURE	INSTINCT	IMPULSE	ACTING-OUT	
PHENOMENOLOGIC DIFFERENTIATION	NO DELAY BETWEEN STIMULUS AND RESPONSE	DELAY BETWEEN STIMULUS AND RESPONSE		PHENOMENOLOGIC DIFFERENTIATION
	──UNINHIBITED ACTION──	──TRANSITION──►INHIBITED ACTION──		
►UNCOORDINATED ACT►─── TRANSITION────►		── SOPHISTICATED COORDINATED ACT──		
PSYCHODYNAMIC DIFFERENTIATION	►TENSION RELIEF──►──DIRECT NEED GRATIFICATION──	──► INDIRECT GRATIFICATION──		PSYCHODYNAMIC DIFFERENTIATION
	──INHIBITED REFLECTION──	──EXCESSIVE REFLECTION──		
	INHIBITED INTENTION	──TRANSITION──	CONSCIOUS INTENTION	UNCONSCIOUS INTENTION

FIG. 3. Episodic dyscontrol (13).

reflection, such actions are occasionally adaptive and may represent the unique contribution of the genius or the man of action. However, more often the abrupt precipitous acts are based on primitive emotions of fear, rage, or sensuous feelings without concern for the effect on the immediate environment or the long-term consequences to the actor or society and are, therefore, self- or socially destructive. These acts are disinhibitions of behavior (in the motor sense) and are often sadistic or bizarre crimes, suicidal attempts, or aggressive or sexual acting out.

These spontaneous or impulsive acts are described as representing a "short circuit" between the stimulus and response. This demands, if only briefly, an analysis of the delay between the stimulus and the act which characterizes most socialized human behavior. The short circuit between the stimulus and the act resulting in precipitous behavior implies that the behavior is not corrected by reflection on past experiences or anticipation of future consequences. It is precisely for this reason that the act is usually self-destructive or self-defeating for the individual, or appears antisocial to the onlooker.

One can identify two facets to this delay between the stimulus and the response. The first I would designate reflective delay (often referred to in the psychoanalytic literature as "thought as trial action"), which is (a) the time necessary for establishing the uniqueness or familiarity of the stimulus by associative connections with past experiences, (b) the time necessary to contemplate alternative courses of action, and (c) the time necessary to project into the future and predict the outcome of alternative actions. The second facet is choice delay, which is possible only following this reflective delay. The choice delay is a decision to postpone immediate action or gratification for long-term rewards, that is, "biding one's time." This choice delay is absent in the extractive sociopathic individual who gives in to his urges, seeking immediate gratification, consequences be "damned," even though he may have made a careful appraisal of the situation and has a good realization of the possible long-term consequences of his action.

The disturbance in reflective delay, characteristic of episodic dyscontrol, depends on a complex interaction among affects, hindsight and foresight, reason, perceptual discrimination, and appropriate generalization. If there is a significant deficiency or inappropriate domination of any one of these mechanisms, the whole process may fail, resulting in a total absence of reflective delay, leading to what I have called primary dyscontrol (see Fig. 3). In such instances there is an immediate reaction to an environmental stimulus, seeking gratification without even the concept that there is an alternative possibility involving delay. This is the true "short circuit" between stimulus and response characteristic of primary dyscontrol. Figure 3 summarizes the phenomenological and psychodynamic differentiation between primary dyscontrol and secondary dyscontrol. Primary dyscontrol is further divided into two subgroups, seizure and instinct dyscontrol. The paradigm of seizure dyscontrol is the postictal confusional state in which behavior is characterized by intense, indiscriminate affects, chaotic and uncoordinated motor patterns, and an indiscriminate selection of the object acted upon, which is often the person closest at hand. There is little specific need gratification, although there is usually a reduction in tension. Such dyscontrol behavior can occur without a prior seizure and, in fact, on rare occasions may not even be a reflection of central nervous system instability.

On the other hand, instinct dyscontrol is characterized by affects that are clearly differentiated and more effectively gratified. Although the motor pattern is lacking in subtlety, it is none the less efficient and coordinated. In this case the object acted upon has at least simple associative links with past experiences. In both instinct and seizure dyscontrol, the behavior is characterized by an explosive, immediate response to an environmental stimulus, which represents a true "short circuit" between stimulus and action.

In secondary dyscontrol there is either conscious or unconscious premeditation between the true stimulus and the act; hence, there is a delay between the stimulus and the act. The reflection, which precedes action, reveals an ambivalent, vacillating attitude regarding the choice to either succumb to or restrain the impulse (Fig. 3). By and large, individuals showing secondary dyscontrol are, in their general life-style, overly inhibited and at some level aware of the true, even though neurotic, intentions of their action. The act itself is more likely to represent a rebellion against an overly strict and inhibiting conscience mechanism, or a devious substitute gratification of unacceptable impulses. As an example, one can think of the explosive act in the overly controlled obsessive character or the hysterical analysand's acting out within the transference neurosis. Figure 3 summarizes the phenomenological and psychodynamic differences between the two subgroups of secondary dyscontrol, that is, impulse dyscontrol and acting out. The primary feature for differentiation is that there is conscious intention in impulse dyscontrol with considerable wavering and doubt, an example of the excessive reflection that accompanies secondary dyscontrol. In the case of acting out this reflection is at an unconscious level.

A simplified dynamic statement often applied to impulsive behavior, or what I have designated as episodic dyscontrol, is that "urges overwhelm controls." This has operational value only if one can determine where an individual falls between the extremes of excessively strong urges overwhelming normal control mechanisms, on one hand, and normal urges uncontrolled by weak or deficient inhibitory mechanisms, on the other. The traditional psychiatric viewpoint stresses weak control mechanisms (9). However, careful clinical evaluation, now supported by growing neurophysiological evidence, reveals that in some instances intense dysphoric affects, associated with excessive neuronal discharges in the limbic system, overwhelm normal control mechanisms, particularly when brain dysfunction in other ways temporarily impairs higher cortical function. Thus, it becomes important to identify the group where intense urges overwhelm normal control mechanisms or transiently impair cortical control. The goal in therapy, then, is not so much to develop stronger inhibitory mechanisms, but in some way to neutralize the intense dysphoria. It is particularly this group that requires a complementary pharmacological regimen in one's psychotherapeutic efforts (10).

Another important dynamic consideration in the evaluation of episodic dyscontrol is the patient's retrospective evaluation of his behavior. During the dyscontrol act itself, the behavior could be called ego-syntonic in that it is an abrupt, often explosive, quick act carried through to immediate completion without any procrastination and doubt. However, in retrospect, often the actor himself is chagrined by his behavior, and hence the act has become ego-alien. This seems to be particularly true if the behavior represents an underlying epileptoid rather than a motivated mechanism, as is usually the case in primary dyscontrol. Of course, if the individual recognizes in retrospect that the act is ego-alien, psychotherapeutic endeavors are considerably facilitated. At other times the act must be seen as ego-alien either at a conscious or unconscious level because responsibility for the behavior is defensively denied. In such instances one finds associated amnesia, projection, or rationalization, so one can assume that the behavior is recognized as unacceptable (secondary dyscontrol). This explains why complete amnesia is more likely to be present during the hysteroid or motivated dyscontrol acts, whereas the epileptoid acts are usually accompanied by a hazy or partial remembering of the events during the dyscontrol act. It is questionable whether any individual manifesting true episodic dyscontrol, as here defined, ever commits acts that are truly ego-syntonic, both at the time the act is committed and also in retrospect. This would much more likely occur in the true psychopath.

Finally, one must consider the intentions of any dyscontrol behavior. As already described, in acting out, the intention is thoroughly disguised, usually representing the symbolic fulfillment of a forbidden impulse. On the other hand, in impulse dyscontrol and instinct dyscontrol the true intention is either directly expressed or only superficially disguised and rationalized. As a simple example of this, one could consider the adolescent boy living in a fatherless family who, in the throes of an oedipal renunciation, kills his mother's lover, usually on some superficial pretense. In seizural dyscontrol (the most primitive level of episodic dyscontrol) the act is so diffuse and uncoordinated that it becomes relatively ineffective. Some patients seem to have the capacity to shift dyscontrol acts from instinct or impulse dyscontrol into this more primitive behavior, which discharges tension but does not lead to more specific (but unacceptable) need gratification. This is one explanation for the frequently reported clinical observation that with an increase in seizures, there is a decrease in other dyscontrol acts. A related defensive maneuver is that the episodic dyscontrol is an episodic inhibition of action. It then protects the individual from the self-destructive consequences of the disinhibited dyscontrol acts, even though the former offers neither need gratification nor release of tension (Fig. 2). It is surprising how often a given patient will demonstrate the whole gamut of dyscontrol acts.

The affects associated with dyscontrol behavior, as already mentioned, are intense. They usually represent discrete fear and rage, but at other times mixtures of the two, sometimes with profound depression. All of these add up to periodic, intense dysphoria from which the patient is compelled to seek immediate relief, often through self-medication. The most common example of this is relief through alcohol. As alcohol suppresses higher cortical function, it ultimately leaves the individual even more susceptible to dyscontrol behavior. Thus, most of the disorders now labeled as pathological intoxication would fit our definition of episodic dyscontrol. Those individuals who deal with the compulsive drug abuser have likewise observed that a number of such users report that they control aggressive impulses through their use of drugs. Hence, a significant number of individuals manifesting episodic dyscontrol might be found in our drug or alcohol clinics.

It has been repeatedly observed that dyscontrol behavior seems almost phase-specific for the adolescent (1). Such behavior represents the complex interaction between the affective turmoil, identity crisis, and undeveloped anticipatory mechanisms characteristic of this age group. Nevertheless, it is important to look carefully at the impulsive adolescent from a phenomenologic, as well as a psychodynamic point of view. Again, a significant number represent a rather specific episodic dyscontrol related to neurological dysfunction. This may represent a neurophysiological maturational lag identifiable with careful neurological and EEG techniques. As such, an identification has specific prognostic and therapeutic implications; this is an important consideration for the clinician.

CASE EXAMPLE: EPISODIC DYSCONTROL

A family referred for therapy because of what appeared to the referring physician as an impending catastrophic dissolution, consisted of a 51-year old father who was a graduate engineer in a middle-level management position at a small but substantial company, a 49-year-old mother, housewife, volunteer worker, now looking for paid employment, and three children. There was a daughter who was a senior in a nearby college, living in her own apartment, a son who was a high school senior with poor academic standing, hence, a confused outlook for the immediate future, and another daughter, a sophomore in high school. They owned their own home in a middle-class suburban community. Both parents had automobiles.

Evidence for the impending family dissolution were the following facts. The older daughter had recently left home because of parental fights, and the youngest had run away on several occasions for the same reason. The son solved the conflict in the family by becoming an avid participant in the high school drug culture, spending as much time away from home as possible. Ultimately, the mother admitted that her recent interest in finding a job was to establish her financial independence so that she could separate and divorce her husband. All members of the family admitted they were afraid of the husband-father's rages. In fact, he also admitted that he was afraid of his rage and was remorseful after the fact. Although he was judged to be severely punishing toward his children, resorting to clubs or sticks to administer physical punishment, he never assaulted his wife.

A typical explosive act was the following. Returning home from work in the evening, the husband would walk up the front driveway to be greeted by the dog jumping on him with muddy paws. The younger daughter would rush out of the house to greet him and grab the car keys so she could drive off. The wife, cooking a meal in the kitchen, would begin belaboring him with a tale of woe regarding the current day and then would turn the children over to him for punishment for the day's list of disobedient behavior. After an unsuccessful confrontation with the children, who "gave me a lot of lip," he would feel his face flushing, heart pounding rapidly, and sparks before his eyes. Rage would well up within him, and he would begin cursing at the top of his voice. The feeling was one of lack of control, and soon he would begin smashing windows, breaking up the furniture, putting his fist through the walls and doors. This could go on for hours. He was aware of what was happening but felt driven to continue. The damage was so severe and frequent enough (several times a month) that it was causing severe financial burden on the family to repair the damage. Several times he drove off recklessly in his car, and, although he occasionally had an accident, he had never seriously hurt himself or anybody else. Several times he fractured his hand by hitting the wall and many times required stitches at the local emergency room. He was described by his family and on the job as a quick-tempered individual with a short fuse. On only two occasions, however, in the past 15 years, had he lost control of himself on the job.

The husband was hospitalized for several days for diagnostic workup. Except for a history of mild hypertension, there was no suggestion of medical problems. Physical, neurological, and laboratory study findings were all within normal limits, and these included a glucose tolerance test and a routine EEG.

The patient was discharged on 400 mg phenytoin (Dilantin) per day with 250 mg to 500 mg primidone (Mysoline) to be taken as desired if he noted mounting tension.

At his first appointment 2 weeks after discharge, he reported another explosive episode following a sequence similar to that described above. However, there was a difference in that he "blew" standing in the middle of the livingroom, cursing at the top of his voice. This lasted no longer than 5 to 10 min and was not accompanied by the characteristic destruction of property. He was followed infrequently for the next 2 years, and it was obvious that the attacks occurred at approximately the same frequency but that the severity was considerably attenuated. On one occasion he discontinued his medicine and a month later had a severe explosive episode so that he voluntarily resumed his pharmacologic regime.

Several years later he called to report that he and his wife had separated. The two older children had left home, and the youngest daughter moved in with her mother. He was living at home alone, no longer taking anticonvulsants and, except for transitory temper outbursts on the job, was not having difficulties.

RENOWNED EXAMPLES OF THE EPISODIC DISORDERS

Example 1. Vincent van Gogh

Early one evening this man approached his roommate Gauguin with an open razor in a menacing way. Gauguin stared him down and commanded that he go back home. He turned on his heels, went to his room, cut off his earlobe and, wrapping it in a handkerchief, presented it to a prostitute whom the two had shared. Later that evening he was found unconscious and bleeding in bed and was rushed to the hospital.

This was the first of seven episodic psychotic reactions that occurred over a period of 1½ years. Most of these lasted a few days to several weeks, but one persisted for more than 2 months. During his life he had several other dyscontrol episodes. One occurred when he was a student and teased by a classmate who pulled his shirttail. He turned and quite uncharacteristically struck his classmate a vicious blow. Another time a colleague teased him by substituting salt for what he thought was sugar. He placed this in his coffee, and when he discovered it he blazed up in fury at all of those involved. A third episode occurred while he was hospitalized after returning from an excursion into the countryside. Halfway up the stairway at the entrance he turned and kicked his attendant in the belly, an attendant who was quite friendly with him. Several other times he attempted suicide in a bizarre way by swallowing small quantities of mildly toxic solutions, whatever was the closest at hand. However, he did terminate his life by suicide with a pistol in what must have been a carefully planned event.

Example 2. Virginia Woolf

After writing farewell notes to her husband and sister, she picked up her walking stick, crossed the meadow and went to the banks of the nearby river. When her husband missed her he feared the worst and ran to the riverbank where he found her walking stick stuck in the mud. Two days later her body washed up on the banks of the river, and the pockets of her jacket were filled with stones.

She had made at least two other suicidal attempts. Once she took a dose of barbiturates insufficient to kill her, and once jumped out of a second-story window that was too low to cause any serious harm. All these suicide attempts occurred during episodic psychotic reactions that were accompanied by hallucinations, delusions, and illusions. Throughout her life she had 20 such psychotic episodes, usually accompanied by severe dysphoric emotions and often by physical attacks on those who were trying to help her. These attacks were preceded by restlessness, sleeplessness, and a number of somatic symptoms, including a rapid and irregular heartbeat, dizziness, and headaches. She was usually confused during the attacks and sometimes would be mute and unresponsive.

Example 3. Edvard Munch

After an evening of heavy drinking, he and his companion returned to the rooming house where they got into a fistfight. He knocked his companion down the stairs and then returned to his room, grabbed his rifle, and shot at his friend at the foot of the stairs. Fortunately, he missed.

During the preceding 3 years he was noted for his frequent barroom brawls, usually with friends or, at least, acquaintances. He had a number of episodic disorders or dyscontrol episodes, mostly panic-phobic reactions with somatic complaints, particularly dizziness. Frequently, he treated himself by alcohol, which sometimes may have quieted the symptoms and at other times probably aggravated them. He had only one hospitalization with acute paranoid panic and hallucinatory, delusional, and illusory symptoms as well as many physical complaints, including a conversion paralysis. The acute symptoms disappeared within several weeks. He admitted himself on several other occasions to spas and sanitoriums. The symptoms at these times were vague but broadly described as nervous exhaustion. Following his one hospitalization, he gave up drinking and retired to a simple rural reclusive life, living for the next 35 years without further episodes but continuing to be creatively productive.

Example 4. Mary Lamb

While setting the dinner table for her family, she began berating her apprentice and throwing forks around the room, one of which struck her father on the head, giving him a scalp laceration. She picked up a kitchen knife and began chasing her apprentice. When her invalid mother protested, she turned on her and stabbed her in the heart, killing her instantly. At this point her brother walked into the room and took the bloody knife from her.

This was the second of 37 episodic psychotic reactions that this individual suffered. Details regarding these psychotic symptoms are sparse, but they were always associated with restlessness, agitation, and finally an attack on somebody in her environment. The earliest symptoms noted were disorganization in her thinking and rambling, disconnected speech. The acute attacks were of short duration early in her life, but became both more frequent and longer as she grew older, until, at the time of her death at age 83, she was continuously ill. It is not clear how much of this terminal illness was senility and how much was chronic residual effect of her frequent episodes.

Example 5. August Strindberg

Frustrated because his married mistress would not divorce her husband and marry him, he decided on the grand renunciation by leaving the country and booking passage on a steamship line. Before the boat was even out of the harbor, he changed his mind and bargained with the pilot to take him back to shore. On shore he decided to kill himself by dying of pneumonia, hoping that this would give his mistress time to get to his bedside. He plunged into the wintry sea and then sat shivering on the shore. To make sure of his pneumonia he then stripped and climbed a tree to expose himself to the cold winds. All of this happened after he had booked a hotel room and had a cigar and a couple of drinks of absinthe. After telegraphing his mistress, he went to bed and took a heavy dose of sedatives. The next morning she arrived at his bedside but he was in good health. The sleeping potion had given him a good night's rest, and apparently his exposure to the elements induced a ravenous appetite.

This man had numerous dyscontrol episodes, many of more primitive nature than the one described above, and five episodic psychotic reactions during one 3-year period. These were characterized by paranoid-panic with confusion, hallucinations, delusions, and some toxic illusory phenomena. Some were preceded by an absinthe spree and at other times by a frustrated love affair. On one occasion, when his mistress deserted him, he ran through the forest pounding on the trees and screaming as if they were his enemies. Another time he locked himself in his room and painted gloomy landscapes while writing to a nearby sanitorium asking for admission because he was losing his mind. However, after the years of his five blatantly psychotic episodes, he gave up his histrionic, dissolute life-style, withdrawing to a somewhat isolated existence, but continuing to produce creative works until his death 15 years later. Although he had three more mild paranoid panics during these last 15 years, they were transitory and did not require institutionalization.

All of these individuals suffered from both episodic dyscontrol and episodic psychotic reactions with circumstantial evidence of an underlying limbic ictus. There is also evidence that their episodic behavioral disorders had considerable influence on their creativity (11).

REFERENCES

1. Ervin, F. R., Epstein, A. W., and King, H. E. (1955): Behavior of epileptic and nonepileptic patients with temporal spikes. *AMA Arch. Neurol. Psychiatry*, 74:488.
2. Monroe, R. R. (1970): *Episodic Behavioral Disorders*, p. 20. Harvard University Press, Cambridge.
3. Heath, R. G. (1954): *Studies in Schizophrenia*. Harvard University Press, Cambridge.
4. Heath, R. G. (1957): Correlations of electrical recordings from cortical and subcortical regions of the brain with abnormal behavior in human subjects. *Confin. Neurol.*, 18:3–6.
5. Goddard, G. U., and Morrell, F. (1971): Chronic progressive eleptogeneses induced by focal electrical stimulation of the brain. *Neurology*, 21:393.
6. Heath, R. G., Mickle, W. A., and Monroe, R. R. (1955): Characteristic recording from various specific subcortical nuclear masses in the brains of psychiatric and non-psychiatric patients. *Trans. Am. Neurol. Assoc.*, 80:17.
7. Lessee, H., Heath, R. G., Mickle, W. A., Monroe, R. R., and Miller, W. H. (1955): Rhinencephalic activity during thought. *J. Nerv. Ment. Dis.*, 122:433.
8. Shapiro, D. (1965): *Neurotic Styles*. Basic Books, New York.
9. Abt, L. E., and Weissman, S. (1965): *Acting out: Theoretical and Clinical Aspects*. Grune & Stratton, New York.
10. Monroe, R. R. (1982): The psychotherapy of the impulsive and acting out patient. *J. Am. Acad. Psychoanal.*, 10:1–26.
11. Monroe, R. R. (1986): *Creative Brainstorms: A Study of Madness and Genius*. Irvington Publishers, New York..
12. Monroe, R. R. (1970): In *Episodic Behavioral Disorders*. Harvard Univ. Press, Cambridge.
13. Monroe, R. R. (1974): Episodic behavioral disorders: An unclassified syndrome. In: *American Handbook of Psychiatry*, edited by S. Arieti and E. B. Brody, Vol. 3, pp. 237–254. Basic Books, Inc., New York.
14. Monroe, R. R. (1982): DSM III style diagnoses of the episodic disorders. *J. Nerv. Ment. Dis.*, 170:664–669.

The Limbic System: Functional Organization and Clinical Disorders, edited by B. K. Doane and K. E. Livingston. Raven Press, New York © 1986.

Carbamazepine in the Treatment of Affective Illness

Robert M. Post and Thomas W. Uhde

Biological Psychiatry Branch, National Institute of Mental Health, Bethesda, Maryland 20205

In an earlier chapter (R. M. Post, *this volume*), we have discussed whether the limbic system might be importantly involved in affective illness. One of the points of leverage in this question focuses on whether drugs which act on limbic and other substrates are effective in manic-depressive illness. In this chapter we review the emerging data on the efficacy of carbamazepine and related anticonvulsants in secondary and primary affective illness and discuss some of the possible mechanisms of action of carbamazepine.

ANTIDEPRESSANT EFFECTS OF CARBAMAZEPINE

We conducted the first double-blind, placebo-controlled clinical trial of carbamazepine in the treatment of acute depression (3,4,38). The results of the first 37 patients studied are summarized in Fig. 1. Slightly more than one-half of the patients showed a pattern of improvement while treated with carbamazepine on a double-blind basis. Seventeen patients showed no evidence of clinical response to the active administration of the drug and, interestingly, showed no evidence of a withdrawal reaction following placebo substitution. In the 20 patients improving during carbamazepine treatment, the clinical onset of improvement appeared after a lag of approximately 1 week. Consistent with the effects of a variety of other antidepressants, improvement in the first week was statistically significant but not clinically robust until the second, third, and fourth weeks of treatment. It is also noteworthy that those patients showing the best response to carbamazepine were significantly more severely depressed at the onset of the clinical trial. They were significantly less depressed by the last week of treatment, further suggesting that improvement in these initially more ill patients did not represent regression to mean. Improvement was noted in both bipolar and unipolar depressed patients, as illustrated in Figs. 2 and 3.

Case #1. Patient #243 was a 40-year-old bipolar I depressed female with a 1.3-year history of continuous illness (predominately depressive with episodic mild hypomania) following the birth of a child. The illness did not respond to desmethylimipramine (300 mg) alone or in combination with lithium or neuroleptics prior to admission to the National

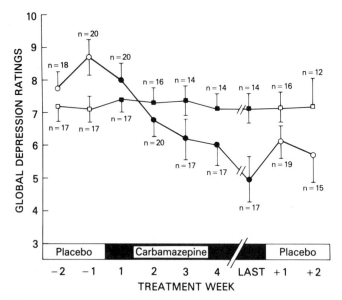

FIG. 1. Antidepressant course in moderate response to carbamazepine: *(circles)* responders; *(squares)* nonresponders.

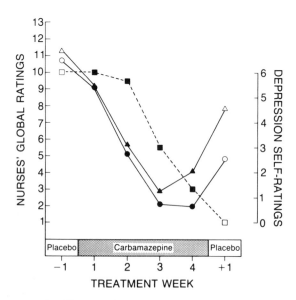

FIG. 2. Time course of antidepressant response to carbamazepine in a treatment-resistant bipolar depressed female: *(circles)* depression; *(triangles)* anxiety; *(squares)* depression (self).

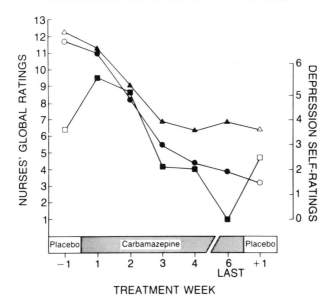

FIG. 3. Time course of antidepressant response to carbamazepine in a unipolar depressed female: *(circles)* depression; *(triangles)* anxiety; *(squares)* depression (self).

Institute of Mental Health (NIMH). She had a classical retarded depression with sleep and appetite disturbance and suicidal hopelessness about her condition and unremitting illness. Her electroencephalogram (EEG) was normal but her computerized axal tomography (CAT) scan, although read as clinically normal, showed a large ventricular-brain ratio (VBR = 11). She had marked cognitive disturbance subjectively and on the Luria-Nebraska battery. Findings from cortisols and dexamethasone suppression tests were also abnormal. She remained severely depressed (ratings less then 9) for an additional 13 weeks, but, as illustrated (Fig. 2), by the second week following blind institution of carbamazepine (initially 200 mg/day raised to 600 mg/day by week 2), she showed dramatic improvement, and by week 3 of treatment there was complete remission of symptoms (Luria-Nebraska impairments normalized during her improved state). Carbamazepine was discontinued because of mild elevations of SGOT and SGPT (bilirubin, alkaline phosphatase, and lactic dehydrogenase (LDH) values were normal). She remained well off active medications for several months, but suffered another severe depressive relapse which again did not respond to routine antidepressants. After reinstitution of carbamazepine treatment, she again showed a rapid antidepressant response.

Case 2. Patient #252 was a 49-year-old unipolar depressed patient with a history of four prior depressions and a chronic depression of 15 months' duration unresponsive to amitriptyline and trazadone. At NIMH she was markedly anxious, depressed, agitated, and somatically preoccupied, but by the second and third weeks of carbamazepine treatment, was substantially improved (Fig. 3). Only mild increases in dysphoria occurred following carbamazepine discontinuation.

When clinical response was observed, it occurred in all aspects of the depressive syndrome, including mood, psychomotor agitation and/or retardation, and in vegetative signs and symptoms. As illustrated in Fig. 4, sleep improved significantly, even by the first week of treatment with carbamazepine, as assessed by half-hourly nurses' sleep checks performed on a double-blind basis.

Carbamazepine was usually administered in doses of 600 to 1,600 mg/day (average below 1,000 mg/day), achieving blood levels between 5 to 12 μg/ml. We observed no relationship of carbamazepine levels in blood or spinal fluid to degree of clinical response, but there was preliminary evidence that the active metabolite carbamazepine-10,11-epoxide correlated with response (Fig. 5) (43). These data are consistent with those in the neurological literature, indicating a relatively poor relationship of carbamazepine levels to degree of anticonvulsant response (5).

CARBAMAZEPINE IN SECONDARY AFFECTIVE ILLNESS AND ITS ASSOCIATED DEPRESSION

Our results in primary affective illness are consistent with preliminary reports in patients with depression associated with other neuropsychiatric illnesses, including epilepsy and alcoholism. Dalby (8) reviewed the literature and indicated in more than 2,500 patients studied that reports of improvement in mood and behavior were noted in approximately 50% of the patients. Dalby's own study in 1971 is edifying in this regard. He reported improvement in the periodic depressions of 11 of 18 patients with complex partial seizures when they were treated with carbamazepine (7). A number of these patients showed improvement in mood despite inadequate seizure control, further suggesting that the psychotropic effects of

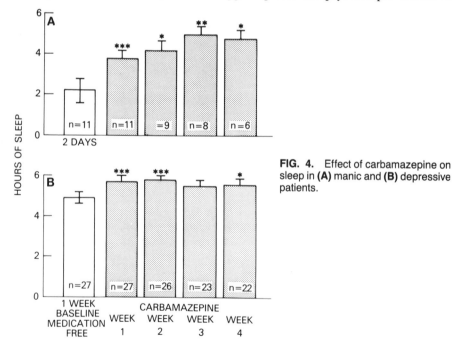

FIG. 4. Effect of carbamazepine on sleep in (A) manic and (B) depressive patients.

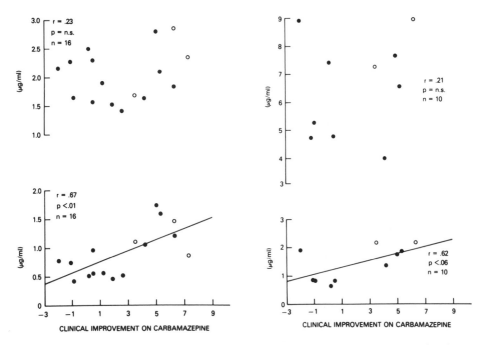

FIG. 5. Carbamazepine **(top)** concentrations in plasma *(right)* or CSF *(left)* were not related to the degree of clinical response, whereas there was a trend for the -10,11-epoxide metabolite **(bottom)** to be correlated with degree of response: (●) depressed; (○) manic.

carbamazepine in this patient population are not necessarily related to better anticonvulsant efficacy. Robertson (47) reported that patients in their epilepsy clinic who were treated with carbamazepine showed less severe depression than epileptic patients treated with other anticonvulsants. Moreover, she reported that patients' Spielberger's Trait Anxiety scores were significantly correlated in an inverse fashion with carbamazepine doses and blood levels; that is, those patients with the highest carbamazepine dose and blood levels showed the lowest levels of trait anxiety. Improvement in mood and anxiety has been reported in many other open studies in epileptic patients and in nonepileptic children treated with carbamazepine (2,9,24).

Particularly in the Scandinavian countries, carbamazepine has been used in the treatment of alcohol withdrawal symptomatology. When used for this purpose, carbamazepine also appears to have useful effects in reducing dysphoria and anxiety in this patient population (50).

ANTIMANIC EFFECTS OF CARBAMAZEPINE

Effects of carbamazepine in mania have been reported in both open and controlled clinical trials (Table 1). Takezaki and Hanaoka (52) reported improvement in a small series of manic patients while treated in an open design with carbamaz-

TABLE 1. *Studies of carbamazepine (CBZ) in acute mania*

Study	N	Diagnosis[a]	Design	Dose of carbamazepine (mg/day) (blood level)	Other drugs	Duration	Results
Takezaki and Hanaoki (52)	10	MD psychosis	Open	200–600	Neuroleptics, tricyclics in some cases	1–11 months	6/10 pts improved in days to weeks
Okuma et al. (33,34)	64	MD psychosis	Open	400–1,200	Neuroleptics	Variable	22/64 pts improved (marked to moderate)
Ballenger and Post, (3,4)	17	MD psychosis	Double blind (B-A-B-A)	600–2,000 [7–15.5]	None	11–56 days	10/17 pts improved—time course similar to neuroleptics
Okuma et al. (32)	32 CBZ 28 chlorpromazine	MD psychosis ICD-9	Double blind comparison w/ chlorpromazine 150–450 mg	300–900 [2.7–11.7 µg/ml] [mean = 7.2 ± 3.4]	Bedtime hypnotics	3–5 weeks	21/32 pts improved on CBZ (marked to moderate) 15/28 pts improved on chlorpromazine
Inoue et al. (18)	5	BP disorder	Open	400–800	Lithium, neuroleptics, tricyclics	Variable	3/5 pts improved
Folks et al. (14)	10	4 BP 3 SA 3 Organic affective	Open	600–1,600	Concomitant medications in 6/10 pts	—	8/10 pts improved—CBZ

Study	n	Diagnosis	Design	CBZ dose [level]	Others	Duration	Results
Kwamie et al. (22)	12	MD	Open	Not specified [8.5–9.5 µg/ml]	Lithium and neuroleptics	Variable	5/12 pts improved
Lipinski and Pope (25)	3	2 BP manic 1 Other[b]	Open; lithium discontinuation	—		—	3/3 pts improved, but all relapsed on lithium discontinuation, suggesting combination needed
Moss and James (27)	1	Major affective disorder, Manic	Open	600–800 [4.5 ± 5.7 µg/ml]	Lithium	—	0/1 pt partial response only; pt improved but relapsed on combination of CBZ + lithium
Yassa (54)	1	MD	Open	600 [8 µg/ml]	Chlorpromazine	26 months	1/1 pt improved
Emrich et al. (10)	6	Maniform psychoses	Double blind	1,800–2,100 OXCBZ	Not stated	Variable	5/6 pts (>25% improvement on IMPS)
Keisling (19)	3	1 SA 1 BP 1 Mania	Open	600–1,400	Lithium (all), tricyclics in one case	2–3 months	3/3 pts improved in combination with lithium
Klein et al. (21)	11	Excited mania or 3 excited SA	Blind	600–1,600 [6–18 µg/ml]	Haloperidol (15–45 mg/day) all patients	5 weeks	10/14 pts improved on CBZ + haloperidol (7/13 pts improved on placebo + halo.)

(continued)

TABLE 1. (continued)

Study	N	Diagnosis[a]	Design	Dose of carbamazepine (mg/day) (blood level) OXCBZ	Other drugs	Duration	Results
Muller and Stoll (28)	48	MD	Open	2.1–3.06 mg/day OXCBZ	Lithium and neuroleptics (7); hypnotics (28)	10–36 days (39 days)	40/48 pt on CBZ > placebo, blind (12) OXCBZ = haloperidol (20)
Sethi and Tawari (49)	5	MD	Open	600–1,600 mg	?	28 days	5/5 pts on CBZ were better than those on chlorpromazine
Grossi et al. (17)	15	MD	Blind vs CPZ randomized	200–1,200 mg	—	21 days	10/15 pts on CBZ had fewer side effects than those on chlorpromazine
Lerer et al. (23)	8	MD	Blind vs lithium randomized		—	21 days	1/8 pts on lithium; trend ($p < .06$) better at 4 weeks
Total	17 Studies		6 Blind		—		153/254 pts (60%) had moderate-marked improvement

[a](MD) manic-depressive; (BP) bipolar; (SA) secondary affective; (OXCBZ) oxcarbazepine.
[b]Hexosaminidase A deficient.

epine. Okuma et al. (34) reported substantial antimanic effects of carbamazepine when added to previously ineffective agents in an open fashion.

In 1978 we reported, in double-blind, placebo-controlled trials, that carbamazepine appeared to have useful acute antimanic effects in lithium-resistant patients (3,4,38). These responses were documented by repeated administration and discontinuation of the drug in an off-on-off-on design. An example of such a clinical response is illustrated in Fig. 6. This patient was a 46-year-old male who had rapid onset of severe manic psychosis while observed during placebo administration. He was extremely disorganized, apparently demonstrating visual hallucinations, and had to be maintained in seclusion during much of the time period. Soon after beginning carbamazepine on a blind basis, improvement in both manic and psychotic components of his illness was observed. However, following dose reduction and placebo substitution, the entire manic syndrome rapidly re-emerged, again necessitating maintenance of the patient in seclusion. With readministration of carbamazepine, improvement was again noted. Some residual psychotic symptomatology remained during this second clinical trial with carbamazepine, such that supplemental treatment with a neuroleptic was begun, leading to further clinical improvement. This observation is of some clinical and theoretical interest, since carbamazepine appears to act by mechanisms other than blockade of dopamine receptors (38,42,45), which is thought to be the primary mode of action of the neuroleptics. This differential mechanism of action of carbamazepine and classical neuroleptics may provide a theoretical rationale for the use of these two classes of agents in combination in some patients who are inadequately treated with either agent alone.

The time course of antimanic effects of carbamazepine in the first 12 patients studied is illustrated in Fig. 7. In similarly diagnosed manic patients [*Research*

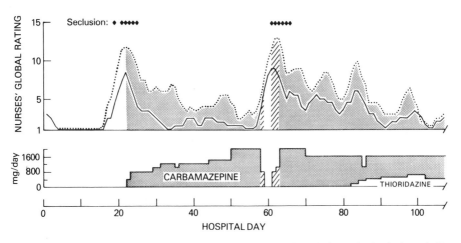

FIG. 6. Therapeutic effect of carbamazepine in a manic patient: (···) psychosis; (—) mania (3-day running means).

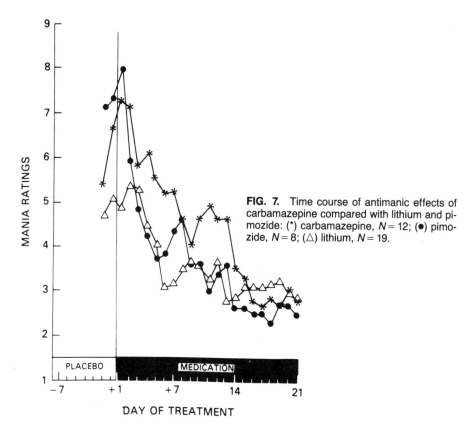

FIG. 7. Time course of antimanic effects of carbamazepine compared with lithium and pimozide: (*) carbamazepine, $N = 12$; (●) pimozide, $N = 8$; (△) lithium, $N = 19$.

Diagnostic Criteria (RDC) (51a) and DSMIII[1]], and utilizing the same rating instruments by our nursing staff who were blind to when and which medications were employed, we observed a roughly parallel time course of antimanic effects compared with neuroleptics such as chlorpromazine or thioridazine or the more pure dopamine receptor blocking agent pimozide. Although other patients were started on lithium carbonate when less severely ill, by weeks 2 and 3, patients did not differ in their mania ratings while treated with either carbamazepine, neuroleptics, or lithium carbonate. Studies using randomized assignment of manic patients to carbamazepine and lithium (and/or a crossover design) would be of considerable importance, particularly in addressing the question about differential responsivity to lithium and carbamazepine.

Okuma et al. (32) followed up on their earlier uncontrolled studies with a double-blind comparison with chlorpromazine, also finding that carbamazepine had equal acute antimanic effects and produced fewer side effects such as sedation compared with chlorpromazine. The other acute studies are summarized in Table 1, and in

---

[1](DSMIII) *Diagnostic and Statistical Manual of Mental Disorders*, 3rd. ed. American Psychiatric Association, Washington, D.C.

both controlled and uncontrolled clinical trials, similar evidence of acute efficacy continues to be reported in 153 of 254 patients (60%).

PROPHYLAXIS

Clinical trials of long-term treatment with carbamazepine are summarized in Table 2. Although our study (4,44) and that of Okuma et al. (32) had been conducted on a double-blind basis, the results of these investigations are similar to those observed in the open clinical trials. In more than 240 patients reported to date, 160, or approximately 67%, have shown substantial improvement on carbamazepine. These rates of improvement are of some considerable significance in light of the fact that most of these patients were unresponsive or inadequately responsive to lithium carbonate. In most of the cases reported, carbamazepine was added onto previously existing treatment regimens. Thus, the overall rate and degree of carbamazepine prophylaxis as a single agent remain to be determined. However, some trials using carbamazepine as the single treatment agent have shown parallel results (31,39).

Moreover, since most patients entered into carbamazepine clinical trials have previously been lithium resistant, it is not known whether or not there is overlap in the responders to lithium and carbamazepine or whether responders to these two agents form rather distinct subgroups. Randomized clinical trials and crossover designs should prove useful in this regard. These findings will be not only of substantial clinical import, but of considerable theoretical interest in suggesting that differential biochemical and physiological mechanisms may underlie the illness in these two populations.

Emrich et al. (12) reported that a small group of patients with lithium-unresponsive manic-depressive illness showed considerable clinical benefit when valproic acid was added on a maintenance basis to their treatment regime. A combination of lithium and valproic acid appeared to be necessary, since several of these patients relapsed when lithium carbonate was discontinued (11). Lipinski and associates (*personal communication*, 1983) observed several patients who seemed to be differentially responsive to carbamazepine and valproic acid. Our first patient to complete a double-blind, placebo crossover to several anticonvulsants was a clearcut responder to carbamazepine on several occasions but unresponsive to valproic acid and phenytoin (39).

It is also of some interest that Chouinard (6) reported that the anticonvulsant clonazepam was effective in treatment of mania, although results of prophylactic clinical trials have not been reported. Clonazepam has also been shown to be a useful anticonvulsant in the treatment of complex partial seizures (26,37). Rather extensive clinical trials would be required to discern whether anticonvulsants with a differential clinical and experimental spectrum of anticonvulsant efficacy on limbic system structures or complex partial seizures would be more effective in manic-depressive illness than those without this clinical profile.

Once the appropriate clinical trials are performed, the interpretation of these data may still be difficult for several reasons. There appears to be some divergence

TABLE 2. *Prophylaxis in manic-depressive illness*

Study	N	Diagnosis[a]	Design	Dose of carbamazepine (mg/day) (blood level)	Other drugs	Duration	Results
Takezaki and Hanaoki (52)	10	MD	Open	200–600	Neuroleptics, tricyclics in some cases	1–11 months	9/10 pts improved
Okuma et al. (33,34)	51	MD	Open	400–1,200	Neuroleptics, lithium, tricyclics	~25 Weeks	34/51 pts improved
Ballenger and Post (4) Post et al. (44)	7	6 MD 1 Confusional psychosis	4 Blind, 3 open	800–2,000 (11.3 µg/ml)	None for 3 patients	6–51 months	6/7 pts improved, esp. lithium nonresponsive cyclers
Okuma et al. (31)	12 CBZ 10 Placebo	MD	CBZ vs. placebo Blind Random assign	400–600 (5.6 ± 2.0 µg/ml)	Acute treatments added during episode breakthroughs	12 Months either Rx	6/10 pts improved on CBZ; 2/9 pts improved on placebo
Inoue et al. (18)	3	MD	Open	400–600	Lithium	18–32 Months	2/3 pts improved
Kwamie et al. (22)	12	MD	Open	—	Others	—	5/12 pts improved (lithium resistant)
Lipinski and Pope (25)	3	2 MD 1 Other[b]	Open	Not specified (8.5–9.5 µg/ml)	Lithium and neuroleptics in one case	3–8 Months	3/3 pts improved, but relapsed on lithium discontinuation—combination necessary?
Yassa (54)	1	MD	Open	600 (8 µg/ml)	Chlorpromazine, decreasing doses from 1,700 mg/day	26 Months	1/1 pt improved

Study	N	Diagnosis	Design	Dose/level	Prior/concomitant medications	Duration	Results
Keisling (19)	3	1 SA 1 BP 1 Manic	Open	600–1,400 (8–9 µg/ml)	Lithium (all), 1 tricyclic	2–8 Months	3/3 pts improved on lithium combination
Kishimoto (20) 1984	32 55	MD	Open	100–1,200 (6–10 µg/ml)	Lithium and others	2–11 yrs $\overline{X}$ = 48.8 months	24/32 pts improved, esp. early onset 43/55 pts and continuous cyclers
Nolen (30)	8	MD	Open	400 (6–12 µg/ml)	Lithium, neuroleptics, antidepressants	6–36 Months	4/8 pts improved (all lithium resistant)
Fawcett and Kravits (13)	34	MD	Open	$\overline{X}$ = 800 (7.4 ± 2.6 µg/ml)	Lithium, antidepressants	4 Months–10 years 54 Months average	22/34 pts improved—17 CBZ alone
Gastpar and Kielholz (15)	13	MD 4 SA 1 UP	Open	200–1,000 $\overline{X}$ = 520	Lithium, neuroleptics, antidepressants	$\overline{X}$ = 14 Months	6/13 pts; 3 SAs relapsed on D/C 9/13 pts lithium resistant (4/19 pts OK CBZ)
Greil et al. (16)	13	MD	Open	600–1,200 (5.5–22 µg/ml)	Lithium	11–15 Months	3/13 pts (1 of 9 on OXCBZ responded)
Placidi et al. (36)	7 8	MD SA	Blind vs lithium random	800–1,600 (7–12 µg/ml)	None	2–92 Months	11/15 pts vs 7/14 on lithium at 2 months 10/15 pts vs 9/14 improved by relapse criteria
Nelson (29)	1	MD	Open	400 (6.8–8 µg/ml)	None	21 Months	1/1 pt improved

[a](MD) manic-depressive; (CBZ) carbamazepine; (OXCBZ) oxcarbazepine; (D/C) discontinued; (SA) secondary affective; (BP) bipolar; (UP) unipolar.
[b]Hexosaminidase A deficient: 160/240, 67%.

in the clinical use of anticonvulsants for complex partial seizures and their rank order of efficacy in experimental models such as that of Albright & Burnham (1). In these investigators' study, they found that carbamazepine followed by valproic acid was the most effective combination agents in inhibiting amygdala-kindled afterdischarges compared with those kindled from the cortex. Clonazepam and phenytoin were intermediate. However, phenytoin and clonazepam are better accepted for their use in patients with complex partial seizures than is valproic acid. In addition, many of the agents that are effective in complex partial seizures are also highly effective in the treatment of generalized seizures (37).

Thus, although a distinction may be easily made among the anticonvulsants that are useful in either complex partial or major generalized seizures compared with those effective only in petit mal, the strategy of using the relative psychotropic efficacy of anticonvulsants to indirectly establish a relationship to area of brain involved may be flawed.

A further complication derives from our recent work on the effects of carbamazepine on the development of amygdala kindling in the rat. In this species, in contrast to the cat and monkey (53), it appears as though doses of carbamazepine that are effective in inhibiting completed kindled seizures do not inhibit the development of kindling (40). These data are also consistent with those of Pinel (35) who reported that agents effective in the completed phase of kindling were not effective in spontaneous kindled seizures and vice versa. For example, they observed that phenytoin was not particularly effective in inhibiting completed amygdala-kindled seizures, whereas it appeared to be a highly effective agent in aborting the spontaneous type. In contrast, diazepam was effective on amygdala-kindled seizures but not on the spontaneous variety. Thus, it would appear that there is substantial difference in the pharmacological responsivity, depending on the longitudinal development of amygdala kindling. Pharmacological manipulations that are effective against completed kindled seizures are not necessarily effective in their development or on the spontaneous type.

Although the data are still inadequate, they are highly suggestive that a similar case may hold for the psychopharmacology of manic-depressive illness where some drugs appear to be effective in one stage but not in another stage of the illness. This principle is most clearly established in parkinsonian patients, where levodopa may initially be adequate to control motor symptoms, but as the illness progresses, a direct dopamine agonist may also be required. Thus, in addition to the possibility that there are different subgroups of lithium and carbamazepine responders, it is also possible that patients may differ in their pharmacological responsivity to these two agents according to their phase of the illness.

There is some preliminary support for this suggestion in that many of our most responsive patients were extremely rapidly cycling patients (41), and Kishimoto (20) recently reported that continuously cycling patients appeared to be most responsive in his series as well. Although a small portion of manic-depressive patients begin to rapid-cycle from the onset of the illness, it is more characteristic for them to develop this at a later stage in the evolution of their illness (48,51). As such, it might suggest that carbamazepine might be more effective in this relatively later and/or more malignant stage of manic-depressive cycling.

The lack of ability of carbamazepine to inhibit the development of amygdala kindling in the rat (38), although it is effective in the cat and monkey (53), raises questions about species differences as well as the possible relevance of this model for manic-depressive illness. Elsewhere we have noted many parallels between the characteristics observed in amygdala kindling and in the development of affective illness (40). In the latter, there are often suggestions of repeated stimuli which are initially inadequate to precipitate the full-blown episodes which, on sufficient repetition, lead to the development of major (affective) episodes. These then recur in a highly reproducible fashion and may ultimately show spontaneity, that is, episodes occur in a regular or rapid-cycling pattern apparently divorced from psychosocial precipitants. Although we did not suggest that there was any parallel in symptomatology or phenomenology between affective episodes and kindled seizures, we thought the temporal and developmental parallels were noteworthy. Moreover, the comparative pharmacology of these processes is of interest.

Preliminary data suggest that the two drugs that now appear to be most useful in the long-term treatment of recurrent bipolar affective illness (lithium and car-bamazepine) have differential effects on animal models of sensitization and kindling (46). Lithium may be effective in blocking behavioral sensitization to psychomotor stimulants, but is ineffective in blocking the development of kindling or in inhibiting completed kindled seizures. In contrast, carbamazepine is a potent anticonvulsant, but does not block stimulant-induced behavior, either acutely or during repeated administration (sensitization).

Thus, if lithium and carbamazepine responders are found to form distinct patient subgroups, the differences in the ability of these drugs to block sensitization and kindling may be of mechanistic interest. Carbamazepine and lithium also differ in many of their biochemical effects (38,45). Comparison and contrast of their be-havioral, physiological, and biochemical effects may help to identify which mech-anisms are important to their therapeutic efficacy in affective illness.

REFERENCES

1. Albright, P. S., and Burnham, W. M. (1980): Development of a new pharmacological seizure model: effects of anticonvulsants on cortical- and amygdala-kindled seizures in the rat. *Epilepsia*, 21:681–689.
2. Arieff, A. J., and Mier, M. (1964): Anticonvulsant and psychotropic action of Tegretol. *Neurology*, 16:107–110.
3. Ballenger, J. C., and Post, R. M. (1980): Carbamazepine (Tegretol) in manic-depressive illness: a new treatment. *Am. J. Psychiatry*, 137:782–790.
4. Ballenger, J. C., and Post, R. M. (1978): Therapeutic effects of carbamazepine in affective illness: a preliminary report. *Commun. Psychopharmacol.*, 2:159–178.
5. Bertilsson, L. (1978): Clinical pharmacokinetics of carbamazepine. *Clin. Pharmacokinet.*, 3:128–143.
6. Chouinard, G., Young, S. N., and Annable, L. (1983): Antimanic effect of clonazepam. *Biol. Psychiatry*, 18:451–466.
7. Dalby, M. A. (1971): Antiepileptic and psychotropic effect of carbamazepine (Tegretol) in the treatment of pscychomotor epilepsy. *Epilepsia*, 12:325–334.

8. Dalby, M. A. (1975): Behavioral effects of carbamazepine. In: *Complex Partial Seizures and Their Treatment*, edited by J. K. Penry and D. D. Daly, pp. 331–343. Raven Press, New York.

9. Donner, M., and Frisk, M. (1965): Carbamazepine treatment of epileptic and psychic symptoms in children. *Ann. Paediat. Fenn.*, 11:91–97.

10. Emrich, H. M., Altmann, H., Dose, M., and von Zerssen, D. (1983): Therapeutic effects of GABA-ergic drugs in affective disorders. a preliminary report. *Pharmacol. Biochem. Behav.*, 19:369–372.

11. Emrich, H. M., von Zerssen, D., Kissling, W., and Moller, H. J. (1982): Antimanic action of propranolol and of sodium valproate. Presented at 13th CINP Congress, Tel Aviv, June 1982.

12. Emrich, H. M., von Zerssen, D., Kissling, W., Moller, H. J., and Windorfer, A. (1980): Effect of sodium valproate in mania. The GABA-hypothesis of affective disorders. *Arch. Psychiatr. Nervenkr.*, 229:1–16.

13. Fawcett, J., and Kravitz, D. O. (1985): The long-term management of bipolar disorders with lithium, carbamazepine, and antidepressants: clinical experience with 90 cases. *J. Clin. Psychiatry*, 46:58–60.

14. Folks, D. G., King, L. D., Dowdy, S. B., Petrie, W. M., Jack, R. A., Koomen, J. C., Swenson, B. R., and Edwards, P. (1982): Carbamazepine treatment of selected affectively disordered inpatients. *Am. J. Psychiatry*, 139:115–117.

15. Gastpar, M., and Kielholz, P. (1984): Carbamazepine treatment in therapy-resistant patients with manic-depressive psychoses. In: *Anticonvulsants in Affective Disorders*, edited by H. M. Emrich, T. Okuma, and A. A. Muller, pp. 148–152. Excerpta Medica, Amsterdam.

16. Greil, W., Kruger, R., Rossnagl, G., Schertel, M., and Walther, A. (1984): Prophylactic therapy of affective disorders with carbamazepine: an open clinical trial. In: *Anticonvulsants in Affective Disorders*, edited by H. M. Emrich, T. Okuma, and A. A. Muller, pp. 153–159. Excerpta Medica, Amsterdam.

17. Grossi, E., Sacchetti, E., Vita, A., Conte, G., Faravelli, C., Hautman, G., Zerbi, D., Mesina, A. M., Drago, F., and Motta, A. (1984): Carbamazepine vs. chlorpromazine in mania: a double-blind trial. In: *Anticonvulsants in Affective Disorders*, edited by H. M. Emrich, T. Okuma and A. A. Muller, pp. 177–187. Excerpta Medica, Amsterdam.

18. Inoue, K., Arima, J., Tanaka, K., Fukui, Y., and Kato, N. (1981): A lithium and carbamazepine combination in the treatment of bipolar disorder—a preliminary report. *Fol. Psychiatr. Neurol. Jpn.*, 35:465–475.

19. Keisling, R. (1983): Carbamazepine and lithium carbonate in the treatment of refractory affective disorders. *Arch. Gen. Psychiatry*, 40:223.

20. Kishimoto, A., Ogura, C., Hazama, H., and Inoue, K. (1983): Long-term prophylactic effects of carbamazepine in affective disorder. *Br. J. Psychiatry*, 143:327–331.

20a. Kishimoto, A. (1984): A follow-up prophylactic study of carbamazepine in affective disorders. In: *Anticonvulsants in Affective Disorders*, edited by H. M. Emrich, T. Okuma, and A. A. Muller, pp. 88–92. Excerpta Medica, Amsterdam.

21. Klein, E., Bental, E., Lerer, B., and Belmaker, R. H. (1984): Carbamazepine and haloperidol v. placebo and haloperidol in excited psychosis. *Arch. Gen. Psychiatry*, 41:165–170.

22. Kwamie, Y., Persad, E., and Stancer, H. C. (1982): The use of carbamazepine in the management of affective disorders. Presented at University of Toronto, Dept. of Psychiatry, Research Day, 1982.

23. Lerer, B., Moore, N., Meyendorff, E., Cho, S-R., and Gershon, S. (1985): Carbamazepine and lithium: different profiles in affective disorder? *Psychopharmacol. Bull.*, 21:18–22.

24. Lerman, P., and Kivity-Ephraim, S. (1974): Carbamazepine sole anticonvulsant for focal epilepsy of childhood. *Epilepsia*, 15:229–234.

25. Lipinski, J. F., and Pope, H. G., Jr. (1982): Possible synergistic action between carbamazepine and lithium carbonate in the treatment of three acutely manic patients. *Am. J. Psychiatry*, 139:948–949.

26. Mikkelsen, B., Berggreen, P., Joensen, P., Kristensen, O., Kohler, O., and Mikkelsen, B. O. (1981): Clonazepam (Rivotril) and carbamazepine (Tegretol) in psychomotor epilepsy: a randomized multicenter trial. *Epilepsia*, 22:415–420.

27. Moss, G. R., and James, C. R. (1983): Carbamazepine and lithium carbonate synergism in mania. *Arch. Gen. Psychiatry*, 40:588–589.

28. Muller, A. A., and Stoll, K.-D. (1984): Carbamazepine and oxcarbazepine in the treatment of

manic syndromes: studies in Germany. In: *Anticonvulsants in Affective Disorders*, edited by H. M. Emrich, T. Okuma, and A. A. Muller, pp. 139–147. Excerpta Medica, Amsterdam.

29. Nelson, H. B. (1984): Cost effectiveness of carbamazepine in refractory bipolar illness (letter). *Am. J. Psychiatry*, 41:465.
30. Nolen, W. A. (1983): Carbamazepine, a possible adjunct to or alternative for lithium in bipolar disorder. *Acta Psychiatr. Scand.*, 67:218–225.
31. Okuma, T., Inanaga, K., Otsuki, S., Sarai, K., Takahashi, R., Hazama, H., Mori, A., and Watanabe, M. (1981): A preliminary double-blind study of the efficacy of carbamazepine in prophylaxis of manic-depressive illness. *Psychopharmacology*, 73:95–96.
32. Okuma, T., Inanaga, K., Otsuki, S., Sarai, K., Takahashi, R., Hazama, H., Mori, A., and Watanabe, M. (1979): Comparison of the antimanic efficacy of carbamazepine and chlorpromazine: a double-blind controlled study. *Psychopharmacology*, 66:211–217.
33. Okuma, T., Kishimoto, A., and Inoue, K. (1975): Anti-manic and prophylactic effects of carbamazepine (Tegretol) on manic-depressive psychosis. (in Japanese) *Seishin-igaku*, 17:617–630.
34. Okuma, T., Kishimoto, A., Inoue, K., Matsumoto, H., Ogura, A., Matsushita, T., Naklao, T., and Ogura, A. (1973): Anti-manic and prophylactic effects of carbamazepine on manic-depressive psychosis. *Folia Psychiatr. Neurol. Jpn.*, 27:283–297.
35. Pinel, J. P. (1983): Effects of diazepam and diphenylhydantoin on elicited and spontaneous seizures in kindled rats: a double dissociation. *Pharmacol. Biochem. Behav.*, 18:61–63.
36. Placidi, G. F., Lenzi, A., Rampello, E., Andreani, M. F., Cassano, G. B., and Grossi, E. (1984): Long-term double-blind prospective study on carbamazepine versus lithium in bipolar and schizo-affective disorders: preliminary results. In: *Anticonvulsants in Affective Disorders*, edited by H. M. Emrich, T. Okuma, and A. A. Muller, pp. 188–197. Excerpta Medica, Amsterdam.
37. Porter, R. J., and Penry, J. K. (1978): Efficacy and choice of antiepileptic drugs. In: *Advances in Epileptology, 1977: Psychology, Pharmacotherapy, and New Diagnostic Approaches*, edited by H. Meinardi and A. J. Rowan, pp. 220–230. Swets & Zeitlinger, Amsterdam.
38. Post, R. M. Ballenger, J. C., Uhde, T. W., and Bunney, W. E., Jr. (1984): Efficacy of carbamazepine in manic-depressive illness: implications for underlying mechanisms. In: *Neurobiology of Mood Disorders*, edited by R. M. Post, and J. C. Ballenger, pp. 777–816. Williams & Wilkins, Baltimore.
39. Post, R. M. Berrettini, W., Uhde, T. W., and Kellner, C. (1984): Selective response to the anticonvulsant carbamazepine in manic-depressive illness: a case study. *J. Clin. Psychopharmacol.*, 4:178–185.
40. Post, R. M., Rubinow, D. R., and Ballenger, J. C. (1984): Conditioning, sensitization, and kindling: implications for the course of affective illness. In: *Neurobiology of Mood Disorders*, edited by R. M. Post, and J. C. Ballenger, pp. 432–466. Williams & Wilkins, Baltimore.
41. Post, R. M., and Uhde, T. W. (1985): Carbamazepine as a treatment for refractory depressive illness and rapidly cycling manic-depressive illness. In: *Special Treatments for Resistant Depression*, edited by J. Zohar, and R. H. Belmaker. Spectrum Press, New York. (*In press.*)
42. Post, R. M., Uhde, T. W., Ballenger, J. C., and Bunney, W. E., Jr. (1982): Carbamazepine, temporal lobe epilepsy, and manic-depressive illness. In: *Advances in Biological Psychiatry, Vol. 8: Temporal Lobe Epilepsy, Mania, and Schizophrenia and the Limbic System*, edited by W. P. Koella, and M. R. Trimble, pp. 117–156. S. Karger, Basel.
43. Post, R. M., Uhde, T. W., Ballenger, J. C., Chatterji, D. C., Green, R. F., and Bunney, W. E., Jr. (1983): Carbamazepine and its -10,11-epoxide metabolite in plasma and CSF: relationship to antidepressant response. *Arch. Gen. Psychiatry*, 40:673–676.
44. Post, R. M., Uhde, T. W., Ballenger, J. C., and Squillace, K. M. (1983): Prophylactic efficacy of carbamazepine in manic-depressive illness. *Am. J. Psychiatry*, 140:1602–1604.
45. Post, R. M., Uhde, T. W., Rubinow, D. R., Ballenger, J. C., and Gold, P. W. (1983): Biochemical effects of carbamazepine: relationship to its mechanisms of action in affective illness. *Prog. Neuropsychopharmacol. Biol. Psychiatry*, 7:263–271.
46. Post, R. M., Weiss, S. R. B., and Pert, A. (1984): Differential effects of carbamazepine and lithium on sensitization and kindling. *Prog. Neuropsychopharmacol. Biol. Psychiatry*, 8:425–434.
47. Robertson, M., and Trimble, M. R. (1983): Depressive illness in patients with epilepsy. A review. *Epilepsia*, 24(Suppl. 2):S109–S116.
48. Roy-Byrne, P. P., Post, R. M., Uhde, T. W., Porcu, D., Davis, D. (1985): The longitudinal course

of recurrent affective illness: Life chart data from research patients at the N.I.M.H. *Acta Psychiat. Scand.*, 71[Suppl. 317]:5–34.

49. Sethi, B. B., and Tiwari, S. C. (1984): Carbamazepine in affective disorders. In: *Anticonvulsants in Affective Disorders*, edited by H. M. Emrich, T. Okuma, and A. A. Muller, pp. 167–176. Excerpta Medica, Amsterdam.

50. Sillanpaa, M. (1981): Carbamazepine—pharmacology and clinical uses. *Acta Neurol. Scand., 64:[Suppl. 88]1–202.*

51. Squillace, K. M., Post, R. M., Savard, R., and Erwin, M. (1984): Life charting of the longitudinal course of affective illness. In: *Neurobiology of Mood Disorders*, edited by R. M. Post and J. C. Ballenger, pp. 38–59. Williams & Wilkins, Baltimore.

51a. Spitzer, R., Endicott, J., and Robins, E. (1975): *Research Diagnostic Criteria*. New York State Department of Mental Hygiene, New York.

52. Takezaki, H., and Hanaoka, M. (1971): The use of carbamazepine (Tegretol) in the control of manic-depressive psychosis and other manic, depressive states. *Clin. Psychiatry*, 13:173–183.

53. Wada, J. A. (1977): Pharmacological prophylaxis in the kindling model of epilepsy. *Arch. Neurol.*, 34:389–395.

54. Yassa, R. (1982): Carbamazepine: an alternative to lithium therapy? *Psychiatr. J. Univ. Ottawa*, 7:252–253.

The Limbic System: Functional Organization and Clinical Disorders, edited by B. K. Doane and K. E. Livingston. Raven Press, New York © 1986.

Clinical Psychiatry and the Physiodynamics of the Limbic System

Benjamin K. Doane

Department of Psychiatry, Dalhousie University, Halifax, Nova Scotia, Canada

HISTORICAL OVERVIEW

Before the psychopharmacological revolution of the 1950s, clinical psychiatry was clearly dominated by psychodynamic and psychosocial theory. The practice of psychiatry was evolving along lines that ran dangerously away from biological medicine. Psychiatrists who adhered to psychodynamic tradition could justify their alienation from the mainstream of medicine on grounds that so little from the realms of anatomy, physiology, or biochemistry was found to be applicable to treatment of the problems of human personality or behavior. A smaller number of biologically oriented psychiatrists, on the other hand, were disquieted by problems in the validation of concepts in psychodynamic theory and believed in the uppermost importance of organic mechanisms underlying major psychiatric illnesses.

A little more than a decade ago, Livingston and Escobar (88) anticipated further advances in overcoming "the crushing burden of otherwise intractable psychiatric illness" through the application of improved surgical techniques. Whereas recent psychiatric history records a decline in the use of surgical procedures for illnesses that are considered to be primarily psychiatric (so-called "psychosurgery"), progress in the field of psychopharmacology has accelerated. This, in itself, substantiates the premise on which the prediction of Livingston and Escobar was based, namely, that physiological brain mechanisms would become increasingly important in the development of psychiatric treatments.

It is predictable that as information about behavioral organization in the brain increases, our capacity to understand, properly classify, and treat abnormal patterns of behavior ("mental illness") will increase. Other papers within this volume signify important developments in our understanding of the human brain as the organ of behavior underlying psychiatric illness. Within the brain, the limbic system is no longer of minor relevance to major psychiatric disorders. Rather, it is evident that the structures comprising the limbic system, along with their connections with neocortex and the rest of the brain, will assume a position of primary importance in future psychiatric theory and practice. One may predict that much of what is useful in psychodynamics will have to accommodate to the physiodynamics of the limbic system.

285

A recurrent theme throughout this volume has been relationships; those between functional units within the limbic system as well as between limbic components and other brain areas. Kenneth Livingston believed firmly in "the limbic system concept," and he referred to "the great enigma—how do the pieces fit together to create a performing whole?" (86). While we move toward the resolution of that enigma, we must avoid the temptation to oversimplify the very apparent complexities and diversities that the limbic system displays, both structurally and functionally. Over the years, differing and changing views have been expressed as to what should be included in the "limbic system" and of the correspondence of that "system" with similar anatomical groupings which, in the past, have been called by different names (73,87,88,92–94,121,128,172,188,189).

Paul Yakovlev (188) recalled (to K. Livingston) that when he had discussed with Papez [whose famous paper in 1937 was entitled, "A Proposed Mechanism of Emotion" (128)] his own ideas of a tripartite division of the central nervous system including an "intermediate system of expression" which functionally resembles current concepts of the limbic system, "emotion" was something that, curiously, could hardly be discussed. Yakovlev said, "I was intrigued by the din and babble on 'emotions' in psychiatry in the 1930's and 1940's, but didn't quite know how to deal with 'emotion' myself without provoking virulent emotions in some of my otherwise genial friends at that time" (189). Yet, he could predict accurately the direction that would be followed, as he said, "From the impact and shock of contradiction, new truths will eventually emerge. Thus the evolving concepts we have nurtured and shared together, may last a long time" (189). It is regrettable that Yakovlev's age and health would not allow him to participate in the symposium upon which this book is based,[1] for we have come a long way since those days which he recalled, and we now deal more readily with emotional behavior and its organic substrates.

Psychiatry's involvement with the neurosciences is increasing rapidly, and there is renewed interest in the concept of neuropsychiatry while, in an allied field, something closely related which is called behavioral neurology is emerging. As new technologies and data further clarify the basis of brain function in psychiatry (especially limbic system dysfunction), the gap between psychiatry and neurology should close. There should be fewer failed consultations requested by psychiatrists or neurologists of each other, wherein problems cannot be properly identified either by the party requesting or answering the consultation. Neuropsychiatric problems will be dealt with more effectively by the two disciplines. In keeping with K. Livingston's prediction (86), the limbic system is providing "bridges that link brain, mind and behaviour in a functional continuum."

When history recognizes the principal shapers of thought leading to the physiodynamics of the limbic system and its relevance to psychiatry, the name of Paul MacLean, who introduced the term "limbic system" (93), will be preeminent. The importance of the relationships between brain evolution and behavior which he has

---

[1]Paul Yakovlev died in October, 1983.

shown should not be underestimated (48). Perhaps MacLean's (94) concept of the "triune brain" may achieve a position of significance among psychiatric concepts equal to that which has been held by Freud's historical concepts of personality structure.

It has been recognized for some time that a number of behavioral parameters, including affect or mood, learning and memory, specific drive-related activities such as sexual behavior, as well as some control of visceral functions, are altered by what Koella has termed "limbic pathoneurophysiology" (82). Experimental work on humans as well as on animals has demonstrated a complexity of interactions within the limbic system which renders the interpretation of some earlier experiments difficult or confusing, e.g., those in which lesions or ablations have involved more than the target structures. There are complex interactions between structures and multiple functions within definable anatomical parts, and many patterns of behavior depend on multiple intact structures for their full functional integrity.

These complexities and, at times, apparently conflicting experimental results have made the data from limbic system research less compelling for everyday clinical psychiatry than would have been the case if the evidence were simpler or more "straightforward." In addition, in the psychotherapeutic interaction, a patient's capacity for introspection into limbic function is poor. Activity controlled by the limbic system may seem largely "irrational" and often is not perceived within one's self in ways that are easily understood or communicated in verbal language. These observations do not detract, however, from the reality of limbic determinism in human psychic functions and psychiatric disorders.

Psychiatry has yet to grasp the full significance of MacLean's elucidation of the relevance of brain evolution to human behavior. As Angevine (7) noted, "We should have a better insight into 'the brain of a snake', 'the appetite of a bird'—and we just might reach a better understanding of ourselves." Similarly, Heimer (66) observed that quantitative studies of interspecific differences in brain areas such as the olfactory system and its connections can be of crucial importance in understanding the functional organization of major brain systems involved in a variety of complex functions, including memory, eating, reproductive behavior, and emotional reactions, to mention just a few. The significance of evolution and the hierarchies of behavioral control within the central nervous system as related to psychiatric illness have been stressed earlier in the chapter by R. M. Post *(this volume)*.

An issue of primary importance in studies of brain evolution and behavior by MacLean and others, which has not yet had its full impact on psychiatry, is the interaction between the more stereotyped behavioral programs of the "reptilian brain" and the plasticity of higher brain structures which characterize mammalian evolution. R. B. Livingston (89, pp. 19–20) has said with regard to brain evolution and human behavior:

> The most remarkable gain . . . upon which cultural capitalization depends, has been that of intergenerational signaling, social imitation, and adoption of complex social styles of life. This is accomplished through the shaping of perception, judgement and behavior

in close accord with given societal circumstances, with that individual's birthright. The fact that early life experiences in all mammals seem to be binding on future value attachments accorded all later experiences suggests that the early witnessing of life becomes imbedded in the growing tissues of the brain in an especially facile and enduring fashion.

LEARNING AND MEMORY

When considering the role of the limbic system in the many complex patterns of human behavior in which learning must play a part, a number of questions arise. To some of these, few answers can yet be offered. One may ask, "In what ways or to what extent can limbic activity which mediates such behaviors as aggression or sexual activity be changed through learning or experience?" For an example of how one important behavioral parameter, aggressiveness/defensiveness, can be altered by lasting changes in electrical activity that is experimentally induced in the amygdala, one may refer to the chapter by R. F. Adamec and C. Stark-Adamec *(this volume)* or to an earlier report by Pinel et al. (130). A second question might be, "How does selective limbic system activity, either spontaneous or in response to stimulation, determine what is learned?" This suggests a third question, "How does the limbic system influence the recall or activation of learned information?" (e.g., in such states as "functional" amnesia and dissociative disorders.) Although the last two questions are especially difficult to approch experimentally, they have implications concerning the physiology underlying basic concepts in psychodynamic theory.

These questions imply that much of human learning and memory recall is an interactive process that involves more than one limbic pathway and connections between limbic structures and neocortex or other brain areas. Amnesia resulting from medial temporal ablations—in particular, as a result of surgical removals in humans—is well known (106,107). Similar data from experiments using monkeys [reviewed by Squire (167) and by Squire and Zola-Morgan (168)] and rats (125) show that in humans and animals hippocampal or combined hippocampal and amygdaloid damage produces amnesic deficits, although the degree of correspondence between animal and human data depends to some extent on the type of material or behavior used to measure memory.

Electrical stimulation of limbic pathways in the temporal lobe in neurosurgical patients may evoke what appear to be memory flashbacks, as described in the chapter by P. Gloor *(this volume)* or may result in interference with recognition or recall (62). Further evidence pointing to the role of limbic structures in human memory function comes from postmortem examination of brains of patients who have died after suffering an Alzheimer-type dementia. Although the effects of Alzheimer's disease are more widespread within the brain than the limbic system, and may also affect more than brain itself (5), biopsy or autopsy material shows that in patients with the disease the biogenic amines, including dopamine, norepinephrine and serotonin, as well as their metabolites, are significantly reduced in the hippocampus, caudate, hypothalamus, and cingulate gyrus (183). Choline acetyltransferase activity has also been reported to be less in the hippocampus, amygdala, caudate, and in most cortical areas of brains of Alzheimer-type patients (28,151).

COMMUNICATION, SOCIAL, AND FAMILY BEHAVIOR

MacLean (94) observed, some time ago, that the reptilian brain "programs" behavior according to instructions based on "ancestral memories," playing a role in what is commonly thought of as instinctual behavior. The paleomammalian or limbic brain, he pointed out, stands in relation to the reptilian and new mammalian brain, where it is of special interest because of its important role in social behavior.

MacLean (94) suggested three major subdivisions of the limbic system: the first fed by the amygdala, the second by the septum, and the third by the anterior thalamic tract. Each has clearly differentiated functions related to such basic classes of behavior as self-preservation or species-preservation, with obvious relevance to human psychiatric entities including disturbances of mood and emotion, feelings of depersonalization, distortion of perception, and paranoid symptoms. In MacLean *(this volume)* elaborates further behavioral categories currently under his investigation which provide further examples of the major role that the limbic system plays in psychiatric problems (see also ref. 96). He has shown that the mammalian cingulate region and thalamocingulate projections are essential for nursing and maternal care, audiovocal communication for maternal–offspring contact, and in play behavior. MacLean refers to the separation call, an activity that is dependent upon cingulate pathways, as the "most primitive vocalization." It would be worthwhile carrying further the studies of Wolff (186) on the ontogenetic differentiation of crying vocalizations as maturation and learning expand the complexity of behavior and emotional expressions from infancy through childhood. "Distress vocalization" or cries have been studied in relation to separation behavior in chicks (127,128) and dogs (157) and are under study by MacLean (95,96,123) in the squirrel monkey, so we may soon learn more about the differentiation of the cries or crying that occurs in states of grief and depression, fear or anxiety, and joy or passion, or in the affectless crying that is seen particularly with damage to the brainstem.

Nonvocal communication that, as MacLean points out, is related to display behavior under the control of the striatal complex, likewise deserves further attention, for there are doubtless meaningful evolutionary roots in the stereotypic postures, movements, and behaviors that are found in depression or certain advanced schizophrenic states, as well as in simple histrionic behavior or normal human reactions under emotional stress. The more we know about expressions or gestures, the more we may know about the organism that controls these, and the more we may add to our skills in treating the illnesses of which they are symptomatic. W. Nauta, some time ago (121), described projections from the limbic system of the forebrain to the midbrain tegmentum of the cat via the medial forebrain bundle, a pathway involved in the mediation of attack behavior elicited by stimulation of the lateral hypothalamus, as shown by Chi and Flynn (24,25). The same or closely situated fibers are involved in feeding behavior, as described by Mogensen et al. (110), who have described the role of limbic structures, including septum, amygdala, and prefrontal cortex, in the initiation and control of such complex movement patterns via connections with nucleus accumbens and globus palidus, as well as the ventral tegmental area. W. J. H. Nauta *(this volume)* and H. J. W. Nauta *(this volume)* have further elaborated on complex interconnections between limbic system and the corpus striatum which provide systems for linking motor activity with cognitive and emotional processes. As H. Nauta observes *(this volume)*, "perhaps neurological illnesses that today appear very dissimilar, such as movement disorders and behavior disorders, may some day be shown to have similar underlying pathological mechanisms."

EPILEPSY, DYSCONTROL, AND KINDLING

As mentioned earlier by R. M. Post *(this volume)*, temporal lobe or complex partial seizures serve as a leverage point in discussing limbic system dysfunction in affective syndromes. It seems odd, in view of the prevalence of various kinds of psychiatric symptoms in epileptic disorders (especially the limbic epilepsies), that the diagnostic classifications most widely used in North American psychiatry only allow for reference to these states as an additional psychiatrically undifferentiated diagnosis along with the code for epilepsy, i.e., as a "residual category" called "atypical or mixed organic brain syndrome" (294.80) in *DSM III*, or among "other specified organic brain syndromes" (294.8) in *ICD-9-CM*.

The various forms of "ictal psychosis" and other "personality disturbances" associated with epilepsy deserve a better method of psychiatric classification. Useful attempts have been made to draw up satisfactory classifications of psychiatric manifestations of epilepsy by a number of authors, including Pond (131), Bruens (19), Betts (15), Fenton (39), and Toone (176). These authors distinguish between those symptoms that are directly related to seizures and those that occur in the interictal and postictal periods, an issue emphasized by G. V. Goddard et al. *(this volume)* and by S. M. Ferguson et al. *(this volume)*. If these time-related factors are then combined with variables such as the type of epilepsy, cerebral locus of the seizure, and symptom type, a more meaningful classification is possible.

Within this schema, the lateralization of the primary epileptic focus is also important, particularly in cases of temporal lobe epilepsy (160,161,178; D. M. Bear, *this volume*; M. Rayport et al., *this volume*) where, as with other conditions such as affective disorders, schizophrenia, and certain of the so-called neurotic disorders, lateralization of function has been shown to relate to symptom patterns, even though there is yet some disagreement concerning both the details and the universality of these effects (13,41–43; C. Stark-Adamec and R. E. Adamec, *this volume*).

M. R. Trimble *(this volume)* suggests that two of the most important subdivisions of epileptic psychosis are the peri-ictal psychoses, associated with ongoing electrical disturbance in the brain, and the chronic forms of interictal psychoses. He is attempting to make possible more precise quantification of the phenomenology of psychopathology in epilepsy, using modern techniques of psychiatric assessment such as Wing's Present State Examination (PSE), as well as computed tomography (CT) scan or positron emission tomography (PET) measurements.

Case histories cited by S. M. Ferguson et al. (this volume) emphasize the importance of carefully distinguishing between seizure-induced symptoms and secondary disturbances of emotion and behavior generated by the epileptic behavior of the patient. They point out that such symptoms may be consistent with psychodynamics. However, a note of caution might also be sounded, for it is often easier to infer psychodynamics than to identify ictal activity deep in the temporal lobe; hence, the one should not rule out the other if a carefully compiled history suggests the likelihood of seizure-related behavior. How many cases like those of B.A.A. or F.E.R. reported by Ferguson and her colleagues exist in mental hospitals, improperly diagnosed because their seizures are too infrequent or unclear to bring them to proper attention? The four cases cited by S. Hirose and S. Endo *(this volume)* likewise draw attention to the real possibility that bizarre psychotic seizure-related behavior might be mistaken for psychiatric illness of different etiology if not adequately investigated.

The discussion of ictal psychosis in this volume raises the perplexing question of why, in some instances, an active seizure focus is associated with psychotic symptoms in the interictal period, whereas in other cases convulsions, especially of "grand mal" variety, render an improvement in the psychiatric state. The latter is a behavioral analog of "forced normalization" in the electroencephalogram (EEG) in association with seizures, as described by Landolt and cited in the case histories presented by S. Hirose and S. Endo *(this volume)*. Although this may be observed with spontaneous seizures, it is most conspicuous in the use of artificially induced seizures [convulsive therapy or electroconvulsive therapy (ECT)], which, although most effective in the treatment of major affective disorders, may also be used in the control of severe and refractory cases of epilepsy (22,30,37,61,74,90,103–105, 149,150,152,153,174,175,185). These effects may be the result of potentiation of inhibition or similar mechanisms as proposed in the discussions by G. V. Goddard et al. *(this volume)* and R. E. Adamec and C. Stark-Adamec (ref. 2 and *this volume*). Clarification of this question could be one of the most important contributions yet to be made in the field of neuropsychiatry.

The usual clinical criteria and diagnostic tests for seizure disorders leave many cases in doubt as to whether the problem is "real" epilepsy or something that, perhaps by exclusion, may be called "functional," and that is often atypical and of uncertain etiology. Cases are observed which continue to be misdiagnosed as "atypical" schizophrenia or depression, or severe borderline personality disorders (as examples) until, finally, an EEG compatible with limbic epilepsy is obtained. Even then there are psychiatrists and neurologists who will make a double diagnosis and ignore obvious and important evidence of a causal relationship between epileptic lesions and disabling psychiatric symptoms. Unfortunately, this deprives the patient of proper treatment. Such treatment might be surgical, but even if pharmacotherapy is possible, it will be to the patient's disadvantage if this is not prescribed on the basis of a proper understanding of the etiology of the behavioral symptoms.

The value of surgical procedures in the treatment of selected cases of limbic epilepsy is borne out of reports such as that given by M. Rayport et al. *(this volume)*. Stereoencephalography is, of course, suited to the detection of seizure discharge activity and hence of value in determining the surgical approach for some cases of epilepsy, with or without major psychiatric manifestations. As technologies improve the means of identifying brain loci of low-intensity ictal or other neuropathological processes underlying psychiatric illness, in the limbic system or elsewhere, one may predict that surgical approaches in the treatment of such conditions will progress, less inhibited by counterminded pressure groups. Such a prediction is strengthened by evidence such as that presented by Rayport and his colleagues.

An added benefit from neurosurgical investigation and treatment of epilepsy in the temporal lobe or elsewhere is the information provided by depth stimulation as shown by P. Gloor *(this volume)* and by M. Rayport et al. *(this volume)*. These methods not only add precision to the determination of foci of seizure origin, but may, in addition, teach much more about the substrates of subjective experience (normal and pathological) than could possibly be determined through animal experimentation.

A behavioral dimension that has received particular attention in this volume is aggression. Although this is absent in a large proportion of cases of limbic epilepsy, and may in some instances be a reaction to fear or panic resulting from the seizure (160), it is more apt to occur interictally in conjunction with other distinctive emotional and behavioral parameters (31). When it does occur, it may be dramatic and violent as illustrated in the cases cited by S. M. Ferguson et al. *(this volume)* and by S. Hirose and S. Endo *(this volume)*. Episodic aggression that stands distinct from an individual's usual behavior will commonly arouse clinical suspicion that the basis for the episodes may be epilepsy. Because the epileptic focus responsible for aggressive outbursts may be difficult to detect electrographically, painstaking methods of diagnosis are necessary through history-taking and psychological measurement.

Despite a sizable literature on the physiology and biochemistry of aggression over the past two decades or more, there is much in clinical states of aggression that is poorly understood. Epileptic discharge is certainly not the only means by which pathological aggression is mediated within the limbic system. Russell R. Monroe *(this volume)* has established a schema for differentiating between episodic dyscontrol (primarily aggressive), which is probably related to ictal discharges, compared with those cases in which the etiology is essentially psychodynamic (112,113). He argues convincingly for the possibility of kindling as the mechanism underlying ictal dyscontrol. M. Girgis *(this volume)* has described the production of lasting aggressive behavior in monkeys following injections of physostigmine into the basal amygdala, accompanied by spike activities in the EEG from the same area for periods lasting several weeks. He suggests that this may represent a form of chemical kindling showing a relationship between the cholinergic system of the amygdala and epileptiform discharges (50). The behavior that he describes in his monkeys appears similar to the savage aggression that we observed in our own work with dogs, in which case reserpine injections were found to induce and sustain aggressiveness in more dominant dogs toward their less dominant experimental partners. This behavior was accompanied by typical parasympathetic hyperactivity with reserpine-induced monoamine depletion, and in its nature closely resembled the aggressiveness that can be produced by stimulating the basal amygdala. In this regard, it is interesting to note the reported facilitation of kindling by either intraperitoneal (8) or intracerebral (47) injections of reserpine.

Having mentioned earlier the closing of the gap between neurology and psychiatry as limbic system research progresses, it might be emphasized that this closure depends not only on a thorough understanding of the genesis of psychiatric disorders in identifiable cases of epilepsy, but also on clarification of disturbed behavior that originates in neuropathological processes that are similar to those that cause seizures, but in which nonepileptic behavioral dysfunction may be the only observable result. These are disorders whose etiologies are still largely hypothetical and which Kenneth Livingston termed the "para-epileptic disorders." Research into these conditions will be aided if the procedure of noninvasive limbic EEG and behavioral activation by procaine hydrochloride injections described by Stark-Adamec et al. (170), Adamec (1), and Adamec et al. (4) progress to a stage where it may be used in clinical investigation.

Into this category might fit certain affective disorders such as those referred to by R. M. Post *(this volume)* as well as cases of episodic dyscontrol described by R. R. Monroe *(this volume)*. Also in this group are the frequent cases in which complex partial seizures are suspected but unproven (in particular, when electrophysiological investigation is limited to the routine scalp EEG without activation).

It is especially for such cases as these that it has been suggested that the kindling model may apply (R. E. Adamec and C. Stark-Adamec; R. M. Post; and R. M. Post and T. W. Uhde, *this volume*; refs. 85,133). Goddard, who with his colleagues first observed the kindling effect in the production of seizure activity (55), states in this volume, "The controversy is whether or not dramatic behavioral changes ever result from covert, or subclinical, seizure activity. We have no direct evidence concerning this matter" (G. V. Goddard et al., *this volume*). For psychiatry this controversy is potentially of outstanding importance. If, indeed, covert or subclinical (i.e., undetectable) seizure activity or similar neuronal processes can have immediate or long-term effects similar to those of overt seizure activity, the carbamazepine-sensitive affective disorders (R. M. Post, *this volume*), cases of episodic dyscontrol (R. R. Monroe, *this volume*), and other psychiatric entities may arise therefrom. As the answer to this question will have profound implications for treatment, research aimed at solving the question should be given high priority.

In the meantime, much excellent research is adding substantially to knowledge about the physiological and biochemical or pharmacological mechanisms for kindling in animal preparations, as is evident within this volume (see chapters by M. Girgis; G. V. Goddard et al.; R. J. Racine and D. McIntyre; W. M. Burnham et al.; R. E. Adamec and C. Stark-Adamec; and P. S. Albright et al., *this volume*). From that research, there is evidence that continues to encourage belief in the relevance of kindling to human psychiatry. For example, as observed by G. V. Goddard et al. *(this volume)* and by others, kindling has a preferential affinity for the limbic system, especially those areas that may be implicated in emotional disorders. R. E. Adamec and C. Stark-Adamec *(this volume)* demonstrated a behavioral balance between aggressiveness and defensiveness, two functions that are known to be affected by stimulation or ablation of the amygdala in various species. They showed that these may be modified over a long term in keeping with changes in amygdaloid afterdischarge thresholds as a result of exposure to repeated kindling.

Until there is more supporting evidence, caution should be exercised when generalizing from the kindling paradigm as it applies to seizure discharges in order to explain nonseizure states. It is not yet established that kindling has a role in human epilepsy. It should be borne in mind that what is analogous may not be identical. Thus, although useful analogies may be drawn between kindling of seizures and the induction of certain nonictal behavioral states, there may be critical differences between what takes place in the kindling of spike discharges and the priming of behavior without a seizure. This topic is particularly relevant to rapid alterations in emotional states, including anger, fear, and manic or depressive affect.

AFFECTIVE DISORDERS

R. M. Post *(this volume)* has presented an excellent discussion and review of affective symptoms, not only in relation to limbic epilepsy but in the light of the structural and functional makeup of the limbic system as a whole. He has warned against the idea that affective representation in the brain is likely to conform to a simple pattern. Major depressive illness has far-reaching effects, involving physiological and biochemical processes outside the central nervous system (117).

A focal point of much of Post's recent work has been the relationship between seizure mechanisms and processes that mediate affective symptoms or behavior, and he has described striking similarities in symptoms reported by patients with complex partial seizures and with major affective illness. Further, Post and his colleagues demonstrated the effectiveness of the anticonvulsant carbamazepine in the control of some affective disorders, especially those that are rapid cycling, which has added another dimension to the management of manic and depressive illness (Post and Uhde, *this volume*).

Post suggests that the kindling model may explain the pathophysiology of some of the major affective disorders (R. M. Post, *this volume*; R. M. Post, and T. W. Uhde, *this volume*; refs. 133, 162). As lithium and carbamazepine have dissimilar effects on amygdaloid kindling in animals, Post et al. (136) hypothesize that two separate physiological mechanisms (kindling and another that is lithium sensitive) determine two groups of patients with bipolar disorders, one of which responds to carbamazepine, the other to lithium carbonate.

M. Rayport et al. *(this volume)* and D. M. Bear *(this volume)* cited the well-known clinical fact that affective expression or anosognosic statements which may be indicative of denial or loss of affect, are related to the side of the brain involved, which in such cases is almost always on the right. In his postulated organizational scheme of interhemispheric differences in corticolimbic functional interaction, Bear provides a hypothetical basis for the influence of laterality on the affective manifestations of stroke, head injury, and epilepsy. His schema also would further explain the observations of Flor-Henry and others (43) regarding the primary involvement of nondominant visuospatial hemispheric systems and their effects on dominant hemispheric systems in the control and balance between opposing "negative" and "positive" mood states.

The affective disorders provide an excellent opportunity to observe some of the implications of behavioral evolution for the psychogenesis of human mental illness. Although there is no experimental animal model of depression that is entirely equivalent to "endogenous" depression in humans, depressive behavior in various species has been produced under laboratory conditions. The majority of examples which closely resemble human behavior which is observed in severe depressive illness have been the result of separation (97), especially of primate offspring from their mothers (63,75,76). It is of interest to note that none of these models have been derived from experiments based on brain stimulation or ablations. These data may be interpreted as manifestations of behavioral patterns which are congenitally "programmed" in the animal brain, presumably with survival value in certain naturally occurring situations. Such behavior resembles grief as experienced by humans and is clearly analogous to the processes involved in separation and loss which have been extensively studied in human children (16,17). Going beyond this analogy, a list may be made of primary signs and symptoms of major affective disorders in humans, and for these one may then impute protective functions that have survival value in behavioral evolution. Such manifestations of depressed behavior include psychomotor retardation or agitation, loss of appetite, loss of sexual drive, insomnia, crying, and subjective dysphoria or "negative" mood, which are listed in Table 1 beside their proposed protective functions in behavioral evolution, together with some of their possible limbic representations.

Earlier, we noted MacLean's elucidation of the separation call as an example of behavior that distinguishes mammals from reptiles (P. D. MacLean, *this volume*; 95). MacLean draws our attention to the possibility that separation feelings, which are subserved by cingulate cortex and thalamocingulate projections, may be involved in at least some forms of clinical depression. This explains why cingulotomy may be a palliative surgical procedure in certain cases of depressive disorder which are refractory to pharmacological or convulsive therapy (81,101,108).

There is strong evidence in the psychiatric literature to suggest that so-called "endogenous" and "reactive" varieties of depressive illness may not always be distinguishable, lying at extreme ends of a continuum (78). Everyday clinical experience suggests that many cases of depressive illness are "mixed," containing elements of both "endogenous" and "reactive" etiology. Many patients in whom

TABLE 1. *Signs/symptoms of depression, possible functional significance in evolution and possible limbic representations*

Signs/symptoms	Functions	Possible limbic representations
Psychomotor retardation	Terminates situationally inappropriate behavior; conserves energy	Septum, hippocampus, caudate, corpus striatum; efferents from nucleus accumbens to tegmentum
Agitation	Reflects increased arousal for defense, flight, recuperation	Septum, hippocampus, amygdala, tegmental projections
Loss of appetite	Decreases exploratory or competitive behavior; slows metabolism	Cingulate gyrus, amygdala, hypothalamus
Loss of sexual drive	Limits competitive behavior; conserves energy	Amygdala, hippocampus, septum, medial forebrain bundle, cingulate gyrus, and thalamocingulate pathway
Insomnia	Maintains vigilance	Amygdala, septum, hippocampus, thalamocortical projections, inputs to hypothalamo-pituitary-adrenal axis
Crying and tearfulness	Represents the "separation call"	Anterior cingulate cortex, tegmental tracts
Subjective mood (negative affect)	Extinguishes attachment behavior	Cingulate cortex, parietal and frontal projections
Irritability	Promotes or maintains defensive or protective behavior in response to threat	Amygdala, hippocampus, lateral hypothalamus

there is substantial evidence of a psychologically determined depressive state (so-called reactive depression) will show some of the physiological concomitants that are typical of "endogenous" depression (sleep loss, appetite loss, etc.). Likewise, patients who unequivocally meet the criteria for "endogenous" depression (unipolar or bipolar type) will also express cognitive correlates of, or rationales (however irrational or colored by depressive delusions) for their depressive state. These observations suggest that two levels of cerebral function are involved: limbic and/or diencephalic in the case of the endogenous features with physiological concomitants, and neocortical (so-called higher learning) in the case of cognitive expressions. The complete picture in any individual case of depression might involve varying proportions of each, in which either level might have a primary role and exert varying degrees of influence over the other and in which the level that has the secondary role might have a higher or lower threshold for activation by the primary site. If one were to accept this sort of paradigm, it would not be difficult then, to apply the kindling model within it.

SCHIZOPHRENIA AND PARANOID STATES

Any new proposals for a unifying or comprehensive theory of the etiology of schizophrenia must now take into account an overwhelming diversity of factors that have positive correlations with the onset or course of schizophrenic disorders. The range runs from macroscopic sociocultural variables, through genetics, brain anatomy, and biochemistry, to histology and histochemistry (109,173).

Schizophrenia is sometimes considered to be primarily a disorder of human higher cerebral activity, for which no convincing analogy exists in animal behavior (either naturally or experimentally produced). However, it is clear from several lines of evidence that schizophrenia involves other levels of brain and the central nervous system (67,71) and may also include systems outside the central nervous system, for example the hemopoietic system (118,187). Within this array the limbic system makes a contribution.

Biochemical factors that have recently been shown to have significant correlations with schizophrenic symptoms and their treatment include the brain catecholamines (72) and, in particular, dopamine receptor activity as demonstrated by Seeman and co-workers (84,158), who have shown that neuroleptic medication, which is at present the principal treatment of schizophrenia, apparently acts specifically to block dopamine receptor activity on the D_2 receptor sites. Reynolds (143,144) recently reported a significant elevation of dopamine levels in the left amygdala of schizophrenics compared with controls. He proposes that this may provide a bridge between the "dopamine hypothesis" and electrophysiological, pathological, and psychological evidence for left temporal lobe function in schizophrenia (41–43,60,119). Reynolds also suggested that phenylethylamine, which has been implicated in schizophrenia and paranoid psychoses as well as in phenylketonuria, may have an influence on the occurrence of psychotic symptoms owing to its high level of activity within the limbic system, which may be related to 5-hydroxytryptamine (5-HT) binding (145). Through more than one chemically mediated mechanism, the limbic system appears to influence the neocortical expression of thought processes as they occur in schizophrenia.

We have already noted the importance of epileptic psychosis in psychiatry. The similarities and differences between epileptic psychosis and some of the symptoms of schizophrenia have received considerable attention (163,164). Excellent examples of ictal psychosis that can be mistaken for schizophrenia are to be found in the chapters by S. M. Ferguson et al. and S. Hirose and S. Endo *(this volume)*. A leading presumption underlying the comparisons between ictal psychosis and schizophrenia is that although the chronological sequence of events as well as the total clinical picture at any one time may differ, essentially the same pathways or structures may mediate similar symptoms in the two diseases. A matter of less certainty is whether similar pathophysiological processes within those pathways or structures may also account for the similarities in symptoms.

Robertson (147) has proposed that because of the similarities between temporal lobe epilepsy and schizophrenia, and because of the postulated role of kindling in temporal lobe epilepsy, perhaps limbic kindling should be examined as a possible useful animal model for studying the neurochemical and neurophysiological changes that take place in the brain in schizophrenia. As Robertson has noted, a number of reports have indicated that dopamine is involved in limbic kindling.

Flor-Henry (41–43) argued the case for left temporal lobe limbic involvement in schizophrenic disorders, based largely on EEG data. Toone et al. (177) and M. R. Trimble *(this volume)* provide evidence that schizophrenia-like symptoms of epilepsy correlate positively but not invariably with data from both CT and PET, indicating atrophic or other pathological changes in the left hemisphere.

D. M. Bear *(this volume)* put forth a schema for cortical-limbic interactions which, if correct, would suggest two different forms of perceptual and ideational activity, one left- and one right-hemispheric, which may be relevant to the paranoid orientation of schizophrenics. Bear's proposal of a dorsal parietofrontal pathway in the right hemisphere, focused peripherally (as if watching for threats from the environment), and a ventral temporofrontal pathway in the left hemisphere, associated with reflective behavior, is compatible with the idea that introverted and autistically elaborated delusions are associated with left-hemisphere function and a more general persecutory orientation toward the world as a whole associated with the right.

Schizophrenic delusional thinking typically differs in certain characteristics from the delusions of affective disorders and temporal lobe epilepsy. Munro (116) proposed that in paranoid (i.e., delusional) states there is dysfunction of a filtering mechanism in the limbic area which is associated with hyperalertness and hyperactive neuronal activity between limbic-cortical systems, the reticular activating system, and the sympathetic system. As his summing up of the literature on delusions shows, many varieties and characteristics of delusional thinking have been described. One of these characteristics is the degree of unreality harbored within the delusion. Depressive delusions, for example, are mood-congruent and typically reflect a feeling of worthlessness on the part of the patient. The delusional thoughts and hallucinations of ictal psychosis may be most bizarre, but are often more readily questioned by the patient who may, in fact, recognize the "as if" quality of hallucinatory experiences (pseudohallucinations). Even the normal individual may have private fantasies which, if they were to be transformed into concepts of reality, would be frankly psychotic. The test of psychosis is not simply the content of the experience, but how well the one having the experience recognizes the unreality or improbability of that experience (i.e., has insight). Hallucinatory perceptual experiences may have a compelling sensory quality of "realness" under various circumstances, as in deafferentation or sensory deprivation (32,34,166) and various organic states (e.g., narcolepsy, focal irritative brain lesions) even though the perceiver—especially if assisted through appropriate communication by a skilled and experienced interviewer—is able to recognize the unreality of the event as belonging to the external environment. In short, the perceiver recognizes the events as "crazy" and the experiences, although very abnormal, are not truly psychotic.

The recognition of reality clearly depends on brain function; so where, indeed, is its physiological locus? Goddard (53) speculated that one's belief that something *is* or *is not* true may be a function of the temporal lobe involving the hippocampus, although there is still no direct evidence to confirm this idea. This concept might be extended to include rudimentary judgments of probability in spatial and time sequences in perception which, in turn, may be governed by limbic-cortical circuits. Such a function would be in keeping with the development of mammalian social behavior which, as noted earlier, has been described by MacLean as an evolutionary step dependent on the limbic system.

A common feature of schizophrenic thought disorder is a failure to perceive improbability, and this would appear to be a feature of schizophrenic delusions. This might be the result of failure of inhibition or extinction of neuronal activity which, although required in early stages of development, normally ceases as development progresses. This would be analogous to Hebb's (64) theory of two kinds of intelligence which operate at early and later stages in perceptual learning or concept formation; the first required in the initial stages of forming cell assemblies in the brain, the second being the intelligence one usually thinks of in everyday behavior. The failure to switch off a learning mechanism that is only required at an early stage of development would allow internal or external stimuli (or "ideas") to be interpreted as if at an earlier stage of life when experience has not yet established what can or cannot be—that is, at a time of life when "anything is possible." Hence, the implausible (perhaps persecutory) idea might be interpreted as possible and quickly progress to the stage where it becomes a belief or a delusion. If such a process exists, one might look at the limbic modulation of cortical activity, including corticolimbic circuits of the type described by Bear *(this volume)*, in search of the pathophysiology involved.

ANXIETY DISORDERS

Anxiety is a pervasive symptom, which may occur secondarily in nearly all psychiatric disorders. Several primary forms are currently recognized in the psychiatric classifications, including obsessional states, phobias, generalized anxiety, panic disorder, and phobic disorders. Learning undoubtedly plays a part in the genesis of these disorders, although R. E. Adamec and C. Stark Adamec *(this volume)* have shown a relationship in cats between fearfulness or defensiveness and the threshold for kindled afterdischarge activity in the amygdala (opposed to the trait of aggressiveness). This suggests a genetically determined temperamental factor that involves the basal amygdala and interconnections with other limbic pathways, including the hippocampus. Subjective feelings of fear or intense anxiety often accompany complex partial seizures (temporal lobe). This, together with Adamec's data, raises the question whether some pathological states of anxiety might be the result of a process similar to kindling.

At present, the most widely used medications in the treatment of anxiety and panic disorders are the benzodiazepines. Robertson (146) and Robertson et al. (148) showed a positive relationship between benzodiazepine receptor activity and emotional reactivity in rats and mice.

W. M. Burnham et al. *(this volume)* demonstrated in rats that the kindling of seizures is associated with changes in benzodiazepine receptor binding, which might have significant implications for postictal or interictal symptoms, including fear or anxiety. In the rat, benzodiazepine receptors are highly concentrated in neocortex, molecular layers of the hippocampus, dentate gyrus, cerebellum, and olfactory bulb (11). Gray (57) and Gray et al. (58) proposed a theory of anxiety based on the γ-aminobutyric acid (GABAergic) action of antianxiety drugs on noradrenergic and serotonergic inputs to the limbic septohippocampal system, especially from the dorsal noradrenergic ascending bundle, which projects widely from the locus ceruleus to the hypothalamus, thalamus, amygdala, olfactory tubercle, septum, hippocampus, and cortex (98). They regard this system as one that responds to discrepancies between expected and perceived stimuli, or to stimuli that are aversive, by inhibiting specific behaviors while increasing attention and arousal. According to their schema, the benzodiazepines and barbiturates, by inhibiting this behavioral-inhibitory system through GABAergic action, not only block the anxiety that is expressed by the system but may also interfere with the development of stress tolerance, a feature that might explain, in part, a psychological dependence that develops with continued administration of such drugs in the clinical setting.

The same authors suggest that their theory of anxiety based on the septohippocampal system is particularly applicable to obsessive-compulsive behavior, especially when it involves excessive checking of potential environmental hazards. They encompass phobic behavior as well within their theory of anxiety, drawing attention to the fact that phobias serve to inhibit specific patterns of motor activity.

We have noted already the decline—perhaps temporary—in the use of surgical procedures in psychiatric disorders. Intractable anxiety and severe obsessive-compulsive states have been among the conditions successfully treated by "psychosurgery" (18,77,108). Gray et al. (58) attribute the success of prefrontal and cingulate leukotomy in part to the fact that these areas are interconnected with the septohippocampal system.

HYSTERICAL DISORDERS

The word hysteria does not refer to an illness. When used in the medical sense, it denotes a group of disorders in which psychological etiologies are assumed to play a part in producing disturbances of perception, motor function, or consciousness. Merskey (99) has reviewed the evidence which, over the years, has consistently pointed to a relationship between physical illness (predominantly, although not exclusively, neurological disorders) and hysterical disorders. The evidence in support of this is particularly convincing in the case of conversion disorders and "hysterical seizures."

By definition, hysterical disorders are involuntary, which distinguishes them from malingering or from the deliberate invention of symptoms for psychological gain. It is clear, however, that many clinicians tend to view hysterical symptoms as "put on," and even in medical circles the adjective "hysterical" has a pejorative connotation. It is reasonable to assume that the division between involuntary hysteria and the willful intentions of malingering is not sharp; in other words, there may be a bit of both. Many symptoms displayed in frank hysteria, however, would be beyond the imitative capacity of the majority of normal individuals, suggesting again that the nervous system may be functioning abnormally.

The physiopathology of hysterical dysfunctions is far from clear. Merskey (99) suggests that there are at least five ways in which the relationship between physical illness and hysterical symptoms might be explained, including the possible elaboration of preexisting illness, owing to independent emotional stress or to the stress of illness, imitation of symptoms of a preexisting illness, regression to hysterical behavior brought about by physical illness, or the possibility that hysterical symptoms may be specifically caused by cerebral damage. He also cites Ludwig's (91) hypothesis that hysteria is due to increased corticofugal inhibition of afferent pathways, which is essentially Pavlov's (129) idea, but notes that there is little direct evidence to support such a theory. Merskey believes that a more fruitful line of approach might be to look at recent evidence concerning gender and lateralization of cerebral functions, as he believes that the differential development of hemispheric specialization in males and females, sometimes combined with brain damage, might contribute to the relative frequency of affective and hysterical syndromes in women, and schizophrenic and psychopathic symptoms in men. He then concludes, "This is not to deny the many other important causal factors in these illnesses, but to recognize that there are indications from systematic studies that we shall know much more in a few years' time about the links between cerebral function and psychiatric illnesses other than just the pure brain syndromes" (99).

One of the strongest lines of evidence concerning the physiopathology of hysteria comes from the frequent observation—noted by Merskey (99)—of an association with epilepsy, particularly of the temporal lobe. Both generalized and focal seizures predispose some individuals to develop "pseudoseizures," which often closely resemble the patient's ictal signs, but which also may deviate clearly from these. Atypical seizures are often suspected of being hysterical, which they may be. However, it is dangerous to assume that behavior is purely psychological just because it is strange. Pseudoseizures, especially when they resemble limbic seizures, again suggest the possibility of "para-epileptic" processes that resemble ictal discharges, although they have not yet been identified electrographically.

A second intriguing association between epilepsy and hysteria is to be found among the dissociative disorders. This, too, has been noted more than once in the literature going back many years (59,99) and applies more specifically to temporal lobe dysfunction. Dissociation, including its more extreme variant of multiple personality, has been noted in association with temporal lobe epilepsy or focal temporal lobe abnormalities in the EEG (100,154). A striking number of patients with dissociative disorder, especially those who approximate the picture of multiple-personality disorder (80,137,138), have been investigated for complex partial seizures before the diagnosis of dissociative disorder or multiple-personality disorder is made. Such patients are apt to manifest symptoms similar to a temporal lobe aura at times when they are most likely to dissociate spontaneously or when they are undergoing hypnotic trance (*personal observation* and ref. 27).

As with the affective disorders, one may suggest that in dissociation (and hypnosis) we are witnessing a function that has significance in behavioral evolution. Dissociation may be derived from normal mechanisms which are needed for survival in the animal kingdom, and it may not be farfetched to suggest that the dissociative function takes part in the play and fantasies of children as well as going unnoticed when it occurs to a minor degree in the day-to-day behavior of normal adults. The observations cited above, noting a relationship between dissociative processes and the temporal lobe, provide reason to suspect that what is observed as dissociative behavior represents a selective filtering of attention which depends on temporal limbic circuits. Hebb (65) suggested that the expressions of behavior that are seen in certain dissociative states and multiple personality may indicate the selective activation of different cell assemblies in the brain. If this is so, the selection or switching on of such specific assemblies would appear to be governed in accordance with affect and the perceptual orientation toward the social environment which, as we have already seen, depend on various components of the limbic system. If this speculation is plausible, so might it be that conversion symptoms have a similar basis.

DISORDERS OF SEXUAL AND REPRODUCTIVE BEHAVIOR

Not all sexual behavior is directly related to reproduction. MacLean (94) described the association that exists, at least in some primates, between male territorial dominance and display behavior including penile erection, the latter having been evoked by electrical stimulation of three limbic circuits, including the spinothalamic tract and medial dorsal thalamic nucleus, with its cortical projections, the mammilothalamic tract and anterior thalamus, fornix, and medial frontal cortex. P. D. MacLean (this volume; 95) notes the involvement of the striatal complex in display behavior from reptiles throughout the mammals. Sexual display in human males may take the pathological form of exposure or exhibitionism which, in the perpetrator, is linked with sexual arousal.

In both sexes, sexual arousal and orgasm are linked with physical pleasure and transient euphoria. However, postorgasmic depression in males has been recorded in the literature dating back for many years—for example, Burton's "The Anatomy of Melancholy," written in the seventeenth century (21) and in deFleury's (29) book on neurasthenic syndromes in 1902—and may have contributed to the belief which was taken seriously in the nineteenth century that a major cause of insanity was sexual excess or "abuse" (masturbation). As already noted, P. D. MacLean (this volume) has suggested a role of the anterior cingulate cortex in depressive feelings which can be likened to feelings of separation, particularly in females. Perhaps there is a counterbalance between the systems that predominate in male and female emotions, such that the same mechanisms that would account for separation-depression in females may be activated with loss of dominance or sexual potency in males, either transiently (postorgastically) or for longer periods in certain clinical depressions. Aberrant sexual behavior in the human male may also include aggression or violence, as in heterosexual or homosexual rape, which raises the question whether lateral limbic pathways concerned with predatory attack or defensiveness including amygdala and hippocampus (R. E. Adamec and C. Stark-Adamec, *this volume*) may be recruited into this kind of sexual aggression.

In the case of the human female, Rémillard et al. (142) and P. Gloor *(this volume)* have shown what appears to be a sex-specific function of limbic portions of the temporal lobe underlying erotic experiences that are somewhat analogous to ictal fear. Their data are derived from reports of sexual auras or ictal experiences in women with temporal lobe seizures and, in the case reported in the chapter by P. Gloor *(this volume)*, from stimulation of the amygdala. Sexual behavior in the human female is more closely linked with familial behavior and bonding than in males. Hence, one may expect to find differences in the patterning of sexual representation in the limbic system between males and females, especially within the cingulate cortex.

Much sexual and reproductive behavior is hormone-dependent (for example, see Meyerson and Eliasson, ref. 102). Although the hypothalamus is known to be a primary site of action of gonadal hormones in both males and females, other areas including mesencephalon and portions of the limbic system may be involved in the uptake of circulating estrogen or progesterone (181,182,191). Significant variations in plasma estrogens and progesterone occur regularly in women throughout the menstrual cycle, and these are known to correlate with mood changes in normal women. More extreme changes of mood and behavior, epecially with heightened irritability, anxiety or defensiveness, and depressive feelings, are found in the so-called premenstrual tension syndrome, which characteristically occurs during the luteal phase of the menstrual cycle, between ovulation and the onset of menses. The etiology of this condition is unclear, although a multiplicity of biochemical hypotheses has been advanced in what amounts to an extensive literature (see review by Reid and Yen, ref. 141). Our own work (33) has shown that in otherwise healthy women with marked symptoms of premenstrual tension, compared with symptom-free controls, there is a significantly greater decline in serum estrogen or progesterone, or both, during the premenstrual week when symptoms are maximal. This suggests that a withdrawal effect may account for such symptoms.

Bäckström et al. (10) reported reductions in spike discharge frequencies in women with partial seizures with intravenous injections of progesterone during the follicular phase of the cycle, which correlated with unbound plasma progesterone levels. Progesterone has been reported to have sedative or anesthetic effects and has been found to raise the threshold for electrically induced seizures, whereas estrogen lowers the seizure threshold (124,171). In the light of our observations of the relationship of premenstrual symptoms to falling hormone levels, the finding of Bäckström et al. (10) provides another instance in which it is tempting to invoke the "kindling model," or an analog thereof, in the physiopathology of severe premenstrual tension symptoms such as outbursts of uncontrollable anger or other emotions. The monthly rise in circulating progesterone and estrogen levels, followed regularly by their decline premenstrually, may stimulate through repeated, spaced withdrawal effects, the intermittent stimulation in the experimental kindling paradigm. This model seems better suited at this time to a progesterone effect than to that of estrogen in view of their opposite effects on seizure thresholds, although more remains to be learned of the localization of action of these and other hormones in the brain. Chemical kindling has been proposed by Post and colleagues (133,162) as a mechanism in the production of psychopathology and is mentioned in the chapter by M. Girgis (*this volume*, cholinergic kindling). Research into the possibility of a kindling effect resulting from rising and falling hormone levels might be worthwhile.

ADDICTIONS AND EATING DISORDERS

The physiology of addictions is still largely a mystery. Recently, attention has been paid to the possible role in addictive mechanisms of endogenous opioid substances which have similar effects (e.g., analgesia, euphoria) to morphine or heroin. The endorphins and enkephalins have lately been studied in relation to a variety of mental illnesses and addictions (14,23,26,35,36,38,56,155,159,180) with interesting and varied results that have yet to clearly establish a role for opioids in particular psychiatric illnesses or in their treatment.

Opioid substances and receptor activity are widely distributed in the brain. More than one type of opioid receptor is found in different areas of the limbic system and its interconnections, e.g., frontal and cingulate cortex, hippocampus and amygdala, thalamus, hypothalamus, caudate, nucleus accumbens and brainstem (68,83,184). As already noted, P. D. MacLean (*this volume*) suggests that the thalamocingulate division may be implicated in drug addiction, based on the view that this anatomical division may be responsible for the euphoriant effects of opioids which relieve the "separation feelings" that promote drug addiction.

The recent literature contains several references to an association between eating disorders (anorexia nervosa and bulimia) and addictive behavior. For example, Garfinkle and Garner (44) quote several reports of a prevalance of alcohol use, excessive smoking or other drug use, in anorexic and bulimic patients. They also cite studies showing a greater than chance correlation between anorexia nervosa and alcoholism in patients' families (fathers>mothers), such that familial alcoholism might even be considered as a predisposing factor in eating disorders. Scott (156) has gone further in suggesting similarities between food and alcohol abuse, including common features in sociocultural elements, familial factors, personality patterns, and responses to various psychological measurements. He concludes that the two groups of disorders may share etiological factors.

Opiate peptides appear to have a role in initiating feeding within the hypothalamic control of appetite and sedation (70). The anterior cingulate region, which also contains opiate receptors, must share a role in the regulation of feeding behavior in mammals as part of its function to subserve mother–infant bonding, as described by MacLean (95,96). Cingulotomy in humans may cause anorexia, again suggesting that this region is important in eating behavior. These observations suggest that the cingulate cortex and its interconnections with other limbic areas might provide a fruitful area for research on addiction and the eating disorders. To date, most research on the organic basis of anorexia and bulimia has concentrated on hypothalamic neurochemical factors.

In addition, one finds other evidence to suggest that the eating disorders have many features of an addiction. Yates et al. (190) presented an intriguing case for the argument that exercise in the form of "obligatory running" is an analog of anorexia nervosa—the former affecting predominantly males, the latter females. It is an interesting observation that in either group both diet and exercise are common features, regardless which is uppermost. Opioids have been suggested as a factor underlying the motivation for distance running.

Further evidence relevant to the possible role of addictive mechanisms in eating disorders may be found in references to the use of naloxone in the treatment of certain manifestations of anorexia nervosa. Moore et al. (115) claimed that intravenous naloxone infusions in anorexic patients assist weight gain by blocking lipolysis, and in Poland, Baranowska et al. (11) reported that naloxone counteracts amenorrhea in some anorexic women, possibly owing to a resulting increase in luteinizing hormone production. Gillman and Lichtigfeld (45,46) believe the effect of naloxone in anorexia nervosa is probably due to inhibition of an excess production of opioids which might act within noradrenergic systems affecting hypothalamic activity. As anorexic and/or bulimic patients struggle against strong appetite, the observation of Atkinson (9) that naloxone in sufficient doses will decrease food intake in seriously obese subjects adds further support to the idea that a neural substrate containing opiate receptors, such as the cingulate cortex, may play a crucial role in eating disorders. Table 2 attempts to show that many of the behaviors in eating disorders are comparable to those seen in addiction.

Although highly speculative at this time, the suggestion is made here that the starvation of anorexia nervosa, along with the excess eating of bulimia, are essentially forms of addiction involving opiate-sensitive neuronal systems which lie, at least in part, within the thalamocingulate division of the limbic system.

CONCLUSIONS

This chapter has touched upon a diversity of topics, calling on points made in other chapters in this volume while glancing into the literature for other evidence from recent research on the limbic system which has implications for clinical psychiatry. Although some parts of this chapter are highly speculative—the precedent for such speculation having been well established already in the literature (79,94,165)—perhaps the whole will serve to promote the thesis that within the brain, the physiodynamics of the limbic system are critical in a comprehensive approach to modern psychiatry.

We now come back to Livingston's question regarding the "limbic system concept," which was quoted near the beginning of this chapter: "How do the pieces fit together to create a performing whole?" Perhaps that question is closer to finding an answer after this volume.

TABLE 2. *Characteristics of behavior in addiction, anorexia nervosa, and bulimia*

Addiction	Anorexia nervosa	Bulimia
Starts as a compensation or escape—for "pleasure" or relief	Starts as a compensation—escape from "fatness"—weight loss is visually "satisfying"	Starts as consummatory compensatory behavior—provides gratification
Leads to habitual activity such as drinking or drug use	Leads to habitual or ritual eating habits	May become a habit or ritual
Is accompanied by social and family disapproval and secretive behavior	Is accompanied by family disapproval—some secretive behavior	May be regarded as socially unacceptable—some secretive behavior
May replace normal patterns of eating/drinking	Replaces normal eating patterns	Replaces normal eating patterns
Becomes a compulsion	Becomes a compulsion	Becomes a compulsion
May be in opposition to "rational" desires of subject	May be in opposition to "rational" motives of subject	May be in opposition to "rational" motives of subject
Efforts to abstain or withdraw produce extreme tension, fear or anxiety, and resistance	Enforced eating or weight gain may produce extreme tension, fear or anxiety, and resistance	Efforts to abstain may produce tension and resistance
Relapses are frequent	Relapses are frequent	Relapses are frequent
Long-term effects may include depression, social restrictions	Long-term effects may include depression, social restrictions	May interfere with normal social behavior

The neocortex is often thought of as providing what is most essential in human behavior. If one tries to "anatomize" the traditional psychodynamic structure of the personality, it is customary to think of what are called the "ego functions" and the "super-ego" as belonging to the higher levels of cortical development. The so-called "Id" and libidinal drives fit more easily, at first glance, with functions subserved by the limbic system, such as love, hate, aggression, and sexual behavior. The evidence we have examined, however, destroys the illusion that such a simplistic formulation can be applied anatomically or physiologically. The limbic system clearly governs, to a degree greater than is often recognized, the processes of human thought and action that are specialized and uniquely human. The limbic system exerts "superego" controls as well as libidinal drives.

In reference to Livingston's question, the limbic system provides a core for mammalian—including human—interaction between organism and environment. It is crucial to the kind of conceptualization that was put forth by Yakovlev (189) before his own ideas were reshaped through his contacts with Papez and the formulation of the emotional brain. In other words, the modern concept of the limbic system, as originally set forth by MacLean and addressed throughout this volume, figures heavily in Yakovlev's "intermediate system of expression," while spanning as well his "innermost system of visceration" and "outermost system of effectuation."

We can view the limbic system as the part of the brain that had to evolve for mammalian (including human) social behavior *in the biological environment*, whereas the neocortex was essential for the behaviors that characterize *culture* and *civilization*. The limbic system is both a driver and a switchman of higher cortical function. Cortical function without the limbic system would have little relevance to daily survival in a biologically ordered world. Perhaps that is why genius is sometimes divorced from social fitness. Without the limbic system, intellect would know no bounds of reality, for the limbic system plays a major role—although not an exclusive one—in determining whether reason or madness prevails.

REFERENCES

1. Adamec, R. E. (1983): Omega analysis and the discrimination of the therapeutic (psychiatric) response to Tegretol. *Perspect. Psychiatry (Univ. Toronto)*, 2:7–8.
2. Adamec, R. E., and Stark-Adamec, C. (1983): Limbic kindling and animal behavior: implications for human psychopathology associated with complex partial seizures. *Biol. Psychiatry*, 18:269–293.
3. Adamec, R. E., and Stark-Adamec, C. (1985): Limbic hyperfunction, limbic epilepsy, and interictal behavior: models and methods of detection. In: *The Limbic System: Functional Organization and Clinical Disorders*, edited by B. Doane and K. Livingston. Raven Press, New York.
4. Adamec, R. E., Stark-Adamec, C., Saint-Hilaire, J-M., and Livingston, K. E. (1985): Basic science and clinical aspects of procaine HCl as a limbic system excitant. *Prog. Neuropsychopharmacol. Biol. Psychiatry*, 9:109–119.
5. Adolfsson, R., Gottfries, C. G., Oreland, L., Wiberg, A., and Winblad, B. (1980): Increased activity of brain and platelet monoamine oxidase in dementia of Alzheimer type. *Life Sci.*, 27:1029–1034.
6. Albright, P. S., Burnham, W. M., and Livingston, K. E. (1985): Seizure patterns and pharmacological responses in the kindling model. In: *The Limbic System: Functional Organization and Clinical Disorders*, edited by B. Doane and K. Livingston. Raven Press, New York.
7. Angevine, J. B. (1978): Embryogenesis and phylogenesis in the limbic system. In: *Limbic Mechanisms: The Continuing Evolution of the Limbic System Concept*, edited by K. Livingston and O. Hornykiewicz. Plenum Press, New York.
8. Arnold, P. S., Racine, R. J., and Wise, R. A. (1973): Effects of atropine, reserpine, 6-hydroxydopamine, and handling on seizure development in the rat. *Exp. Neurol.*, 40:457–470.
9. Atkinson, R. L. (1982): Naloxone decreases food intake in obese humans. *J. Clin. Endocrinol. Metab.*, 56:196–198.
10. Bäckström, T., Zetterlund, B., Blom, S., and Romano, M. (1984): Effects of intravenous progesterone infusions on the epileptic discharge frequency in women with partial epilepsy. *Acta Nurol. Scand.*, 69:240–248.
11. Baranowska, B., Rozbicka, G., Jeske, W., and Abdel-Fattah, M. H. (1984): The role of endogenous opiates in the mechanism of inhibited lutenizing hormone (LH) secretion in women with anorexia nervosa: the effect of naloxone on LH, follicle-stimulating hormone, prolactin and β-endorphine secretion. *J. Clin. Endocrinol. Metab.*, 59:412–416.
12. Bear, D. M. (1985): Hemispheric asymmetries in emotional function: a reflection of lateral specialization in cortical-limbic connections? In: *The Limbic System: Functional Organization and Clinical Disorders*, edited by B. Doane and K. Livingston. Raven Press, New York.
13. Bear, D. M., and Fedio, T. (1977): Quantitative analysis of interictal behaviour in temporal lobe epilepsy. *Arch. Neurol.*, 34:454–467.
14. Berger, P. A., and Barchas, J. D. (1982): Studies of β-endorphin in psychiatric patients. *Ann. NY Acad. Sci.*, 398:448–459.
15. Betts, T. A. (1981): Depression, anxiety and epilepsy. In: *Epilepsy and Psychiatry*, edited by E. H. Reynolds and M. R. Trimble. Churchill Livingstone, Edinburgh.
16. Bowlby, J. (1973): *Attachment and Loss, Volume II. Separation; Anxiety and Anger*. Hogarth Press, London.

17. Bowlby, J. (1980): *Attachment and Loss, Volume III. Loss; Sadness and Depression.* Hogarth Press, London.
18. Bridges, P. K., and Bartlett, J. R. (1977): Psychosurgery: yesterday and today. *Br. J. Psychiatry,* 131:249–260.
19. Bruens, J. H. (1974): Psychoses in epilepsy. In: *Handbook of Clinical Neurology,* Volume 15, edited by P. J. Vinken and G. W. Bruyn. Elsevier, New York.
20. Burnham, W. M., Niznik, H. B., and Kish, S. J. (1985): Biochemical changes in the limbic system following kindling: assay studies. In: *The Limbic System: Functional Organization and Clinical Disorders,* edited by B. Doane and K. Livingston. Raven Press, New York.
21. Burton, R. (1907): *The Anatomy of Melancholy.* (Original published in 17th century) Reprinted by Chatto and Windus, London.
22. Caplan, G. (1945): Treatment of epilepsy by electrically induced convulsions: a preliminary report. *Br. Med. J.,* (April 14), 511–512.
23. Catlin, D. H., Gorelic, D. A., and Garner, R. H. (1982): Clinical pharmacology of β-endorphins in depression and schizophrenia. *Ann. NY Acad. Sci.,* 398:434–447.
24. Chi, C. C. and Flynn, J. P. (1971): Neuroanatomic projections related to biting attack elicited from hypothalamus in cats. *Brain Res.,* 35:49–66.
25. Chi, C. C., and Flynn, J. P. (1971): Neural pathways associated with hypothalamically elicited attack behaviour in cats. *Science,* 171:703–706.
26. Clouet, D. H. (1982): A biochemical and neurophysiological comparison of opioids and antipsychotics. *Ann. NY Acad. Sci.,* 398:130–139.
27. Curtis, J. (1984): (Dr. John Curtis, Nova Scotia Hospital, Dartmouth, N.S., Canada). *(Personal communication).*
28. Davies, P. (1979): Neurotransmitter related enzymes in senile dementia of the Alzheimer type. *Brain Res.,* 171:319–327.
29. deFleury, M. (1902): *Les grands symptômes neurastheniques (pathogenie et traitement).* Félix Alcan, Paris.
30. Delay, J., Puech, P., and Maillard, J. (1945): Confusion mentale périodique. Resultats de l'électrochoc et d'insufflation ventriculaire. *Ann. Méd. Psychologiques.* (Séance du 11 Juin), 58–60.
31. Devinsky, O., and Bear, D. M. (1984): Varieties of aggressive behavior in temporal lobe epilepsy. *Am. J. Pychiat.,* 141:651–656.
32. Doane, B. K. (1955): Changes in visual function with perceptual isolation. Unpublished Doctoral Thesis, McGill University.
33. Doane, B. K., Longley, W. J., and Cox, K. (1986) Serum estrogen and progesterone levels in relation to premenstrual symptoms. *(in preparation)*
34. Doane, B. K., Mahatoo, W., Heron, W., and Scott, T. H. (1959): Changes in perceptual function after isolation. *Canad. J. Psychol.,* 3:210–219.
35. Emrich, H. M. (1984): Endorphins in Psychiatry. *Psychiatr. Dev.,* 2:97–114.
36. Emrich, H. M., Vogt, P., And Herz, A. (1982): Possible antidepressive effects of opioids: actions of buprenorphine. *Ann. NY Acad. Sci.,* 398:108–112.
37. Erb, A., and Pozniak, J. (1939): Versuch einer Cardiazolbehandlung der Epilepsie. *Z. Gesamte Neurologie.,* 166:581–587.
38. Extein, I., Pottash, A. L. C., and Gold, M. S. (1982): A possible opioid receptor dysfunction in some depressive disorders. *Ann. NY Acad. Sci.,* 398:113–119.
39. Fenton, G. W. (1981): Psychiatric disorders of epilepsy: classification and phenomenology. In: *Epilepsy and Psychiatry,* edited by E. H. Reynolds and M. R. Trimble. Churchill Livingstone, Edinburgh.
40. Ferguson, S. M., Rayport, M., and Corrie, W. S. (1985): Brain correlates of aggressive behavior in temporal lobe epilepsy. In: *The Limbic System: Functional Organization and Clinical Disorders,* edited by B. Doane and K. Livingston. Raven Press, New York.
41. Flor-Henry, P. (1969): Psychosis and temporal lobe epilepsy; a controlled investigation. *Epilepsia,* 10:363–395.
42. Flor-Henry, P. (1976): Lateralized temporal-limbic dysfunction and psychopathology. *Ann. NY Acad. Sci.,* 280:777–795.
43. Flor-Henry, P. (1983): *Cerebral basis of psychopathology.* John Wright, Bristol.
44. Garfinkle, P. E., and Garner, D. M. (1982): *Anorexia Nervosa: a multidimensional perspective.* Brunner/Mazel, New York.

45. Gillman, M. A., and Lichtigfeld, F. J. (1981): Naloxone in anorexia: role of the opiate system. *J. Roy. Soc. Med.*, 74:631–632.
46. Gillman, M. A., and Lichtigfeld, F. J. (1984): Opioid involvement in anorexia nervosa. *S. Afr. Med. J.*, 65:4.
47. Girgis, M. (1978): Neostigmine activated epileptiform discharge in the amygdala: electrographic-behavioral correlations. *Epilepsia*, 19:521–530.
48. Girgis, M. (1980): Paul Maclean and the limbic system of the brain. In: *Limbic Epilepsy and the Dyscontrol Syndrome*, edited by M. Girgis and L. G. Kiloh. Elsevier/North Holland Biomedical Press, Amsterdam.
49. Girgis, M. (1985): Biochemical patterns in limbic circuitry: biochemical-electrophysiological interactions dsplayed by chemitrode techniques. In: *The Limbic System: Functional Organization and Clinical Disorders*, edited by B. Doane and K. Livingston. Raven Press, New York.
50. Girgis, M., and Hofstatter, L. (1979): Amygdala cholinergic hypersensitivity; implications for psychomotor (limbic) seizures and episodic behavior disorders. In: *Modern Concepts in Psychiatric Surgery*. edited by E. R. Hitchcock, R. H. Ballantine Jr. and B. A. Myerson. Elsevier/North Holland Biomedical Press, New York.
51. Gloor, P. (1985): The role of the human limbic system in perception, memory and affect: lessons from temporal lobe epilepsy. *The Limbic System: Functional Organization and Clinical Disorders*. edited by B. Doane nd K. Livingston. Raven Press, New York.
52. Goddard, G. V. (1980): The kindling model of limbic epilesy. In: *Limbic Epilepsy and the Dyscontrol Syndrome*, edited by M. Girgis and L. G. Kiloh. Elsevier/North Holland Biomedical Press, Amsterdam.
53. Goddard, G. V. (1983): Unpublished transcripts of free discussion at International Symposium: Patterns of Limbic System Dysfunction; Seizures, Psychosis and Dyscontrol. Univ. of Toronto, May, 1983.
54. Goddard, G. V., Dragunow, M., Maru, E., and Macleod, K. (1985): Kindling and the forces that oppose it. In: *The Limbic System: Functional Organization and Clinical Disorders*, edited by B. Doane and K. Livingston. Raven Press, New York.
55. Goddard, G. V., McIntyre, D. C., and Leech, C. K. (1969): A permanent change in brain function resulting from daily electrical stimulation. *Exp. Neurol.*, 25:295–329.
56. Gold, M. S., Pottash, A. C., Sweeney, D., Martin, D., and Extein, I. (1982): Antimanic, anti-depressant and antipanic effects of opiates: clinical, neuroanatomical and biochemical evidence. *Ann NY Acad. Sci.*, 398:140–150.
57. Gray, J. A. (1977): Drug effects on fear and frustration: possible limbic site of action of major tranquilizers. In: *Drugs, Neurotransmitters and Behavior: Handbook of Psychopharmacology, Vol. 8*, edited by L. Iversen, S. D. Iversen and S. H. Snyder. Plenum Press, New York.
58. Gray, J. A., Holt, L., and McNaughton, N. (1983): Clinical implications of the experimental pharmacology of the benzodiazepines. In: *The Benzodiazepines: From Molecular Biology to Clinical Practice*, edited by E. Costa. Raven Press, New York.
59. Greaves, G. B. (1980): Multiple personality 165 years after Mary Reynolds. *J. Nerv. Ment. Dis.*, 168:577–596.
60. Gruzelier, J. H. (1983): A critical assessment and integration of lateral asymmetries in schizo-phrenia. in: *Hemisyndromes: Psychobiology, Neurology, Psychiatry*. edited by M. Myslobodsky. Academic Press, New York.
61. Guirard, P., and Mallet, J. (1948): A propos d'un état stuporeux prolongé survenu chez une épileptique et de sa disparition par électro-choc. *Ann. Méd. Psychologiques* (séance du 12 Jan.), 202–204.
62. Halgren, E., Engel, J., Wilson, C. L., Walter, R. D., Squires, N. K., and Crandall, P. H. (1983): Dynamics of the hippocampal contribution to memory: stimulation and recording studies in humans. In: *Neurobiology of the Hippocampus*, edited by W. Seifert. Academic Press, New York.
63. Harlow, H. E., Wadsworth, R. O., and Harlow, M. K. (1965): Total social isolation in monkeys. *Proc. Natl. Acad. Sci. USA*, 54:90–97.
64. Hebb, D. O. (1949): *The Organization of Behavior*. Wiley and Sons, New York.
65. Hebb, D. O. (1984): (Donald O. Hebb, Honorary Professor, Dept. of Psychology, Dalhousie University, Halifax, N.S. Canada) *(personal communication)*.
66. Heimer, L. (1978): The olfactory cortex and the ventral striatum. In: *Limbic Mechanisms: The Continuing Evolution of the Limbic System Concept*, edited by K. Livingston and O. Hornykiewicz. Plenum Press, New York.

67. Henn, F. A., and Nasrallah, H. A. (1982): *Schizophrenia as a Brain Disease*. Oxford University Press, New York.
68. Henriksen, S. J., Chouvet, G., McGinty, J., and Bloom, F. E. (1982): Opioid peptides in the hippocampus: anatomical and physiological considerations. *Ann. NY Acad. Sci.*, 398:207–219.
69. Hirose, S., and Endo, S. (1985): Clinical pictures and courses of four cases of limbic epilepsy: a special reference to their relation to EEG patterns. In: *The Limbic System: Functional Organization and Clinical Disorders*. edited by B. Doane and K. Livingston. Raven Press, New York.
70. Hoebel, B. G. (1984): Neurotransmitters in the control of feeding and its rewards: monoamines, opiates and brain-gut peptides. In: *Eating and its Disorders. Research Publications: Ass'n for Research in Nervous and Mental Disease. Vol. 62*, edited by A. J. Stunkard and E. Stellar. Raven Press, New York.
71. Holzman, P. S. (1983): Smooth pursuit eye movements in psychopathology. *Schizophr. Bull.*, 9:33–36.
72. Hornykiewicz, O. (1982): Brain catecholamines in schizophrenia—a good case for noradrenaline. *Nature*, 299:484–486.
73. Isaacson, R. L. (1982): The Limbic System (2nd ed.). Plenum Press, New York.
74. Kalinowsky, L. B., and Kennedy, F. (1943): Observations in electric shock therapy applied to problems of epilepsy. *J. Nerv. Ment. Dis.*, 98:56–67.
75. Kaufman, I. C. (1973): Mother-infant separation in monkeys: an experimental model. In: *Separation and Depression: Clinical and Research Aspects*, edited by J. P. Scott and E. C. Senay. Westview Press, Washington. Reprinted in J. D. Keehn, *Origins of Madness: Psychopathology in Animal Life*. Pergamon Press, New York.
76. Kaufman, I. C., and Rosenblum, L. A. (1967): The reaction to separation in infant monkeys: anaclitic depression and conservation-withdrawal. *Psychosom. Med.*, 29:648–675.
77. Kelly, D., Richardson, A., and Mitchell-Heggs, N. (1973): Technique and assessment of limbic leucotomy. In: *Surgical Approaches in Psychiatry*, edited by L. V. Laitinen and K. E. Livingston. Medical and Technical Publishing Co., Ltd., Lancaster.
78. Kendall, R. (1968): *The Classification of Depressive Illness* (Institute of Psychiatry; Maudsley Monographs, No. 18). Oxford University Press, London.
79. Kiloh, L. G. (1980): Psychiatric disorders and the limbic system. In: *Limbic Epilepsy and the Dyscontrol Syndrome*, edited by M. Girgis and L. G. Kiloh. Elsevier/North Holland, New York.
80. Kluft, R. P. (1984): An introduction to multiple personality disorder. *Psychiatr. Ann.*, 14:19–24.
81. Knight, G. (1973): Additional stereotactic lesions in the cingulum following failed tractotomy in the subcaudate region. In: *Surgical Approaches in Psychiatry*, edited by L. V. Laitinen and K. E. Livingston. Medical and Technical Publishing Co., Ltd., Lancaster.
82. Koella, W. P. (1984): The limbic system and behavior. *Acta Psychiatr. Scand.*, 69 [*Suppl. 313*]:35–45.
83. Kosterlitz, H. W., and McKnight, A. T. (1980): Endorphins and encephalins. *Adv. Int. Med.*, 26:1–36.
84. Lee, T., Seeman, P., Tourtellotte, W. W., and Farley, I. J., and Hornykiewicz, O. (1978): Binding of ³H-neuroleptics and ³H-apomorphine in schizophrenic brains. *Nature*, 274:897.
85. Livingston, K. E. (1977): Limbic system dysfunction induced by "kindling"; its significance for psychiatry. In: *Neurosurgical Treatment in Psychiatry, Pain and Epilepsy*, edited by W. H. Sweet, S. Obrador and J. G. Martin-Rodriguez. University Park Press, Baltimore.
86. Livingston, K. E. (1978): The experimental-clinical interface: kindling as a dynamic model of induced limbic system dysfunction. In: *Limbic Mechanisms: The Continuing Evolution of the Limbic System Concept*, edited by K. E. Livingston and O. Hornykiewicz. Plenum Press, New York.
87. Livingston, K. E. (1980): Limbic connections: the limbic system as a substrate for epileptic disorder. In: *Limbic Epilepsy and the Dyscontrol Syndrome*. edited by M. Girgis and L. G. Kiloh. Elsevier/North Holland Biomedical Press, Amsterdam.
88. Livingston, K. E., and Escobar, A. (1973): Tentative limbic system model for certain patterns of psychiatric disorders. In: *Surgical Approaches in Psychiatry*, edited by V. Laitinen and K. E. Livingston Medical and Technical Publishing Co., Ltd. Lancaster.
89. Livingston, R. B. (1978): A casual glimpse of evolution and development relating to the limbic system. In: *Limbic Mechanisms: The Continuing Evolution of the Limbic System Concept*, edited by K. E. Livingston and O. Hornykiewicz. Plenum Press, New York.

90. Logre, B. J. (1949): Epilepsie et intermittence. La notion de l'électro-choc préventif. *Sem. Hôp. Paris*, 25:3622–3623.
91. Ludwig, A. M. (1972): Hysteria—a neurobiological theory. *Arch. Gen. Psychiatry*, 27:771–777.
92. MacLean, P. D. (1949): Psychosomatic disease and the "visceral brain": recent developments bearing on the Papez theory of emotion. *Psychosom. Med.*, 11:338–353.
93. MacLean, P. D. (1952): Some psychiatric implications of physiological studies on frontotemporal portion of limbic system (visceral brain). *EEG Clin. Neurophysiol.*, 4:407–418.
94. MacLean, P. D. (1973): *A Triune Concept of the Brain and Behavior.* (Hincks Memorial Lectures, 1969), edited by T. Boag and D. Campbell. Univ. of Toronto Press, Toronto.
95. MacLean, P. D. (1985): Brain evolution relating to family, play and the separation call. *Arch Gen. Psychiatry*, 42:405–417.
96. MacLean, P. D. (1985): Culminating developments in the evolution of the limbic system. In: *The Limbic System: Functional Organization and Clinical Disorders.* edited by B. K. Doane and K. E. Livingston. Raven Press, New York.
97. McKinney, W. T., and Bunney, W. E. (1969): Animal models of depression, I. Review of evidence: implications for research. Arch. Gen. Psychiatry, 21:240–248. Reprinted in: *Origins of Madness: Psychopathology in Animal Life.* edited by J. D. Keehn. Pergamon Press, Oxford.
98. McNaughton, N., and Mason, S. T. (1980): The neuropsychology and neuropharmacology of the dorsal ascending noradrenergic bundle—a review. *Prog. Neurobiol.*, 14:157–219.
99. Merskey, H. (1979): *The Analysis of Hysteria.* Baillière Tindall, London.
100. Mesulam, M. M. (1981): Dissociative states with abnormal temporal lobe EEG: multiple personality and the delusion of possession. *Arch. Neurol.*, 38:176–181.
101. Meyer, G., McElhaney, M., Martin, W., and McGraw, C. P. (1973): Stereotactic cingulotomy with results of acute stimulation and psychological testing. In: *Surgical Approaches in Psychiatry*, edited by L. V. Laitinen and K. E. Livingston. Medical and Technical Publishing Co., Ltd., Lancaster.
102. Meyerson, B. J., and Eliasson, M. (1977): Pharmacological and hormonal control of reproductive behavior. In: *Handbook of Psychopharmacology, Vol. 8: Drugs, Neurotransmitters and Behavior*, edited by L. L. Iversen, S. D. Iversen, and S. H. Snyder. Plenum Press, New York.
103. Michaux, L., Buge, A., and Lebourges, J. (1955): Accès confuso-oniriques répétés chez une épileptique. Déclenchement des accès après crises convulsives spontanées. Action favorable de la sismothérapie. *Ann. Méd. Psycholog.*, 113:873–879.
104. Michaux, L., Escourolle, R., Widlocher, D., and Saulnier, M. (1955): Epilepsie temporale séquelle de'encéphalopathie infantile. Etat obtusionnel quasi-schizophrénique. Intercurrence de phases oniriques et de phases obsessionnelles. Rémissions exclusivement sismothérapiques. *Ann. Méd. Psycholog.*, 113:266–272.
105. Michaux, L., and Tison, M. (1943): Etat confuso-onirique prolongé post-critique chez une épileptique. Guérison par l'électro-choc. *Ann. Méd. Psycholog.*, (séance du 26 Mai) 103–107.
106. Milner, B. (1970): Memory and the medial temporal regions of the brain. In: *Biology of Memory*, edited by K. H. Pribram and D. E. Broadbent. Academic Press, New York.
107. Milner, B. (1972): Disorders of learning and memory after temporal lobe lesions in man. *Clin. Neurosurg.*, 19:421–446.
108. Mitchell-Heggs, N., Kelly, D., and Richardson, A. E. (1977): Stereotactic limbic leucotomy: clinical, psychological and physiological assessment at 16 months. In: *Neurosurgical Treatment in Psychiatry, Pain and Epilepsy.* edited by W. H. Sweet, S. Obrador and J. G. Martin-Rodriguez. University Park Press, Baltimore.
109. Mitsuda, H., and Fukuda, T. (1974): *Biological Mechanisms of Schizophrenia and Schizophrenia-like Psychoses.* Igaku Shoin, Ltd., Tokyo.
110. Mogenson, G. J., Jones, D. L., and Yim, C. Y. (1980): From motivation to action: functional interface between the limbic system and motor system. *Prg. Neurobiol.*, 14:69–97.
111. Möhler, H., and Richards, J. G. (1983): Benzodiazepine receptors in the central nervous system. In: *The Benzodiazepines From Molecular Biology to Clinical Practice.* edited by E. Costa. Raven Press, New York.
112. Monroe, R. R. (1970): *Episodic Behavioral Disorders.* Harvard Univ. Press, Cambridge.
113. Monroe, R. R. (1974): Episodic psychotic reactions: an unclassified syndrome. In: *Biological Mechanisms of Schizophrenia and Schizophrenia-like Psychoses*, edited by H. Mitsuda and T. Fukuda. Igaku Shoin, Ltd., Tokyo.
114. Monroe, R. R. (1985): Episodic behavioral disorders and limbic ictus. In: *The Limbic System:*

Functional Organization and Clinical Disorders, edited by B. Doane and K. Livingston. Raven Press, New York.

115. Moore, R., Mills, I. H., and Forster, A. (1981): Naloxone in the treatment of anorexia nervosa: effect of weight gain and lipolysis. *J. Roy. Soc. Med.*, 74:129–131.

116. Munro, A. (1982): Delusional hypochondriasis: a description of monosymptomatic hypochondriacal psychosis (MHP). *Clark Institute of Psychiatry Monograph Series, No. 5*, Toronto.

117. Murphy, D. L., and Wyatt, R. S. (1972): Reduced monoamine oxidase activity in blood platelets from bipolar depressed patients. *Am. J. Psychiatry*, 128:1351–1357.

118. Murphy, D. L., and Wyatt, R. S. (1972): Reduced monoamine oxidase activity in blood platelets from schizophrenic patients. *Nature*, 238:225–226.

119. Myslobodsky, M. S., Mintz, M., and Tomer, R. (1983): Neuroleptic effects and the site of abnormality in schizophrenia. In: *Hemisyndromes: Psychobiology, Neurology, Psychiatry*. edited by M. S. Myslobodsky. Academic Press, New York.

120. Nauta, H. J. W. (1985): A simplified perspective on the basal ganglia and their relation to the limbic system. In: *The Limbic System: Functional Organization and Clinical Disorders*, edited by B. Doane and K. Livingston. Raven Press, New York.

121. Nauta, W. J. H. (1958): Hippocampal projections and related neural pathways to the midbrain in the cat. *Brain*, 81:319–340.

122. Nauta, W. J. H. (1985): Circuitous connections linking cerebral cortex, limbic system and corpus striatum. In: *The Limbic System: Functional Organization and Clinical Disorders*, edited by B. Doane and K. Livingston. Raven Press, New York.

123. Newman, J. D., and MacLean, P. D. (1982): Effects of tegmental lesions on the isolation call of squirrel monkeys. *Brain Res.*, 232:317–330.

124. Newmark, M. E., and Penry, J. K. (1980): Catamenial epilepsy: a review. *Epilepsia*, 21:281–300.

125. Olton, D. S. (1983): Memory functions and the hippocampus. In: *Neurobiology of the Hippocampus*, edited by W. Seifert. Academic Press, New York.

126. Panksepp, J., Meeker, R. and Bean, N. J. (1980): The neurochemical control of crying. *Pharmacol. Biochem. Behav.*, 12:437–443.

127. Panksepp, J., Vilberg, T., Bean, N. J., Coy, D. H., and Kastin, A. J. (1978): Reduction of stress vocalization in chicks by opiate-like peptides. *Brain Res. Bull.*, 3:663–667.

128. Papez, J. W. A. (1937): A proposed mechanism of emotion. *Arch. Neurol. Psychiatry*, 38:725–743.

129. Pavlov, I. P. (1932): Essay on the physiological concept of the symptomatology of hysteria. In: *I.P. Pavlov: Psychopathology and Psychiatry—Selected Works*, edited by Y. Popov and L. Rokhlin. Foreign Languages Publishing House, Moscow.

130. Pinel, J. P. J., Treit, D., and Rovner, L. I. (1977): Temporal lobe aggression in rats. *Science*, 197:1088–1089.

131. Pond, D. A. (1957): Psychiatric aspects of epilepsy. *J. Ind. Med. Prof.*, 3:1441–1451; cited by Toone, B., Psychoses of epilepsy In: *Epilepsy and Psychiatry*, edited by E. H. Reynolds and M. R. Trimble. 1981. Churchill Livingstone, Edinburgh.

132. Post, R. M. (1985): Does limbic system dysfunction play a role in affective illness? In: *The Limbic System: Functional Organization and Clinical Disorders*, edited by B. Doane and K. Livingston. Raven Press, New York.

133. Post, R. M., and Ballenger, J. C. (1981): Kindling models for the progressive development of psychopathology: sensitization to electrical, pharmacological and psychological stimuli. In: *Handbook of Biological Psychiatry, Part IV: Brain Mechanisms and Abnormal Behavior-Chemistry*, edited by H. M. van Praag. Marcel Dekker, Inc., New York.

134. Post, R. M., and Uhde, T. W. (1985): Carbamazepine in the treatment of affective disorders. In: *The Limbic System: Functional Organization and Clinical Disorders*, edited by B. Doane and K. Livingston. Raven Press, New York.

135. Post, R. M., Uhde, T. W., and Wolff, E. A. (1984): Profile of clinical efficacy and side effects of carbamazepine in psychiatric illness: relationship to blood and CSF levels of carbamazepine and its 10, 11-epoxide metabolite. *Acta Psychiat. Scand.*, 69[Suppl. 313]:104–120.

136. Post, R. M., Weiss, S. R. B., and Pert, A. (1985): Differential effects of carbamazepine and lithium on sensitization and kindling. *Prog. Neuropsychopharmacol. Biol. Psychiatry*, 8:425–434.

137. Putnam, F. W. (1984): The psychophysiologic investigation of multiple personality disorder: a review. *Psychiat. Clin. North Am.*, 7:31–39.

138. Putnam, F. W. (1984): The study of multiple personality disorder: general strategies and practical considerations. *Psychiatr. Ann.*, 14:58–61.
139. Racine, R., and McIntyre, D. (1985): Mechanisms of kindling: a current view. In: *The Limbic System: Functional Organization and Clinical Disorders*, edited by B. Doane and K. Livingston. Raven Press, New York.
140. Rayport, M., Ferguson, S. M., and Corrie, W. S. (1985): Contributions of cerebral depth recording and electrical stimulation to the clarification of seizure patterns and behavior disturbances in patients with temporal lobe epilepsy. In: *The Limbic System: Functional Organization and Clinical Disorders*, edited by B. Doane and K. Livingston. Raven Press, New York.
141. Reid, R. L., and Yen, S. S. C. (1981): Premenstrual syndrome. *Am. J. Obstet. Gynecol.*, 139:85–104.
142. Rémillard, G. M., Andermann, F., Testa, G. F., Gloor, P., Aubé, M., Martin, J. B., Feindel, W., Guberman, A., and Simpson, C. (1983): Sexual ictal manifestations predominate in women with temporal lobe epilepsy: a finding suggesting sexual dimorphism in the human brain. *Neurology*, 33:323–330.
143. Reynolds, G. P. (1983): Increased concentrations and lateral asymmetry of amygdala dopamine in schizophrenia. *Nature*, 305:527–529.
144. Reynolds, G. P. (1984): Lateral asymmetry of amygdala dopamine in schizophrenia. *Canad. Coll. Neuropsychopharmacol. Abstracts.* Seventh Annual Scientific Meeting, Halifax, p. 35.
145. Reynolds, G. P. (1984): Phenylethylamine in mental and neurological disorders. *Canad. Coll. Neuropsychopharmacol. Abstracts.* Seventh Annual Scientific Meeting, Halifax, p. 58.
146. Robertson, H. A. (1979): Benzodiazepine receptors in 'emotional' and 'nonemotional' mice: comparison of four strains. *Europ. J. Pharmacol.*, 56:163–166.
147. Robertson, H. A. (1984): Epilepsy, kindling and the schizophrenias. *Canad. Coll. Neuropsychopharmacol. Abstracts.* Seventh Annual Scientific Meeting, Halifax, p. 56.
148. Robertson, H. A., Martin, I. L., and Candy, J. M. (1978): Differences in benzodiazepine receptor binding in Maudsley reactive and Maudsley non-reactive rats. *Europ. J. Pharmacol.*, 50:455–457.
149. Robinson, L. (1943): Electroshock therapy for psychotic epileptic. *Dis. Nerv. Syst.*, 4:253–255.
150. Rondepierre, J., and Vié, J. (1943): Essais de traitement de l'épilepsie par l'électro-choc. *Rev. Neurol.*, (séance du 3 Dec, 1942) p. 329.
151. Rossor, M. N., Emson, P. C., Iversen, L. L., Mountjoy, C. O., Roth, M., Fahrenkrug, J., and Rehfeld, J. F. (1982): Neuropeptides and neurotransmitters in cerebral cortex in Alzheimer's Disease. In: *Aging, Vol. 19. Alzheimer's Disease: A Report of Progress in Research.* edited by S. Corkin, K. L. Davis, J. H. Growdon, E. Usdin, and R. J. Wurtman. Raven Press, New York.
152. Sal y Rosas, F. (1939): El tratamiento de la epilepsia por el cardiazol. *Rev. Neuropsiquiatr.*, 2:81–99.
153. Sargent, W., and Slater, E. (1972): *Treatment in Psychiatry*, (5th edition). Churchill Livingstone, London.
154. Schenk, L., and Bear, D. M. (1981): Multiple personality and related dissociative states in patients with temporal lobe epilepsy. *Am. J. Psychiatry*, 138:1311–1316.
155. Schulz, R., Wüster, M., Duka, T., and Herz, A. (1980): Acute and chronic ethanol treatment changes endorphin levels in brain and pituitary. *Psychopharmacology*, 68:221–227.
156. Scott, D. W. (1983): Alcohol and food abuse: some comparisons. *Br. J. Addiction*, 78:339–349.
157. Scott, J. P. (1974): Effects of psychotropic drugs on separation distress in dogs. *Proc. IX Int. Cong. Neuropsychopharmacology*, (Excerpta Medica International Congress Series No. 359).
158. Seeman, P., Lee, T., Chau-Wong, M., and Wong, K. (1976): Antipsychotic drug doses and neuroleptic/dopamine receptors. *Nature*, 261:717–719.
159. Seizinger, B. R., Bovermann, K., Maysinger, D., Höllt, V., and Herz, A. (1983): Differential effects of acute and chronic ethanol treatment on particular opioid peptide systems in discrete regions of rat brain and pituitary. *Pharmacol. Biochem. Behav.*, 18[Suppl. 1]:361–369.
160. Sherwin, I. (1980): Specificity of psychopathy in epilepsy, significance of lesion laterality. In: *Limbic Epilepsy and the Dyscontrol Syndrome*, edited by M. Girgis and L. G. Kiloh. Elsevier/North Holland Biomedical Press, Amsterdam.
161. Sherwin, I. (1984): Differential psychiatric features in epilepsy; relationship to lesion laterality. *Acta Psychiat. Scand.*, 69[Suppl. 313]:92–103.
162. Silberman, E. K., and Post, R. M. (1980): The march of symptoms in a psychotic decompensation: case report and theoretic implications. *J. Nerv. Ment. Dis.*, 168:104–110.

163. Slater, E., Beard, A. W., and Glitheroe, E. (1963): The schizophrenia-like psychoses of epilepsy, Parts i-v. *Br. J. Psychiatry*, 109:95–105.
164. Slater, E., and Moran, P. (1969): The schizophrenia-like psychoses of epilepsy: relation between ages of onset. *Br. J. Psychiatry*, 115:599–600.
165. Smythies, J. R., Adey, W. R., Brady, J. V., and Walter, W. G. (1966): *The Neurological Foundations of Psychiatry*. Blackwell Scientific Publications, Oxford.
166. Solomon, P., Kubzansky, P. E., Leiderman, P. H., Mendelson, J. H., Trumbell, R., and Wexler, D. (1961): *Sensory deprivation: a symposium held at Harvard Medical School*. Harvard Univ. Press, Cambridge.
167. Squire, L. R. (1983): The hippocampus and the neuropsychology of memory. In: *Neurobiology of the Hippocampus*, edited by W. Seifert. Academic Press, New York.
168. Squire, L. R., and Zola-Morgan, S. (1983): The neurology of memory: the case for correspondence between human and non-human primate. In: *The Physiological Basis of Memory*, edited by J. A. Deutsch. Academic Press, New York.
169. Stark-Adamec, C., and Adamec, R. E. (1983): Psychological methodology versus clinical impressions: different perspectives on psychopathology and seizures. Chapter 18. In: *The Limbic System: Functional Organization and Clinical Disorders*. edited by B. Doane and K. Livingston. Raven Press, New York.
170. Stark-Adamec, C., Adamec, R. E., Graham, J. M., Bruun-Meyer, S., Perrin, R. G., Pollock, D., and Livingston, K. E. (1982): Analysis of facial displays and verbal report to assess subjective state in the non-invasive detection of limbic system activation by procaine hydrochloride. *Behav. Brain Res.*, 4:77–94.
171. Stitt, S. L., and Kinnard, W. J. (1968): The effect of certain progestins on the threshold of electrically-induced seizure patterns. *Neurology*, 18:213–216.
172. Swanson, L. W. (1983): The hippocampus and the concept of the limbic system. In: *Neurobiology of the Hippocampus*, edited by W. Seifert. Academic Press, New York.
173. Tatesu, S. (1974): On histologic findings in schizophrenia and schizophrenic state. In: *Biological Mechanisms of Schizophrenia and Schizophrenia-like Psychoses*. edited by H. Mitsuda and T. Fukuda. Igaku Shoin, Ltd. Tokyo.
174. Taylor, J. H. (1943): Complications of and contraindications to electroshock therapy. *Arch. Neurol. Psychiatry*, 49:789–790.
175. Taylor, J. H. (1946): Control of grand mal epilepsy with electroshock. *Dis. Nerv. Syst.*, 7:284–285.
176. Toone, B. (1981): Psychoses of epilepsy. In: *Epilepsy and Psychiatry*, edited by E. H. Reynolds and M. R. Trimble. Churchill Livingstone, Edinburgh.
177. Toone, B. K., Garralda, M. E., and Ron, M. A. (1982): The psychoses of epilepsy and the functional psychoses: a clinical and phenomenological comparison. *Br. J. Psychiatry*, 141:256–261.
178. Trimble, M. R. (1984): Interictal psychoses of epilepsy. *Acta Psychiatr. Scand.*, 69[Suppl. 313]9–19.
179. Trimble, M. R. (1985): Radiological studies in epileptic psychosis. Chapter 15. In: *The Limbic System: Functional Organization and Clinical Disorders*. edited by B. Doane and K. Livingston. Raven Press, New York.
180. Volavka, J., Anderson, B., and Koz, G. (1982): Naloxone and naltrexone in mental illness and tardive dyskinesia. *Ann. NY Acad. Sci.*, 398:97–102.
181. Walker, R. F., and Wilson C. A. (1983): Changes in hypothalamic serotonin associated with amplification of LH surges by progesterone in rats. *Neuroendocrinology*, 37:200–205.
182. Whalen, R. E. and Luttge, W. G. (1971): Differential localization of progesterone uptake in brain. Role of sex, estrogen pretreatment and adrenolectomy. *Brain Res.*, 33:147–155.
183. Winblad, B., Adolffson, R., Carlsson, A., and Gottfries, C. G. (1982): Biogenic amines in brains of patients with Alzheimer's Disease. In: *Aging, Vol. 19. Alzheimer's Disease: A Report of Progress in Research*, edited by S. Corkin, K. L. Davis, J. H. Growdon, E. Usdin, R. J. Wurtman. Raven Press, New York.
184. Wise, S. P., and Herkenham, M. (1982): Opiate receptor distribution in the cerebral cortex of the rhesus monkey. *Science*, 218:387–389.
185. Wolff, G. E. (1956): Electroconvulsive treatment—a help for epileptics. *Am. Practitioner Dig. Treatment*, 7:1791–1793.

186. Wolff, P. H. (1969): The natural history of crying and other vocalizations in early infancy. In: *Determinants of Infant Behavior IV*, edited by B. M. Foss. Methuen & Co., Ltd., London.

187. Wyatt, R. J., Murphy, D. L., Belmaker, R., Cohen, S., Donnelly, C. H., and Pollin, W. (1973): Reduced monoamine oxidase activity in platelets: A possible genetic marker for vulnerability to schizophrenia. *Science*, 179:916–918.

188. Yakovlev, P. I. (1948): Motility, behavior and the brain: stereodynamic organization and neural co-ordinates of behavior. *J. Nerv. Ment. Dis.*, 107:313–335.

189. Yakovlev, P. I. (1978): Recollections of James Papez and comments on the evolution of limbic system concept. In: *Limbic Mechanisms: The Continuing Evolution of the limbic System Concept*, edited by K. E. Livingston and O. Hornykiewicz. Plenum Press, New York.

190. Yates, A., Leehey, K., and Shisslak, C. M. (1983): Running—an analogue of anorexia? *N. Engl. J. Med.*, 308:251–255.

191. Zigmond, R. E., and McEwen, B. S. (1970): Selective retention of oestradiol by cell nuclei in specific brain regions of the overiectomized rat. *J. Neurochem.*, 17:889–899.

The Limbic System: Functional Organization and Clinical Disorders, edited by B. K. Doane and K. E. Livingston. Raven Press, New York © 1986.

Epilogue: Reflections on James Wenceslas Papez, According to Four of His Colleagues (Compiled by Kenneth E. Livingston*)

Robert B. Livingston

Department of Neuroscience, University of California at San Diego, La Jolla, California 92093

Kenneth Livingston had intended to present a paper in tribute to James W. Papez at the symposium on which this volume is based, but he was unable to attend because of illness. Ken was interested primarily in what the antecedents were to Papez's 1937 paper (15), why Papez did not pursue the problem further, and why Papez's theory of emotion, which enjoys considerable prominence now, took several years to attract attention. Ken's paper was to have been based in part on material from approximately a dozen personal interviews that he conducted from 1981 to 1982 with people who had had close professional contact with Papez. Transcriptions from four of those whom Ken interviewed (*Paul C. Bucy*, neurosurgeon; *Webb Haymaker*, neuropathologist; *Paul D. MacLean*, neurophysiologist; and *William Stotler*, neuroanatomist) were made available to Ken's brother, Robert B. Livingston, M.D., who edited them for this epilogue, and they are presented here.

INTERVIEW WITH PAUL C. BUCY, M.D.†

P.C.B.: When we witnessed the symptomatology that developed when we removed both temporal lobes in the monkey, we wanted to determine the extent of the extirpations and corresponding degenerations. So we sectioned all of the brains serially and stained alternate sections for myelin and cells. I studied all the material and reached conclusions as to what anatomical changes had taken place, and they were extensive.

When I got in touch with Papez and asked if he would contribute to this study, he replied, "Of course!" I gathered all the material together and took it down to Ithaca to go over it with him. I spent a week there discussing with Papez the slides and their interpretation in light of the symptomatology exhibited by the monkeys.

When questions came up, Papez would get out his slide material, animal and human. We would go over all this together and analyze it to establish just what

---

*Deceased.

†P.O. Box 1457, Tryon, North Carolina 28782. (Interviewed in Boston, 8 April 1981.)

anatomical changes were manifested in our series of monkeys. We were able to establish firm conclusions as to what the changes were. Although I had contact with Papez thereafter, from time to time, there was nothing as detailed or prolonged as that first visit.

Papez was very cordial and receptive, but he was a strange man in many ways. At first glance, he impressed you as being a farmer rather than a scientist. Although distinguished people—like Mettler—studied with Papez, by and large he worked alone, even when he was training graduate students. He was distinctly a loner.

K.E.L.: Did he talk with you about his paper on emotion? (15).

P.C.B.: Oh, yes. Of course, that was the main reason I went there.

K.E.L.: As far as we can determine, he made no reference to that paper in any of his later publications, from 1937 through 1951, when he retired.

P.C.B.: He probably thought he had said it all.

K.E.L.: Papez's paper came out at a time when there was growing concern about surgical interventions in patients with mental illness. Moniz (14) first published on frontal lobotomy in Europe in 1935 and 1936. For some reason, there was little response. Do you think that people were not interested, or perhaps that they disagreed with Moniz?

P.C.B.: No, no. Neither. Some may have disagreed with doing lobotomy, but they accepted Moniz's thesis that mental processes were affected by lobotomy, and that mental symptoms might be appropriately ameliorated.

The same thing was true when [Heinrich] Klüver and I presented our temporal lobe studies to the faculty at the University of Chicago. This was an informal group known as the Neurology Club. It consisted of people at the University of Chicago who were interested in the nervous system in one way or another. There was Ajax Carlsson, Ralph Gerard, Arno Luckhart, C. Judson Herrick, Ben Kling, George Bartholmetz, and clinicians Roy Drinker, Percival Bailey, Earl Walker, and myself. It was a stimulating group.

Each month we would meet, and one of the group would present work in progress or completed work, and the rest would give it hell. I recall that when we presented this material on bilateral temporal lobectomy, Arno Luckhart said, "This is incredible. You have created psychopathic disease!"

Well, that was the trouble: We had! Or course the psychologists didn't like that, and most of the psychiatrists didn't believe that emotional diseases, psychiatric disorders, had any organic basis. They weren't about to buy it. This was absolutely contrary to their beliefs. It was received by them on a very emotional basis, but it was received.

I'm sure that Papez experienced the same thing. The difference was that Papez had an hypothesis, a good, sound idea. But we had lesions in monkeys and reproducible changes in their behavior.

When we started out, we were not trying to find out what removal of the temporal lobe would do, or what changes in behavior of the monkeys it would produce. What we found out was completely unexpected! Heinrich had been experimenting with mescaline. He had even taken it himself and had experienced hallucinations. He had written a book about mescaline and its effects (9,10). Later, Heinrich gave mescaline to his monkeys. He gave everything to his monkeys, even his lunch! He noticed that the monkeys acted as though they experienced paraesthesias in their lips. They licked, bit, and chewed their lips. So he came to me and said, "Maybe we can find out where mescaline has its action in the brain." So I said, "OK."

We began by doing a sensory denervation of the face, but that didn't make any difference to the mescaline-induced behavior. So we tried motor denervation. That didn't make any difference, either. Then we had to sit back and think hard about *where to look*. I said to Heinrich, "This business of licking and chewing the lips is not unlike what you see in cases of temporal lobe epilepsy. Patients chew and smack their lips inordinately. So, let's take out the uncus." Well, we could just as well take out the whole temporal lobe, including the uncus. So we did.

We were especially fortunate with our first animal. This was an older female that had been in the laboratory of George Bartholmetz. She had become vicious—absolutely nasty. She was the most vicious animal you ever saw: It was dangerous to go near her. If she didn't hurt you, she would at least tear your clothing. She was the first animal on which we operated. I removed one temporal lobe (we found out later that it didn't matter which temporal lobe you took out first). The next morning my phone was ringing like mad. It was Heinrich, who asked, "Paul, what did you do to my monkey? She is tame!" Subsequently, in operating on nonvicious animals, the taming effect was never so obvious.

That stimulated our getting the other temporal lobe out as soon as we could evaluate her. When we removed the other temporal lobe, the whole syndrome blossomed.

K.E.L.: That, of course, was what became known as the *Klüver–Bucy syndrome*, a remarkable example of serendipity—something important yet entirely unexpected developing from Klüver's curiosity about mescaline!

P.C.B.: We never returned to the mescaline problem. The temporal lobe business took up so much of our time and attention that we couldn't get back to that again.

Papez was fascinated with that whole story. He relished the temporal lobes. He had lots of relevant human pathological and animal comparative material that we could refer to. He was so familiar with his material that he could walk over and pick out a particular box and particular slide that he knew dealt with the certain pathway pertinent to the problem we wanted to comprehend.

You knew, of course, that he had a remarkable collection of brains of distinguished people: the Burt Green Collection. These were brains of prominent scientists, politicians, etc.; people who had shown some unusual intellectual capability one way or another. The assumption was that it would be possible to find out on what basis of brain structure they might be exceptional. What was surprising was that each of those brains had some abnormality, a small infarct here or there, evidence of old trauma, or something else. Whether there were characterological distinctions or not, Papez could nevertheless study the effects of those lesions.

K.E.L.: You suggested that something akin to Papez's ideas about brain mechanisms relating to emotion had been implicated earlier by C. Judson Herrick.

P.C.B.: Yes. Papez pointed out in his 1937 paper (15) that Herrick and others recognized that the medial wall of the cerebral hemisphere in lower vertebrates is functionally related to the hypothalamus and that the lateral wall is similarly related to the dorsal thalamus.

Herrick's formulation (7) was based on anatomical observations, and it lacked physiological or psychological evidence. People knew little about functional neuroanatomy, and a theoretical formulation with implications for visceral or emotional control didn't impress them. Herrick's evidence was based on animal work and appeared in an anatomical journal that did not have much impact on clinical thinking. Papez was additionally concerned with incorporating psychological and clinical evidence relating to emotion.

K.E.L.: I wonder where the great schism between neurology and psychiatry arose? Hughlings Jackson, David Ferrier (2), and other leaders in neurology in England and on the continent, and S. Wier Mitchell in the U.S., tried to include all mental and psychological phenomena with the brain as manifestations of brain functions. What interfered with that monistic view of the brain?

P.C.B.: Ignorance, largely. Don't blame Freud for all of that: Freud was just the tail on the donkey. His acceptance and popularity put a final kibosh on the idea that the brain organ produced ideation, emotion, and behavior.

Have you read Percival Bailey's book on Freud? Bailey read carefully everything in German, French, and English that Freud had published. He wrote a critical appraisal of Freud's interpretations and called it *Sigmund the Unserene* (1). Bailey's book is also available in a French translation, including a preface written by a Frenchman which is not in the English version.

K.E.L.: I wonder how much Sherrington had to do with the schism between psychiatry, psychology, and neurology? He claimed that mental processes could not be examined in terms of energy, and therefore that [the] mind moves more ghostly than a ghost.[1]

Sherrington's mind–brain commentaries were written late in life, e.g., *Man on His Nature* (16). Sherrington was a revered figure and carried great influence. Some of his students, e.g., Wilder Penfield and Jack Eccles, took much the same position.[2]

Do you suppose that a return to Cartesian dualism was favored by the pessimism experienced during Sherrington's lifetime, which arose from the fact that the new

---

[1]Sherrington's position was enunciated prior to anyone's recognition that *information* is neither matter nor energy, it is an emergent property of highly complex systems and is mutually interactive with matter and energy. [R.B.L.]

[2]The separation between psychological and neurological approaches, which assumed total disparateness and incommensurability between brain and mind, was not so evident in the thinking of the leaders of the preceding generation, although that had been the celebrated view of Rene Descartes in the seventeenth century. [R.B.L.]

microscopic neuroanatomy did not immediately reveal anatomical correlates of mental illness?[3]

Do you think that the split was perhaps also influenced by pessimism following comparable technical advances in neurophysiology?[4]

Ebbe Hoff told me that when he was working in Sherrington's laboratory, he expressed an interest in learning more about Pavlov's work and even in going to Russia to visit Pavlov's laboratory. Sherrington replied, "If it is just a matter of curiosity, that's all right, but if you are doing that because you are interested in physiology of the nervous system, it's a waste of time."

You worked in John Fulton's laboratory at Yale. Perhaps you saw the two famous chimpanzees, Becky and Lucy?

P.C.B.: Yes, I knew Becky and Lucy. Fulton (4) reported on them in London at the *International Neurological Congress* in 1935. They had become neurotic at the time I was in Fulton's lab in 1933. Carlyle Jacobsen was doing discrimination testing with them and was making the tests progressively more difficult. The choices became so difficult that finally the chimps broke down. They refused to go into the testing room. They would lie down on the floor, throw themselves around, and have temper tantrums, just like small children. They would bite and scratch and fuss to avoid being tested.

Fulton removed their frontal lobes. Their behavior immediately smoothed out. But, unexpectedly, they were neither better nor worse in performing the tests than they had been before. They made the same mistakes, *only now they weren't emotionally bothered by their failures.* They would perform the tests at about the same failure rate, but they simply didn't mind making errors. This is what attracted Egaz Moniz. He said, *"If you can do that for chimpanzees, why wouldn't it work on my compulsive and overanxious patients?"*

INTERVIEW WITH WEBB HAYMAKER, M.D.*

K.E.L.: There is a bit of contrast between Paul Yakovlev's experience at Harvard and James Papez's experience at Cornell. Neither university wanted them to take their slide materials and specimens with them when they retired. Yakovlev fortunately was able to move his entire collection, two tons of mounted whole human brain sections, to the Armed Forces Institute of Pathology, in Washington, D.C., and to continue working with the collection.

---

[3]When the microtome was invented and aniline dyes were introduced in the nineteenth century, there was immediate hope that mental illnesses could soon be explained on the basis of anticipated anatomical differences. Therefore a number of distinguished neuroanatomists and neurophathologists were put in charge of mental hospitals. Sherrington himself was an excellent histologist; in fact, he invariably combined structure and function in research and teaching (e.g., by insisting on having histology and physiology taught in the same department). [R.B.L.]

[4]Electrical stimulation and methods of recording (the EEG, the cathode ray oscilloscope, and other instruments) could localize physiological processes in space and time much better but did not apparently reveal mental processes or emotions or mechanisms of subjective control of behavior. [R.B.L.]

*16181 Greenwood Lane, Los Gatos, California 95030. (Interviewed in Los Gatos, 18 March 1981.)

Cornell apparently would not let Papez take his slide materials and specimens with him when he left. A great deal of his collection was later lost or destroyed. Some of it ended up in the Museum of Medicine at Cincinnati. This was accomplished through intercessions by A. R. Vonderahe, with the assistance of Frank Mayfield.

W.H.: Papez wasn't fully appreciated at Cornell. He left, as you know, before retirement.

K.E.L.: Yes. He left Cornell in 1951, apparently rather abruptly. He simply walked out and closed the door, leaving everything in his laboratory and office just as it was at that moment. Glenn Russell, who was a graduate student in Papez's laboratory at that time, packed all the loose material, letters, sketches, notes, and papers into two large cardboard boxes. He sent the boxes to us, intact, some 18 years later. That became the nucleus of our collection of Papez memorabilia.

W.H.: I met Papez in 1942. I had read his 1937 paper on emotion sometime earlier and had written him for a reprint. We had a brief exchange of letters. When I was inducted into the army in the spring of 1942, I went to Riverside for induction and had orders to proceed without delay to Washington, D.C. This was the usual thing with army orders, so I thought, "Why not visit Papez en route to Washington?"

Travel in those days was by railway. I got off in Ithaca and went directly to Papez's laboratory. I spent about a week there. He put me up at the University Club, not far from his home, and picked me up so that we could walk back and forth to his lab.

Immediately on meeting Papez, I knew that he was a person with whom I could talk. He was very pleasant to be with. We seemed to be on the same "wavelength." He would chatter and talk along, with his little smile. He would get rather close and speak in a quiet voice, as though we were exchanging great confidences.

Now and then I would have dinner at the Papez home. His wife cooked and participated in conversation in the kitchen and at the table. She was a homemaking person—plain, simple, honest, very unpretentious. They were both delightful. So it was a very happy period that I spent there.

He noticed that I was smoking cigarettes and commented, "You know, I was smoking cigarettes, until a month ago. Pearl began telling me all the time that my vest was getting full of ashes. I thought it was a filthy habit anyway, so I stopped. It was awful for a while."

I sent you a copy of Papez's lecture notes. I have the impression that his students didn't appreciate him every much. He wove into his lectures ideas about psychology and behavior which didn't seem to interest the students. They couldn't somehow fit those ideas into neuroanatomy. He was a bit up in the sky as far as they were concerned.

Papez was a great man, a very important person. I think he was a kind of saint. The person who knew him best and who is very articulate is Fred Mettler. He probably sent you his recollections of Papez and the article he wrote on Papez for the *Founders of Neurology* (1970). It is a most lucid account.

K.E.L.: What prompted you to visit Papez? Was it his 1937 article?

W.H.: Yes, I had read it several times. My first contact with Papez was through that reprint request. When the opportunity finally arrived, he was quite agreeable to my coming to visit him. There was no doubt that he thought the message of his 1937 paper was important. He told me he was disappointed that he had received so few requests for reprints. He said, "I thought it was a pretty good paper."

As we looked at slides, he would move from pathway to pathway, linking things together, talking about synaptic organization, speculating about functions, just on a plain slide.

Papez was born, you know, in Glencoe, Minnesota, a little town not far from where S. W. Ranson was born. They got to be friends. He said, "We often had arguments. Sometimes Ranson would win; sometimes I would." He would link up the Ranson encounters with the thalamus, saying, "These things have to be connected somehow."

At the time of my visit, Papez was making experimental lesions to study the connections of the substantia nigra, particularly the connections to the caudate and striatum. He would talk about the arguments that he and Ranson had had and then smile. He had won the battle between them over where these fibers from the substantia nigra were going.

You asked whether I had seen him since. Yes, he came to a meeting of the American Neurological Association and presented an exhibit on his "blue bodies." Professor Schultz was with us then at the Armed Forces Institute of Pathology, so Schultz and I looked at the Papez exhibit very carefully. Papez came around and talked with us a bit later. It had become an obsession with him, late in his career. The same blue-bodies study got him into some trouble in Columbus, Ohio.

After my visit, Papez asked me to send him some brain material in which he would look for the blue bodies. I sent him about six blocks from very diverse neuropathologies, such as Cushing's disease. He wrote back that he had found blue bodies in all the specimens I had sent, "except possibly one."

When I was in Ithaca, I cautioned him to not publish this material until he had shown with suitable controls that the blue bodies were indicative of something particular and significant. Criticism didn't seem to bother him; he just continued blithely along.

K.E.L.: Did he sustain the dialogue with you mainly on the blue bodies?

W.H.: Oh, no! During daytimes, he would talk about anything; in the evening it was always about the thalamus. The blue-bodies discussions were certainly not very prominent.

Subsequently, I had extensive correspondence with Papez, particularly because he suggested that we write a book together on neuroanatomy. I would send a chapter to him, but usually it was the other way around. He sent me a great bulk of material. Electron microscopy was coming in about that time, and a great deal of exciting new material was beginning to be interpreted and understood in relation to the rest of neuroanatomy. Anyway, nothing ever came of our book project, but the material sent by Papez was superb.

Sometime ago, I sent you a copy of the book on the hypothalamus (5). A number of illustrations in that volume were originally intended for the Papez–Haymaker book on brain anatomy. Papez was meticulous in his work and a master at description. Once in a while, he would get into difficult technical material in pathology, but his main thrust was always on localization of function in anatomical terms: *What pathways were involved? What might be their functional implications?*

INTERVIEW WITH PAUL D. MACLEAN, M.D.*

P.D.M.: My earliest recollection of Papez's thesis on emotion is that I went to the library looking for another particular article in the *Archives of Neurology and Psychiatry.* As I recall, I found the Papez article on emotion in the same volume and was absolutely fascinated with it, terribly excited. What I was striving to understand was some idea of how the different sensory systems carrying feeling could get into the hypothalamus. These would be cortico–cortical connections, to be sure, but it was important to have some idea as to how sensory feeling might be feeding into the hippocampus.

Originally, my interest was in psychosomatic medicine. The thinking, then, was that everything of this sort went on in the hypothalamus. So I wanted to record electrical activity from the base of the brain near the midline, hoping to pick up activity from the hypothalamus. I was working with a new style of nasopharyngeal electrodes that were easy to introduce and from which we got nice quiet recordings. But I discovered that they were umpteen centimeters away from the hypothalamus— quite close to the medial parts of the temporal lobe. We thought we were recording activity from the fusiform gyrus and the hippocampal area.

I haven't been able to reconstruct how I got into this recording mode with patients with psychomotor epilepsy and became so fascinated by their symptomatology. I worked with Stanley Cobb at the Massachusetts General Hospital for two years during 1947 and 1948. I ran into the Papez paper pretty early; 1947 I think. I was working in Bob Schwab's laboratory—a great bunch—completely surrounded and steeped in EEG experiences.

K.E.L.: Did Stanley Cobb know Papez personally? Did he suggest you go and see Papez?

P.D.M.: Oh, he knew Papez! I had the feeling that the "leaders" in neurology all recognized Papez as a person who had a great fund of knowledge and information. But they also thought he was a little bit "touched." He didn't exactly fit in; he didn't quite make it with the Eastern Ivy League!

I think I went to Cobb with a kind of anatomical question, "How [do we] account for all of these sensory auras (visual, auditory, etc.) that we encounter in patients who have psychomotor epilepsy?" These patients had all sorts of different sensory experiences associated with their auras: auditory, visual, somesthetic, and visceral. I talked about Papez's article, and I guess Cobb must have said, "Why don't you go up to see him?"

---

*9916 Logan Drive, Potomac, Maryland 20854. (Interviewed in Potomac, 1–2 February 1981.)

We had had this correspondence beforehand. He picked the dates. It must have been when he had a letup in teaching. I drove to Ithaca with Dr. Arellano, a neuroscientist and cellist from Peru. On our way out of Boston we narrowly escaped from having a bad automobile accident; in that event I wouldn't have gotten to meet Papez.

We went straight to his lab and talked with him about the things we would like to see. I don't recall seeing any students around. I think it may have been the Easter holidays. He just took off time from his usual routines and devoted himself to talking with us about these questions. We did go over to his house one evening and had an interesting time there, too.

Papez had access to a large collection of vertebrate brain material, including the Wilder Collection of primate brains. He had many comparative brain series, but we concentrated on the macaque. We were there about two and a half days, I guess, and went through an entire brain. With Papez, that was like walking through a grand park! It was just a lot of fun! My brain was like a sponge, sopping it up. I learned more anatomy in that short time than in all the rest of my life.

Take for example, Muratoff's bundle. How many people worry about a topic like that? About Muratoff's bundle, the ancient commissures, the subcallosal bundle, the supraoptic commissure, etc. We spent quite a bit of time discussing many such tracts and their possible origins and where they were going. We went into quite a bit of depth about things you don't have time to do that often or that thoroughly, anywhere. It was quite a remarkable experience.

Papez gave us a continuing discourse. He would keep seeing fiber tracts that he "had always wondered about" and would stop to ponder and discuss them.

In addition, we looked at some gross specimens: human and other primates. It must have been with the whole human brain material that he began to point out fibers that might be coming to the hippocampus from visual, auditory, and other sensory areas. Then I got extremely excited! This was the only thing I would have added to what he had said in 1937—that there were other possibilities for information to get into the hippocampal formations. That was all that I added in the way of anatomical ideas in my 1949 paper, which came out in *Psychosomatic Medicine* (11).

K.E.L.: How did he react to your 1949 paper? Did you get a letter from him about that?

P.D.M.: Yes, I think so. I didn't send him proofs or anything beforehand. I did check things with him to be sure I wasn't misquoting him. He was very gracious and generous and said how pleased he was with it.

K.E.L.: Did you talk with Papez about his motivation in writing the 1937 paper on emotion?

P.D.M.: Yes, we talked about that quite a lot. Papez spoke to us at some length about how he happened to write it. He said he had read an announcement from an English foundation, offering a grant of $150,000 for "significant investigations on the mechanisms of emotion." It would be interesting to see whether we could find that announcement. Papez said it made him mad—those were his words (the only time when I was there that his language seemed to get a little rough). He was provoked at people offering such a large sum when we already know a lot about these mechanisms. He implied that he had dashed the paper off rather quickly. That was one thing Lester Aaronson explained to me later; that the 1937 paper of Papez was not dashed off all of a sudden. Papez had been worrying about that problem for years already in the early 1930s when Aaronson was in Papez's laboratory. Papez had evidently long been interested in the brain mechanisms of emotion, really wrestling with that idea.

K.E.L.: In some of Papez's early correspondence with Vonderahe, Papez said how great it would be if we could establish the anatomic mechanisms of emotion inasmuch as emotion had historically been treated as if it were something almost magical.

K.E.L.: Did Aaronson say why Papez never referred to that paper in his subsequent writings?

P.D.M.: No, he didn't say anything about that. Papez must have had some strange feelings about that paper, that he might be showing a soft side by talking about emotion—perhaps by not being a sufficiently hard scientist. But he didn't show any of that feeling when we were there. He knew I had come up because of the paper, so I suspect he may have been rather glad to talk to somebody who was really interested in that paper. I didn't have any hesitation in talking about it, so he could enjoy that and feel less guilty.

I think Raymond Dart may have been a little put out at Papez because Papez never referred to a paper published by Dart in 1935 on the whole structure of the neopallium, its history and significance. In that paper, Dart made the pitch that the parahippocampal gyrus (he called it neopallium when it might more appropriately have been called the parahippocampal gyrus—part of Yakovlev's mesopallium) controls the muscular display of emotion. Dart's paper recognizes the prepyriform area and the parahippocampal areas, which are forward in the dorsal convexity of the reptilian brain. Striatal history offers us a clue as to the divergent activities of the two divisions of the mammalian neopallium.

Of course, having been a student of Elliott Smith, Dart would regard only the pyriform area and the hippocampal formation as paleopallium or, I should say, old pallium. Elliott Smith, in a paper on the natural subdivision of the pallium (17), introduced the word neopallium. Pallium was apparently introduced by Reichert in 1859. Elliott Smith takes off from Turner's paper of 1890, in which Turner mentions the rhinal and hippocampal fissures as being the dividing line between the old and the new pallium. He felt that the old pallium corresponds to Schwalbe's falciform lobe, which would take in the hippocampal rudiment, the induseum griseum, the hippocampal formation, and the pyriform lobe. The globus hippocampi is the way Turner referred to it.

K.E.L.: What does globus hippocami mean?

P.D.M.: Well, there are many definitions. According to Elliott Smith, it meant the pyriform temporal lobe. So the old pallium for both Smith and Dart applied only to the falciform lobe of Schwalbe. The cingulate gyrus was neopallium for them. I have found a good many people who regard the cingulate gyrus as neo-pallium and don't go along with Paul Yakovlev's (21) designation of it as transitional cortex, mesocortex.

K.E.L.: What about your paper (13) on the stream of interoceptive information coming in through the hypothalamus and septum and going to the basal dendrites of the hippocampal pyramids while exteroceptive information goes to the apical dendrites of the same pyramidal cells?

P.D.M.: Well, that may not be so crazy! Along these lines, I am puzzled to this day about the cingulate gyrus. I had expected that the cingulate would light up with visual, auditory, and other sensory stimuli, but the only thing that elicited cingulate responses was the vagus. The cingulate gyrus may be rather parallel to the hippocampus, receiving an unconditional message to which may be added exteroceptive signals to make the picture whole. The posterior part of the cingulate, area 23, has primarily sensory connections, whereas the anterior part, area 24, has primarily downstream motor connections. It talks particularly to the striatum.

K.E.L.: You brought Papez back to the attention of the neuroscience world. That was very important.

P.D.M.: Actually, it is rather shameful if that is the case.

K.E.L.: It is the shame of the rest of the world, not of Papez or you.

P.D.M.: At least while I was there, Papez was very animated. I suspect he may not have been so animated much of the time. I think his relations with the outer world were not very joyful or cordial. He may have had to be rather self-contained. I think that like a lot of people who work on the brain, Papez felt sort of sorry for the rest of the world because of its ignorance and lack of curiosity about the brain!

K.E.L.: What I can't account for is why Papez left that important paper and that subject lying fallow.

P.D.M.: That question is hard to answer. The reason was not apparent through any of my contacts with him. He came to visit us later in New Haven. He was there for the New Year in 1950. Alison [Mrs. P. D. MacLean] remembers that visit and enjoyed both Papez and his wife, Pearl.

Papez's kind of laboratory operations will have to be revived someplace. We have something of the needed kind here[5] where there is convergence and symbiosis among structural and functional disciplines. There aren't many such laboratories elsewhere, including Europe. For example, Konrad Lorenz and his people, in Seewiesen, don't have the brain side going; their work is altogether on behavior.

A lot of people made kites and model airplanes before they got an airplane that could fly. You can see the direction the world is going. The world has got to get into the brain, though there is the potential there of having too much manipulative knowledge.

I don't think the world wants necessarily to get this message all at once. I think there are ways to come at it indirectly. Certainly you can approach it through

---

[5]Laboratory of Brain Evolution and Behavior, National Institute for Mental Health, Poolesville, Maryland 20837.

epilepsy, as we have been discussing, if you use epilepsy as Hughlings Jackson did, as a display of brain function.

You can look at history, which is pretty short, and begin to throw in this limbic business, and appreciate that limbic mechanisms constitute a powerful operating force in the world. For better or for worse, the limbic brain is not the brain for reading, writing, and arithmetic. The limbic brain has a different code, and the exchange is on a different level.

This is not to deny the world out there, but time and space are not out there, they are up here in our heads. *If we knew more about these mechanisms, people might begin to realize that our universe and everything in it is up here, in our noggin, including all the values we attach to things and people.*

INTERVIEW WITH WILLIAM STOTLER*

W.S.: Papez received his medical degree from the University of Minnesota and stayed on a year with J. B. Johnson, (8) a great comparative neuroanatomist, who was especially interested in the amygdala.

K.E.L.: That's interesting because in his 1937 paper, Papez doesn't include the amygdala except to say that its function was unknown. Indeed, he doesn't mention the amygdala, insula, uncinate fasciculus, or even temporal lobe. Those were added to the "limbic system" by MacLean (11,12) and by Yakovlev (21).

W.S.: Following his experience with Johnson, Papez went into medical practice, concentrating on neurology. Largely because of his work with Johnson, Papez was shortly invited to teach at the Atlanta College of Physicians and Surgeons (later part of Emory University) as Professor and head of the Department of Anatomy. Papez taught at Emory for eight years.

Papez then went to Cornell, as Assistant Professor, attracted there because of the greater opportunity for research. Cornell was strong on academic rank. They didn't have Associate Professors, just Assistant Professors and Professors. Papez was quickly advanced and served as Professor of Anatomy at Cornell from 1920 to 1951.

Papez used to tell with amusement that he sometimes had dreams about the embalmer who prepared bodies for dissection. This diener somewhat resembled a cadaver himself. Papez dreamt that the diener and the cadavers were plotting against him.

Bateman was one of Papez's students. Lake Cayuga froze over sometime before my arrival. Bateman, Papez, and some others, skated all the way across. When Papez retired from Cornell, it was Bateman who invited Papez to continue working in Columbus, Ohio, where he became Director of Biological Research at the State Hospital.

I was with Papez at Cornell from 1937 to 1941. I began my neuroanatomical studies with Albert Kuntz at St. Louis University. At that time, St. Louis awarded

---

*University of Oregon School of Medicine, Portland, Oregon. (Interviewed in Portland, 16 March 1981.)

masters degrees but did not have a doctoral program in anatomy. For the Ph.D., they farmed out graduate students to Cornell, with Papez, and to Minnesota, with Johnson and Rasmussen. I think I was the first student sent to Cornell. Kuntz told me that he had created the opportunity for me to go.

I was very impressed by Papez, from his publications. When I got the chance to do graduate studies at Cornell, I thought it was wonderful. When I arrived, I talked with Professor Kerr, the chairman. He was quite a formal Scotsman who headed the graduate training program. He told me that I was going to work with Dr. Papez.

It was summer, and Papez came in from his cottage on Lake Cayuga. He had a cigarette hanging on his lip, looking rather like someone from the Left Bank of the Seine. I thought, "What am I getting into here?"

K.E.L.: From 1937, when you arrived at Cornell, you worked up to become Papez' chief lieutenant—you became his alter ego in some ways, did you not?

W.S.: Yes. I first came to Cornell when Papez was getting that 1937 paper together. He had a great deal of material that wasn't included, a big volume of things he had abstracted from the literature as background information. He gave all that to me to read. It was somewhat overwhelming. I had to go to the library to verify his references.

I also did some cingulate lesions in cats. We were looking for behavioral changes. We found a type of akinetic mutism. Some of the cats would sit there and lap milk, but they really didn't seem to "give a damn": You had to start them by putting their noses into the milk.

One of them had a seizure and went flying across the room. At that time I did not realize what an epileptogenic region we were dealing with. Arthur Ward in Seattle soon heard about this. He had published a paper on cingulectomy. I had done that with Papez, more or less on the side. It was not published. The only comment on that work was in a review in one of the neurological journals, by Papez, where he mentioned that I had done the work.

Soon after the paper on emotion came out, about 1938 or 1939, *Life* magazine became very interested in emotion. They sent a science editor, and Fritz Goro came along to take pictures. *Life* had quite a spread on that subject. *Life* had apparently approached other people about emotions and had been referred to Papez.

K.E.L.: What did Papez do for recreation or avocation?

W.S.: He built quite a nice cabin on the shores of Lake Cayuga. He did some canoeing on the lake. During the summer, he would disappear a lot of the time. He would come in, often on weekends, and I would see him then. During the academic year, he would work late into the night. Pearl would call up and say, "Send Jim home." We were quite informal. I used to smoke cigars then. I found a quite good Cuban cigar that wasn't very expensive. Papez and Vonderahe would come in and steal my cigars!

One of Papez's students went to the Department of Anatomy at Cincinnati. He wrote a paper on the basal ganglia, which Papez decided needed a lot of revision.

I believe that this was the beginning of Papez's close association with Vonderahe, a very remarkable man who taught anatomy, neurology, and psychiatry.

K.E.L.: We have many of Vonderahe's letters and correspondence with Papez. In several letters, Vonderahe wrote in detail about two patients who had explosive rage attacks and at autopsy had small tumors in the hypothalamus. Papez was very interested and discussed these cases thoroughly. In one of his letters Papez wrote, "I think we are on the track of something very important." This was prior to publication of the 1937 paper.

W.S.: One of the papers Papez published related to a woman physician who was a graduate of Cornell. She had willed her brain to the Burt Green Collection. She had developed a tumor in the uncinate fasciculus or thereabouts; I don't remember exactly. She began using very foul language—completely out of her character. In order to protect her, her children tried to hide the facts. Papez studied her brain and published his interpretation of it.

K.E.L.: What did Papez think about his 1937 paper on emotion?

W.S.: He thought it was the best paper he had ever written. He told me that it was going to be a landmark. Although he received quite a few requests for reprints, the ideas in the paper didn't take hold outside of a rather erudite group that really understood it.

Among other people, he discussed it with John Fulton before it was published. Fulton was certainly sympathetic. At Creighton, I gave a talk on Papez's work in relation to psychosomatic medicine. In her neuroanatomy course at Michigan, for faculty from all around the country, Elizabeth Crosby gave a great deal of credit to Papez's ideas, including his thesis on the neuroanatomical substrate of emotion. Papez and Crosby had different approaches to comparative neurology, but she fully recognized the value of his contributions.

At the time of Webb Haymaker's visit, I had been working on the basal ganglia with Papez. Haymaker was quite impressed with connections we demonstrated in the prerubral field: fasciculus lenticularis, ansa lenticularis, and an adjacent bundle that became the fasciculus thalamicus. This ascended to the ventralis anterior of the thalamus and was relayed on to the motor cortex. It gave off collaterals to the red nucleus. The red nucleus contributed a major input to the inferior olive. Haymaker was keenly interested in that work.

K.E.L.: Who else do you recall visiting Papez while you were at Cornell?

W.S.: Bucy had come to Cornell before Haymaker, bringing serial sections of the temporal lobe resections he and Heinrich Klüver had done in monkeys, at the time they discovered the Klüver–Bucy syndrome.

These were bilateral temporal lobectomies, which had gotten into Meyer's loop, leading to a good deal of degeneration in the striate cortex. There was a question whether abnormalities of recognition (lack of fear at the sight of snakes and the like) might have been the result of not *seeing* well enough. Although the animals did have some loss of visual fields, from what I saw, I don't believe that injury to the optic radiations had any effect on the altered behavior of these monkeys.

Bucy was greatly interested in neostriatal projections to the globus pallidus and back through the ventralis anterior of the thalamus. At that time, Bucy had been making premotor ablations of cortex in pursuit of his studies on spasticity, rigidity, and flaccidity in relation to notions about the pyramidal tract.

K.E.L.: An impression we have is that Papez seldom referred to the 1937 paper in his subsequent writings. For example, Paul Yakovlev met Papez in 1946. Over the next 12 years or so, they were in close communication. Papez came and spent a full week with Paul on two separate occasions while they worked together on brain material in the Yakovlev Collection. But Paul says that during that entire long period of active exchange of ideas and working together, Papez never mentioned the neuroanatomical mechanisms of emotion, nor did he once refer to his 1937 paper.

W.S.: At the *ARNMD Meeting* in New York on the extrapyramidal tract, there was much talk about obtaining financial backing for more research on the brain in relation to mental illnesses. Professor Walter Freeman (psychiatrist) came by and said, "Dr. Papez, there are a couple of ladies I would like to have you meet." I was tagging along. These ladies had diamonds and jewelry and the appearance of great elegance, so I thought this was going to be an approach for money to do research. Suddenly, Dr. James Watts (neurosurgeon), an associate of Freeman's, came by with a couple of young fellows and said, demonstrating on the foreheads of the two ladies, "This is where we made the incisions." Nothing else had been said. That was the first inkling that they were lobotomized patients.

This took place at about the beginning of the lobotomy period, before Freeman and Watts had published their book on frontal lobotomy (3).

K.E.L.: Do you think Papez was concerned or embarrassed that some of his work and research was being used in that kind of clinical application?

W.S.: No, I don't believe so. Anyway, this was a bad time for him at Cornell, and he had become distracted by things going on there. You see, they moved the basic sciences part of the medical school from Ithaca to New York, consolidating the medical school at one location. Papez didn't go with the move. Kerr, who was Head of Anatomy in Ithaca, made arrangements that the departments in Ithaca would remain autonomous for a while and carry on graduate work as they had been doing. Kingsbury, who was the head of the histology portion of Anatomy, took over as Acting Dean when Kerr became incapacitated with cardiac problems. Then, Kingsbury retired.

In the time I was at Cornell, I often asked why they didn't make Papez chairman of the department. He was finally made chairman, but then they introduced a man from the Poultry Department of the School of Agriculture to take Papez's place. That man wasn't an anatomist at all. He wasn't even a geneticist, but they gave him the title of Professor of Animal Genetics and made him head of the whole thing. He brought over a considerable number of faculty from the Zoology Department. So the entire scene had changed.

But the thing that got me was to see Papez, that great and distinguished scientist and human being, being humiliated and obliged to do all the laboratory scut work himself.

The graduate students rebelled at this poultry fellow. They threatened to resign in a body if he were not replaced. He was replaced by Odelman, who was a distinguished embryologist, and also and primarily, a distinguished classical scholar who had translated many of the classics. That made things a little better. But they were exceedingly rough on Papez.

Even before that, he was upset by the fact that they lost the medical students. He stopped going to meetings of the American Association of Anatomists. After I came to the University of Oregon, Olof Larsell, who was chairman of the Department of Anatomy, had a good deal to do with nomination of anatomists for positions on national societies. Since the British–American Association of Anatomists was registered in the State of New York, one member of the Board had to be from New York. Larsell asked my opinion whether Papez would like to be that person. I said I thought he certainly would. Then Papez started coming to the meetings again, and his colleagues nationally and internationally brought him out of that shell. I thought that was a fine contribution.

Then, there were papers dealing with emotion and psychic functions of the brain. I remember Professor Walle Nauta, chairing one of the sessions, asking whether Professor Papez would care to comment on some presentation or discussion. I was sitting next to him and had to nudge him to get him to react. He was a little indifferent to it. He did occasionally have to chair sessions at the Anatomy Association meetings.

K.E.L.: Do you remember when Papez began to be interested in the "blue bodies"?

W.S.: Yes. Ellie Henschell was a technician for Spielmeyer in Germany. She was Jewish. She had a brother who was a physician. They were trying to get her out of Germany and trying to get her into Papez's laboratory. When she began as a technician for Papez, I didn't have my degree yet, but she always called me "Doctor," which was a great embarrassment. She stained those little blue bodies and got Papez interested in them. Ellie Henschell came out of Germany about 1940. She came to the lab about 1940 or 1941. I think she did the staining that demonstrated the blue bodies as early as 1941. I didn't think much of them, and whenever Papez and I met, that subject never came up. We didn't talk about the blue bodies.

K.E.L.: Did they appear only in the brains of psychotic patients?

W.S.: They were supposed to be a sign of mental illness, but I don't know. I didn't approve of the uncontrolled assumptions. Papez recognized my reservations, and we discussed other things. We discussed the connections of the limbic system and many other parts of the brain.

K.E.L.: What did you call the limbic system in those days? Did you refer to it as *Broca's limbic lobe*?

W.S.: No, we just referred to it as *limbic*.

K.E.L.: Was the subject of emotion and, specifically, the Papez circuit ever actually on the program at the anatomical meetings?

W.S.: No, but of course there were things that came up on the organization of the thalamus and its connections which had a bearing on Papez's concept. *The subject of the anatomical basis of emotion probably should have been on the anatomists' program.*

ACKNOWLEDGMENTS

Partial support for this endeavor (through Peter D. Olch, M.D.) from the National Library of Medicine is gratefully acknowledged. The audio tapes of the interviews were transcribed by Mrs. Elisabeth Marsland, Librarian Emeritus of The Wellesey Hospital in Toronto. Her help in gathering together the Collection of Papez Memorabilia is also gratefully acknowledged.

REFERENCES

1. Bailey, P. (1966): *Sigmund the Unserene: A Tragedy in Three Acts.* Charles C Thomas, Springfield, Illinois.
2. Ferrier, D. (1876): *The Functions of the Brain.* Smith, Elder and Co., London.
3. Freeman, W., and Watts, J. W. (1942): *Psychosurgery: Intelligence, Emotion and Social Behavior Following Prefrontal Lobotomy for Mental Disorders.* Charles C Thomas, Springfield, Illinois.
4. Fulton, J. F., and Jacobsen, C. F. (1935): The functions of the frontal lobes: A comparative study in monkeys, chimpanzees and man. *Adv. Mod. Biol. (Moscow),* 4:113–123.
5. Haymaker, W., Anderson, E., and Nauta, W. J. H., eds. (1969): *The Hypothalamus.* Charles C Thomas, Springfield, Illinois.
6. Haymaker, W., and Schiller, F. (1970): *The Founders of Neurology.* Charles C Thomas, Springfield, Illinois.
7. Herrick, C. J. (1933): Morphogenesis of the brain. *J. Morphol.,* 54:233–258.
8. Johnston, J. B. (1906): *The Nervous System of Vertebrates: The Evolution of the Cerebral Hemispheres.* Blakiston's Son & Co., Philadelphia.
9. Klüver, H. (1928): *Mescal.* The "Divine" plant and its psychological effects. Kegan Paul, Trench, Trubner & Co. London.
10. Klüver, H. (1942): *Mescal and Mechanisms of Hallucinations.* University of Chicago Press, Chicago.
11. MacLean, P. D. (1949): Psychosomatic disease and the "visceral brain." *Psychosom. Med.,* 11:338–353.
12. MacLean, P. D. (1952): Some psychiatric implications of physiological studies on frontotemporal portion of limbic system (visceral brain). *EEG Clin. Neurophysiol.* 4:407–418.
13. MacLean, P. D. (1958): The limbic system with respect to self-preservation and the preservation of the species. *J. Nerv. Ment. Dis.,* 127:1–11.
14. Moniz, E. (1936): *Tentatives Operatoires dans le Traitement de Certaines Psychoses.* Masson et Cie., Paris.
15. Papez, J. W. (1937): A proposed mechanism of emotion. *Arch Neurol. Psychiatry (Chicago),* 38:725–743.
16. Sherrington, C. S. (1963): *Man on His Nature.* 2nd ed. Cambridge University Press, Cambridge. (The Oxford Lectures, Edinburgh, 1937–1938; 1st ed., 1940.)
17. Smith, G. E. (1907): A new topographical survey of the human cerebral cortex; Being an account of the distribution of the anatomically distinct cortical areas and their relationship to the cerebral sulci. *J. Anat. (London),* 41:237–254.
18. Smith, W. K. (1943): The representation of respiratory movements in the cerebral cortex. *J. Neurophysiol.,* 6:349–360.

19. Spencer, W. G. (1894): The effect produced upon respirations by faradic excitation of the cerebrum in the monkey, dog, cat and rabbit. *Phil. Trans.*, B185:609–657.
20. Ward, A. A. Jr. (1947): The cingular gyrus: Area 24. *J. Neurophysiol.* 11:13–23.
21. Yakovlev, P. I. (1948): Motility, behavior and the brain; stereodynamic organization and neural co-ordinates and behavior. *J. Nerv. Ment. Dis.*, 107:313–335.

Subject Index